Dietary Supplement Test Methods

Liquid Chromatography Separation Techniques and Application

Dietary Supplement Test Methods

Liquid Chromatography Separation Techniques and Application

David (Dajing) Ji
Analytical Laboratories in Anaheim, USA

Darryl Sullivan
Eurofins Scientific, USA

World Scientific

NEW JERSEY • LONDON • SINGAPORE • BEIJING • SHANGHAI • HONG KONG • TAIPEI • CHENNAI • TOKYO

Published by

World Scientific Publishing Co. Pte. Ltd.

5 Toh Tuck Link, Singapore 596224

USA office: 27 Warren Street, Suite 401-402, Hackensack, NJ 07601

UK office: 57 Shelton Street, Covent Garden, London WC2H 9HE

Library of Congress Cataloging-in-Publication Data
Names: Ji, David Dajing, author. | Sullivan, Darryl M., author.
Title: Dietary supplement test methods : liquid chromatography separation
techniques and application / David (Dajing) Ji, Darryl Sullivan.
Other titles: Bao jian pin de ce shi fang fa. English
Description: Hackensack, NJ : World Scientific, [2022] | Includes index.
Identifiers: LCCN 2022000601| ISBN 9789811249242 (hardcover) |
ISBN 9789811249259 (ebook for institutions) | ISBN 9789811249266 (ebook for individuals)
Subjects: | MESH: Dietary Supplements--analysis | Chromatography,
Liquid--methods | Laboratory Manual
Classification: LCC RM258.5 | NLM QU 25 | DDC 613.2 23/eng/20220--dc09
LC record available at https://lccn.loc.gov/2022000601

British Library Cataloguing-in-Publication Data
A catalogue record for this book is available from the British Library.

《保健品的测试方法: 液相色谱的分离技术与应用》
Originally published in Chinese by Shanghai Scientific & Technical Publishers

For any available supplementary material, please visit
https://www.worldscientific.com/worldscibooks/10.1142/12643#t=suppl

Typeset by Stallion Press
Email: enquiries@stallionpress.com

Contents

Chapter 1
Introduction

Testing for dietary supplements is a very challenging task, and includes quantitatively measuring of all ingredients listed on the products label claim (including herbs and herb extracts) with different formulas, dosage forms and complex matrixes.

At present, there are many kinds of dietary supplements on the market with all kind ingredients in different formulas. The products quality and safety are critical. Unqualified adulterants and substitute products are sometimes appearing on the market. Also, the new products and ingredients are constantly appearing in the market. Scientific, accurate testing methods with high selectivity are the basis for product quality control and market regulation.

Currently, the most authoritative test methods are US Pharmacopoeia method (USP), AOAC International (AOAC) and Codex methods, among others. Due to the diversity of formulas, complex matrixes and numerous compounds need to be tested, it is difficult for a single test method to properly test all products on the market. Some methods can accurately test certain components in certain formulas, but for products with different formulations, due to different ingredients, different dosage forms and other factors alternative methods may be required. Some of the ingredients may have some unpredictable interferences, resulting in the deviation of the results. There are some ingredients that may not even be able to be tested at all. Therefore, relying on a single authoritative method is not enough. In addition, there are many products and ingredients that have no authoritative test methods at all. The adjustment, improvement, establishment of alternative test methods and development of new test methods are very important and necessary in the dietary supplements industry.

The testing of dietary supplements also includes the analysis of some selected contaminates that may be present in the products. For example, some sports nutrition products may contain illegal compounds, such as synthetic compounds or prescription drugs. This type of testing also requires a strong set of test methods.

Some authoritative test methods were developed in the past 20 or 30 years or even earlier. These include titration, gravimetric, colorimetric and thin-layer chromatography technologies. The accuracy and specificity of these older test methods may need to be improved and updated.

The United States Pharmacopoeia is currently working on a modernization of test methods aimed at replacing older gravimetric, titration and colorimetric methods. The intent is to replace these techniques with modern instruments and technology to obtain more accurate and reliable test methods. But progress has been slow and the testing methods for dietary supplements have not been greatly impacted yet. In 2002, the National Institute of Health (NIH) in United States established the Office of Dietary Supplements (ODS) to develop scientific and high-quality dietary supplements test methods and reference standards for use in researching dietary supplement products. ODS commissioned and funded AOAC to develop number of scientific, high-quality test methods. So far, 16 test methods have been validated and published, and some methods are still in progress. There is still a long way to go to satisfy the testing needs of the industry.

The dietary supplement testing requirements in the FDA Good Manufacturing Practice (GMP) adopted by the US Congress underlines two points, it must be a scientifically valid method and the test methods must be verified. It is not necessary to use official or compendial test methods. This provision took into consideration the uniqueness and complexity of testing of dietary supplements.

The methods provided in this book were developed based on scientific principles and rely on advanced instrumentation and technology. Some methods are validated by a single laboratory, and a few methods are undergoing multiple laboratory validation procedures through AOAC. These methods can be used as alternatives to help solve problems for compendial methods in laboratory. Many of the methods in this book do not have any compendia methods to compare with. These methods could be considered as best practice industry test methods. After these methods undergo verification, they can be submitted to relevant organizations to be considered as official test methods.

This book is not simply to provide test methods, but more importantly, through the demonstration of the development of the methods and discussion, it is designed to give readers some idea on how to develop and establish test methods. This will aid significantly in future development work, as well as dietary supplement research.

The liquid chromatographic separation technology descripted in this book can be used not only in the testing of the dietary supplements but also in medical research, food and food safety testing, as well as agriculture and environmental testing.

Dietary supplement testing also includes safety testing, such as heavy metals, microorganisms, pesticides and other residues. This type of testing is not included in the book.

1 Liquid Chromatography Separation Techniques and Application

Different compounds, when introduced in a mobile phase solution, will interact differently with stationary phases of the analytical column. These differences in interactions result in different levels of retention on the stationary phase, and different retention times. This activity facilitates the separation of different compounds of interest.

The following is an introduction to the different types of stationary phases and how they work.

1.1 *Types of stationary phases*

(i) *Reversed phase column*

Non-polar compounds with a certain number of straight carbon chains bonded to the surface of a silicone gel or other similar materials are used to form reversed stationary phase. The non-polar molecules that are bonded to the surface of the stationary phase materials could be $C_{18,}$ C_8, C_{30}.

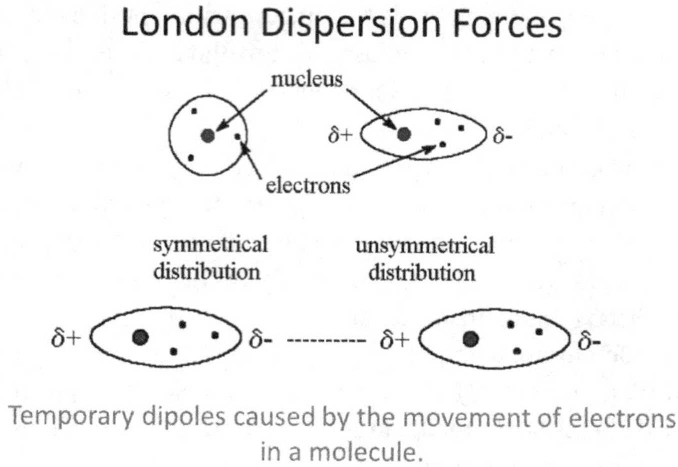

Figure 1.1: Diagram of dispersion force.

The longer the carbon chain is, the greater the non-polarity; C_{18} is the most widely used column.

The interaction force between the analytes and the reversed phase column is called the dispersion force (London force).

Non-polar molecules produce instantaneous dipole moments and induce adjacent non-polar molecules to also produce instantaneous dipole moments, resulting in mutual affinity (see Figure 1.1).

The phenomenon of similar compatibility in daily life is the role of dispersal forces between substances. For example, non-polar vitamin E can only be dissolved in non-polar oils or other non-polar solvents, polar salts can only be dissolved in polar water.

The stronger the non-polarity analytes, the stronger the attraction to the reversed phase column, and the longer the retention time in the column.

Conversely, the more the polar molecules, the lesser the attraction to the column, and result in shorter retention times.

In Figure 1.2, the TMS (Trimethylsilane) is a molecule that bonded to the silicone surface to reduce the activity of silanol in chromatography.

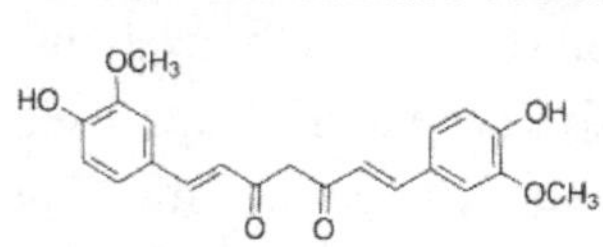

curcumin

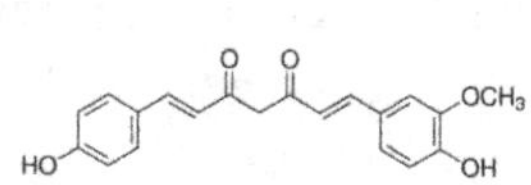

demethoxycurcumin

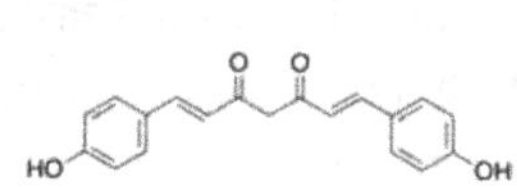

bisdemethoxycurcumin

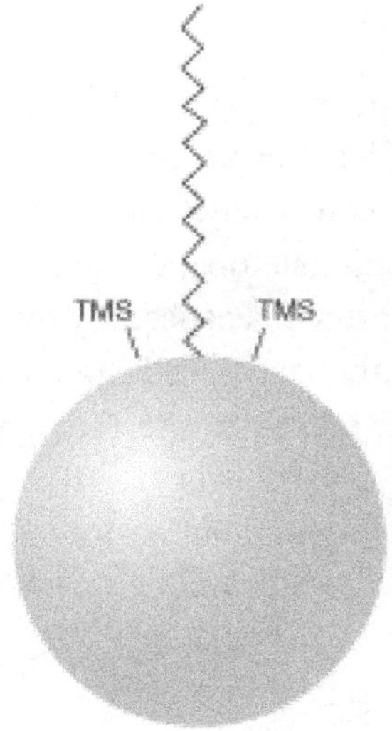

Figure 1.2: Illustration of C18 stationary phase.

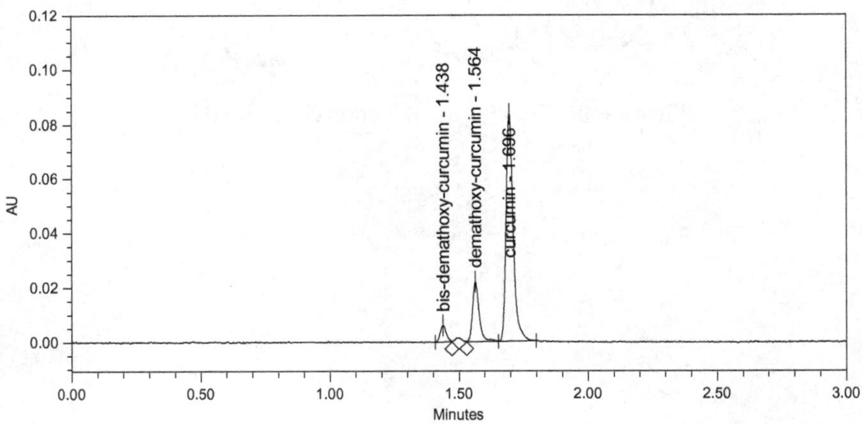

Figure 1.3: Chromatogram of curcumins, with reversed phase column.

Figure 1.3, the non-polarity of curcumin > demethoxycurcumin > bisdemethoxycurcumin because curcumin contains two non-polar methoxy groups, demethoxycurcumin only one and bisdemethoxycurcumin none. Therefore, the least non-polar bisdemethoxycurcumin eluted first, and then demethoxycurcumin and finally curcumin.

(ii) *Phenyl column*

Aromatic non-polar compounds bounded to the surface of silica gel or other material form phenyl stationary phase. Besides the dispersion force, the interaction force between phenyl stationary phase and analytes contains aromatic rings or conjugate double bonds called the π–π interaction force. The π–π interaction force is caused by overlapping of low energy π electron clouds of both stationary phase and analytes.

As showed in Figure 1.4, there are three types of overlap between stationary phase and analytes electron clouds.

Due to the additional π–π interaction force, the aromatic analytes get longer retention time than other analytes with similar non-polarity in a phenyl column.

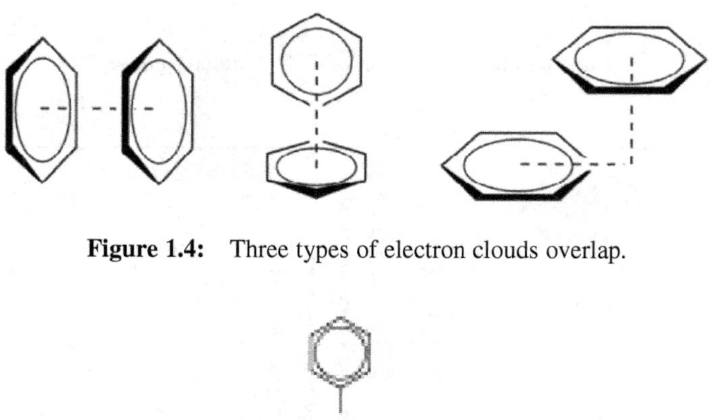

Figure 1.4: Three types of electron clouds overlap.

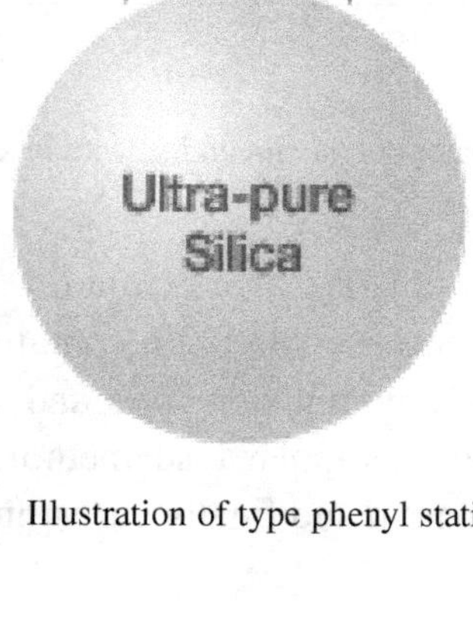

Figure 1.5: Illustration of type phenyl stationary phase.

For example, lutein and zeaxanthin are co-existing in nature, due to similarity in molecules; using a reversed phase C_{18} column is difficult to separate them, though C_{30} can separate them with long run time. But a phenyl column can easily separate them, because of the additional π–π interaction force (Figure 1.6).

Consider one more example. Figure 1.7 is a chromatogram and UV spectrum of a pure corosolic acid reference standard tested using a C_{18} column, at 4.23 min corosolic acid was eluted, and the UV spectrum at 4.23 min shows the spectrum characteristic of pure corosolic acid. Figure 1.8 is the chromatogram of corosolic acid with sample matrix, also tested using a C_{18} column. But the UV spectrum at 4.23 min is varied as shown in the display of UV absorption at 280 nm. It means there is an interfering compound, with a maximum UV absorption at 280 nm, as in the sample matrix. The interfering compound should contain aromatic group or conjugate double bond, due to the specific absorption at 280 nm.

In order to separate the interfering compound, instating of C_{18} column, a phenyl column is used. The un-polarity of corosolic acid and interfering compound could be similar, so reversed phase column cannot separate them easily. However, the interfering compound contains low energy

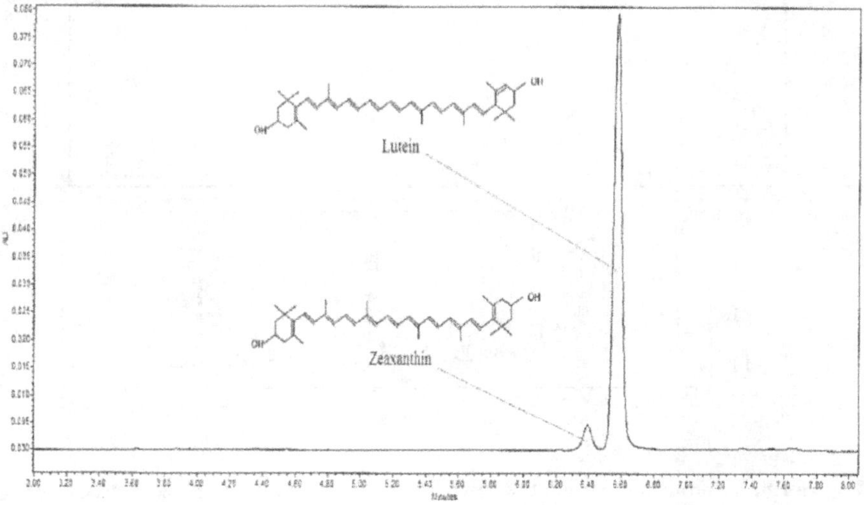

Figure 1.6: Chromatogram of lutein and zeaxanthin with phenyl column.

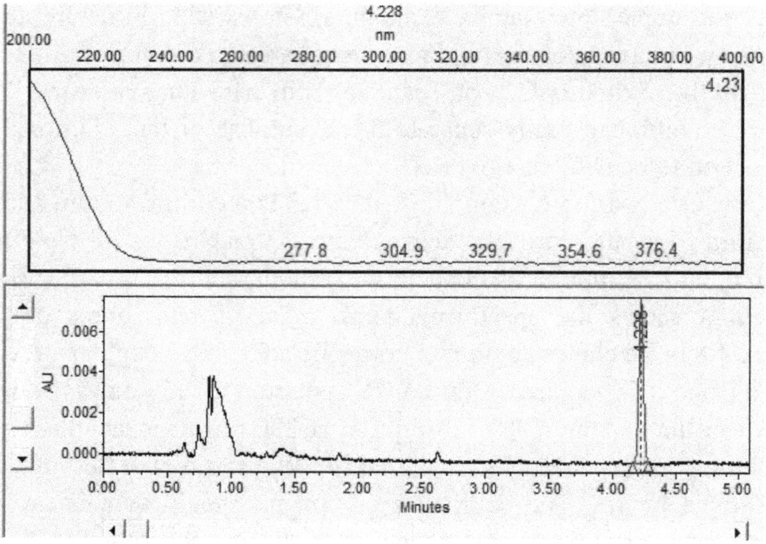

Figure 1.7: Chromatogram and UV spectrum of pure corosolic acid with C_{18} column.

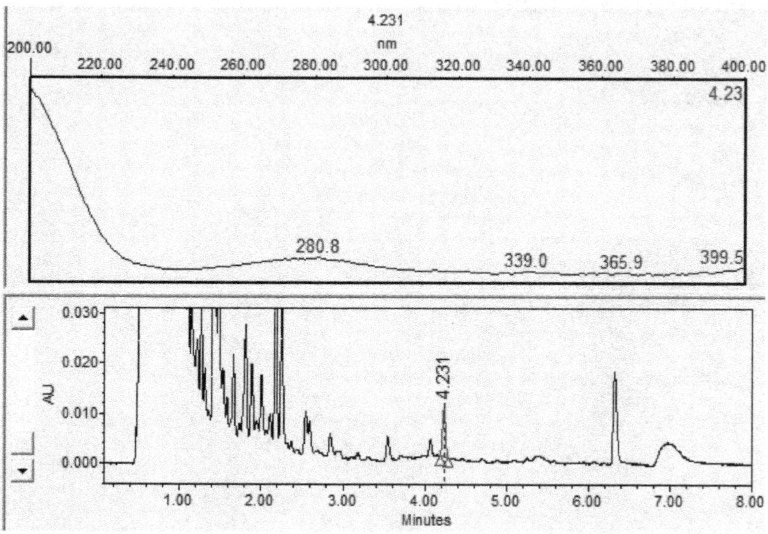

Figure 1.8: Chromatogram and UV spectrum of corosolic acid in sample matrix with C_{18} column.

π electron that can interact with phenyl column, cause additional π–π interaction force, and get longer retention than corosolic acid.

See Figures 1.9 and 1.10, with phenyl column the retention time of corosolic acid is 6.20 min. However, based on the UV spectrums in Figure 1.10 the interfering compound was delayed by 6.31 min; it conformed the truth of π–π interaction.

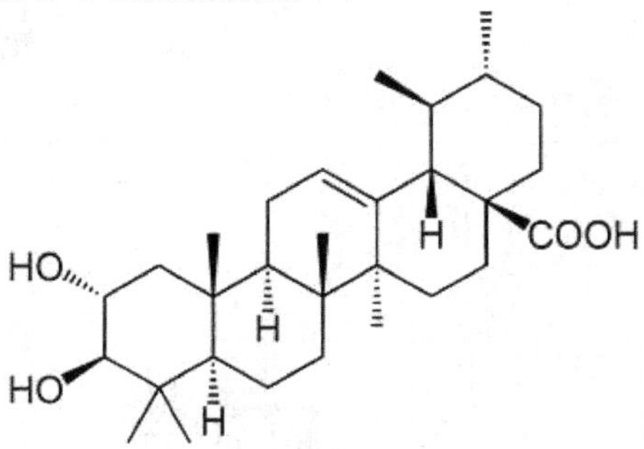

Corosolic Acid

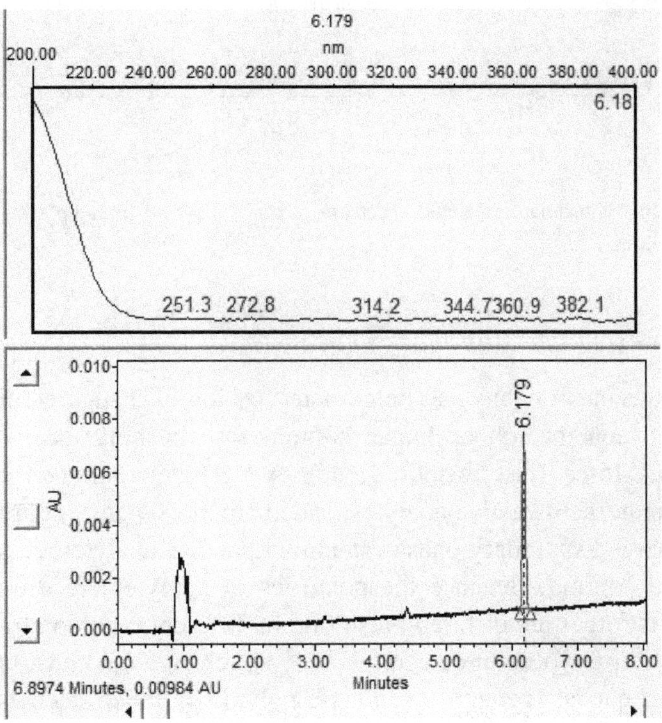

Figure 1.9: Chromatogram and spectrum of pure corosolic acid assayed with a phenyl column.

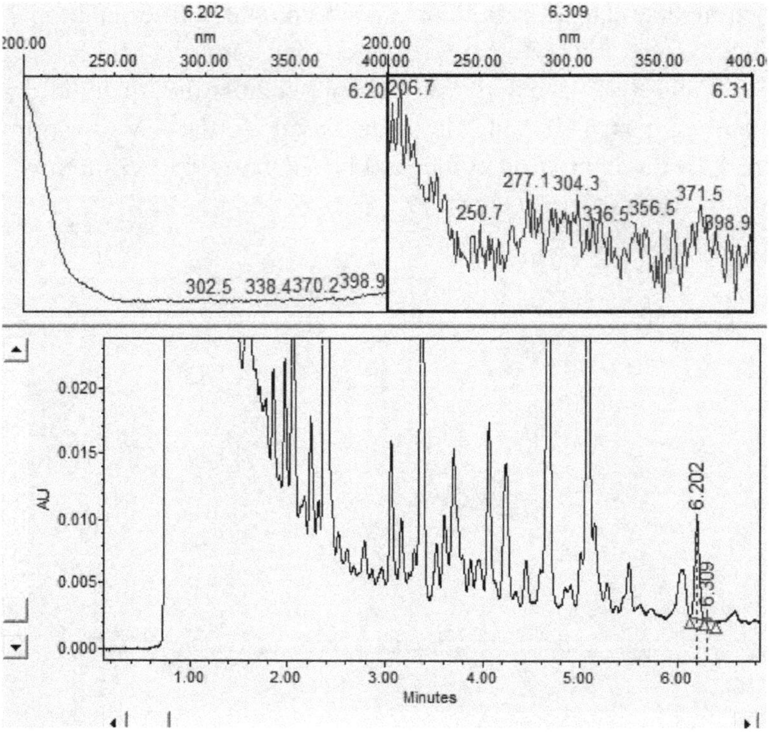

Figure 1.10: Chromatogram and spectrum of corosolic acid in sample matrix with a phenyl column.

(iii) *Ion exchange stationary phase*

Polar molecules or ions can be attracted by ion exchange columns. The force between the ion exchange column and the polar analytes is the Columbus force (electrostatic force). A positively charged stationary phase can attract negative analytes, called anion exchange column; negatively charged stationary phase can attract positive analytes, called cation exchange column. Because the polarities of analytes are different, the Columbus forces are different, resulting in different retention times.

There are two main categories of ion exchange columns. One is the surface of carrier (generally synthetic polymers) which itself is charged under certain mobile phase conditions (see Figure 1.11). The other one is

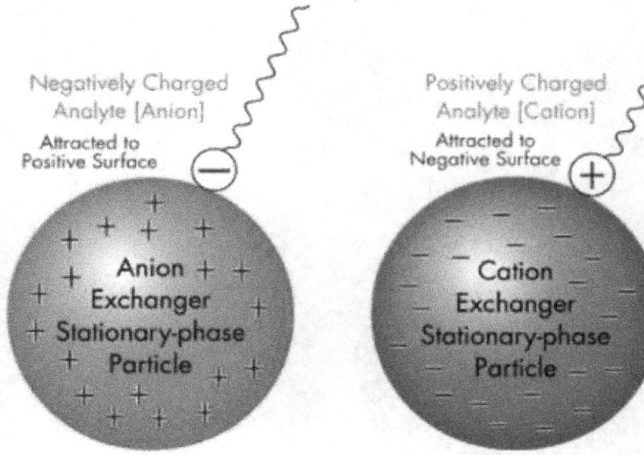

Figure 1.11: Polymer base ion exchange stationry phase.

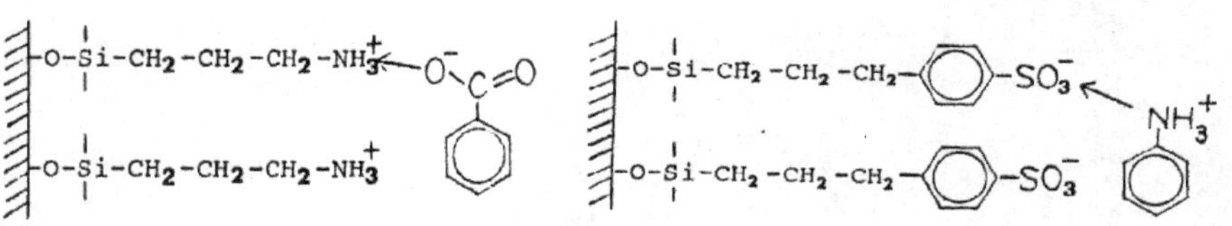

Figure 1.12: Silica bonded ion-exchange stationary phase.

polar compounds or ions bounded to the surface of carrier (usually silica) (see Figure 1.12).

For example, choline is an organic cation and can be separated by the cation exchange column (Figures 1.13 and 1.14).

(iv) *Hydrogen bond stationary phase*

Stationary phase contains a hydroxy group (–OH) that can interact with analytes containing hydroxy (–OH) or amine (–NH_2) group due to hydrogen bond interaction.

Hydrogen bound column can separate analytes containing hydroxy and amine groups from the matrix or other compounds (Figure 1.15).

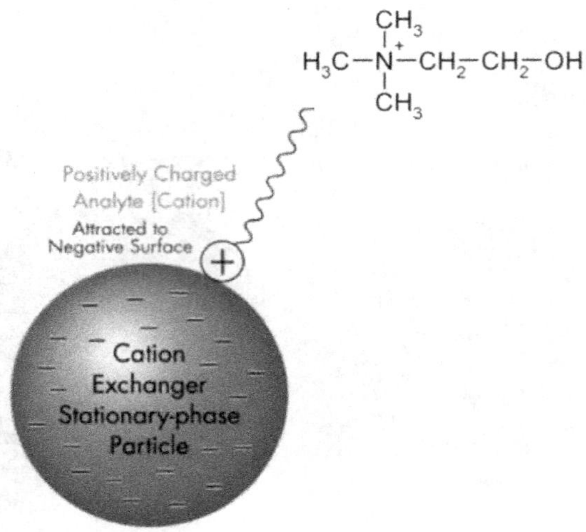

Figure 1.13: Schematic diagram of cation exchange column.

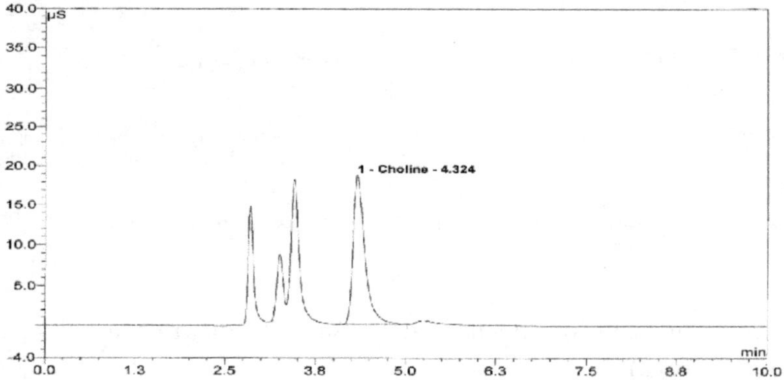

Figure 1.14: Chromatogram of choline run by cation exchange column.

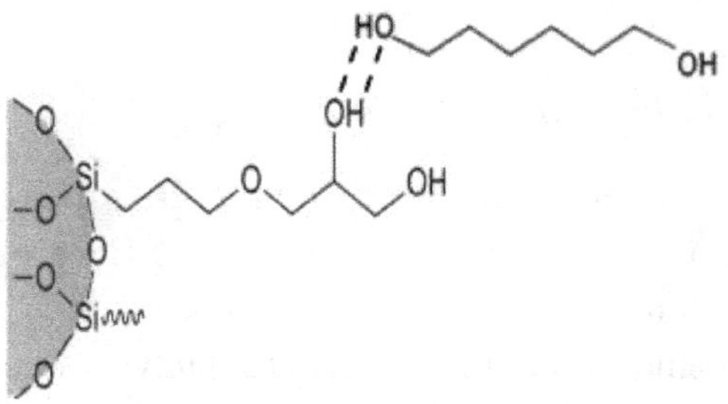

Figure 1.15: Illustration of hydroxy bond stationary phase.

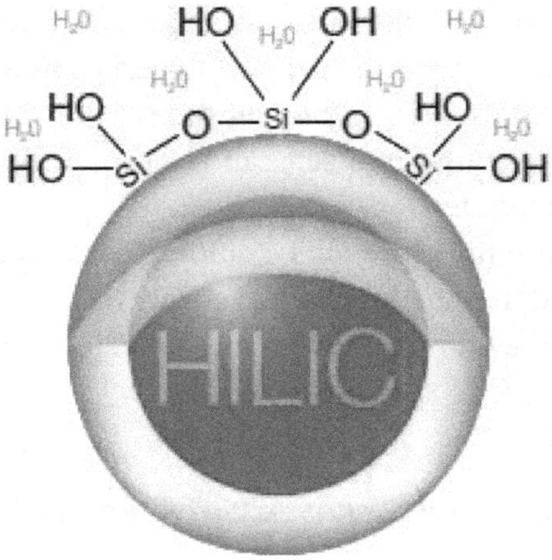

Figure 1.16: Kinetex Hlica normal phase stationary phase.

(v) *Normal phase*

Polar molecules coated carriers or bare silica form a normal stationary phase (as shown in the Figure 1.16).

Normal phase can interact with polar analytes based on the principle of similar compatibility. Under low pH mobile phases, additional hydrogen bond interaction forces may be created. The more non-polar the mobile phase is, the longer the retention time for polar analytes is, but there is less retention time for non-polar analytes.

Normal phase columns are commonly used to separate polar compounds, but non-polar mobile phase (such as 99%, 100% organic solvents) can be used to separate certain non-polar compounds also. For example, α, β, γ, δ tocopherols and tocotrienol are difficult to separate by reversed phase column, especially β and γ isomers. By using normal phase columns with non-polar mobile phase allα, β, γ, δ tocopherols and tocotrienols can be separated.

(vi) *Affinity column*

A special bio-affinity force can be applied to chromatography. The interaction forces usually are a biological biochemical affinity forces such as enzymes and substrates, antigens and antibodies, etc. The bio-macromolecules can be bonded to the support materials as an affinity stationary phase. The corresponding bio-substance will be attracted to the stationary phase, resulting in a separation or a purification application. In dietary supplement testing, avidin bounded support particles can be used to attract biotin molecules in a complex formula during the sample preparation procedure, i.e., after a reagent wash, use an acid to dissociate biotin from the avidin bounded material, and lastly inject it into the HPLC to quantify the biotin amount.

(vii) *Chelate and ligand exchange chromatography*

There are two kinds applications of chelating exchange chromatography. One is used to separate or preconcentrate different metal ions, specifically called chelate exchange chromatography. The other one, the most common application, is used to separate ligand compounds, even goes further to separate ligand enantiomers, specifically called ligand exchange chromatography.

Figure 1.17 shows, a chelating exchange stationary phase.

Different metal ions have different stability constants with chelating stationary phases. The more stable the chelating is, the longer is the retention time.

Proper metal ions can be selected and added to the mobile phase. Once the chelating column reaches equilibrium, the metal ion is attracted evenly on the column. The equilibrated column now becomes a "new stationary phase", specially called a ligand exchange column.

Different ligand analytes have different stability constants with the metal ion attached on the stationary phase. Again, the more stable the

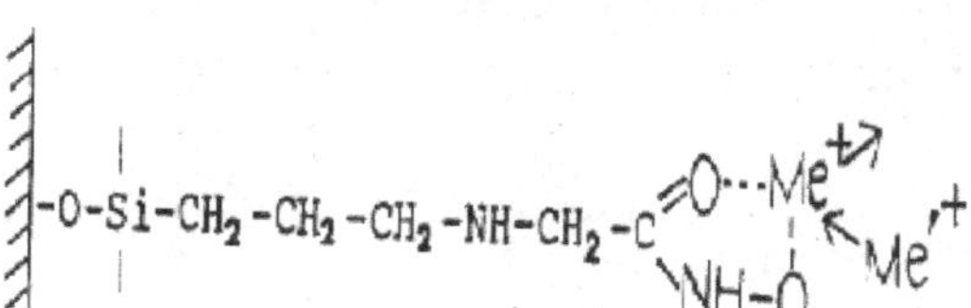

Figure 1.17: Chelating stationary phase.

chelating is, the longer is the retention time, resulting in ligands separation. Due to the different chelate stability, the ligand enantiomers could be separated by the ligand exchange chromatography.

The aforementioned chelate column is not popular, and difficult to find. Cation exchange columns actually can replace the chelate exchange column. The cation exchange column can attract metal ions. Once the column is in equilibrium with the selected metal ions, it exhibits the same chromatography function as ligand exchange column.

The following is one example of using cation exchange column equilibrium with Cu^{2+} to separate hydroxybutyric acid enantiomers (Figure 1.18).

A reverse phase column, such as C_{18}, also can be used as a ligand exchange column to separate the ligand analytes and even their enantiomers. A selected metal ion and suitable ligand (e.g., EDTA) can be added to the mobile phase to form a chelate molecule and be attracted on the C_{18} reversed phase column. When you achieve equilibrium, inject the ligand analyte to chromatography system, the ligand, under test, is going to chelate with the metal ion in the mobile phase, and compete with the original ligand. The more stable chelate formed by the ligand analyte, the longer retention time will be obtained. The chelate stability constants of ligand enantiomers at times are different, thus causing different retention times and resulting enantiomers separation.

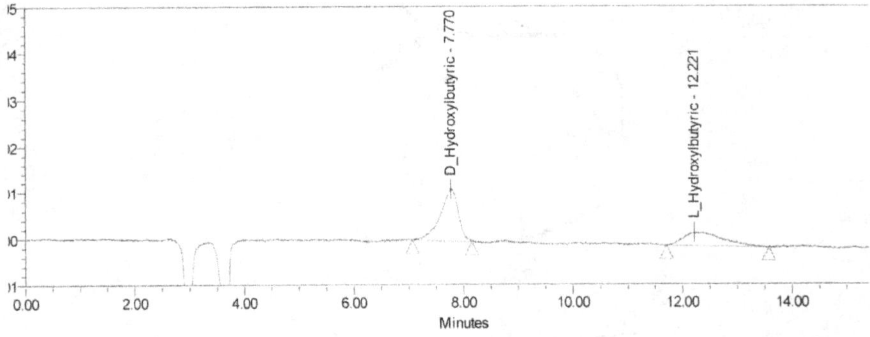

Figure 1.18: Chromatogram of D/L hydroxybutyric acid. Column: cation exchange column; mobile phase: 2.0mM Cu^{2+}, pH 2.0.

1.2 *Mobile phase application*

In liquid chromatography, mobile phase application directly affects the separation efficiency and chromatograms feature.

(i) *The pH of the mobile phase*

The pH of the mobile phase can affect both the stationary phase and the analytes. If the stationary phase is silica base, the silanol on the surface of silica gel will be dissociated while increasing the pH of mobile phase, and turn into negative charge, which creates additional electrostatic forces for the analytes, especially for those acidic and alkaline analytes.

The surface of silica gel has many pores with different diameter sizes (as shown in the Figure 1.19).

If the analytes are negatively charged, they may be excluded outside of the pore, irregularly changing the flow path of the analytes, reducing the column efficiency and peak symmetry. If the analytes are positively charged, the analytes could be attracted to the pores, cause peak tailing, as well reduce the column efficiency.

Therefore, it is recommended that the pH of mobile phase should not exceed 4 in general, when a silica-based reversed column is used.

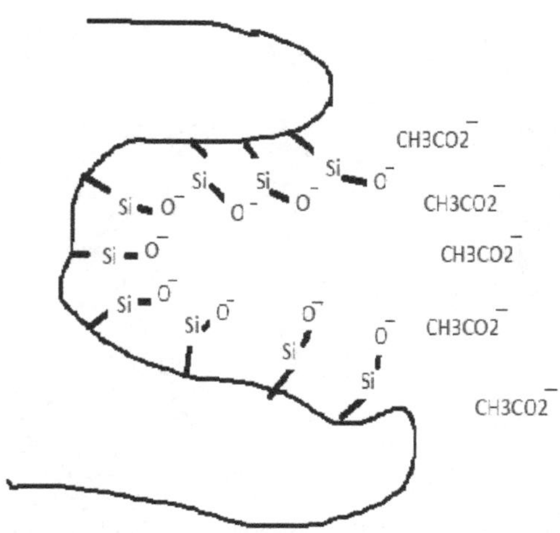

Figure 1.19: The surface of silica gel has many different dimeter wholes.

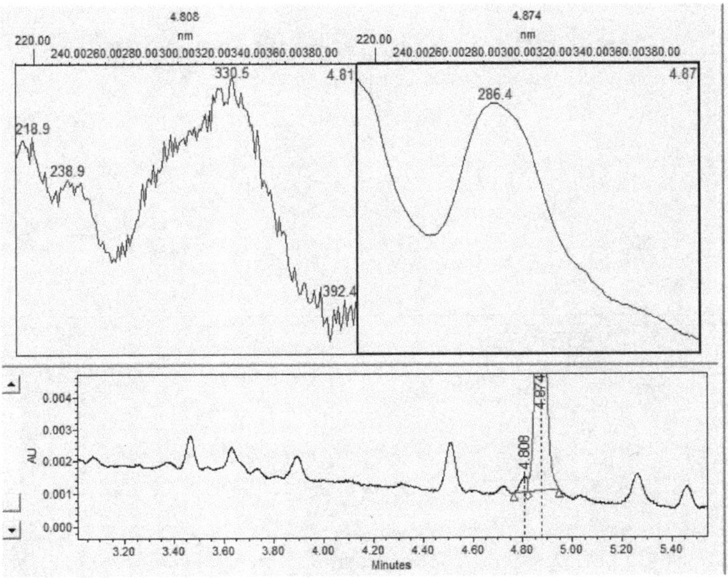

Figure 1.20: Chromatogram of folic acid, chromatography condition: C_{18} column, mobile phase pH 3.0.

The mobile phase with low pH will reduce the polarity of acidic compounds and thus increase the interaction force with the reversed phase column and prolong the peak retention time. This is beneficial for the separation of acidic compounds and possibly eliminate interference. Compare Figures 1.20 and 1.21, while mobile phase pH reduced to 2.0, the interfere compound was completely separated from folic acid peak, because the folic acid peak was relatively delayed.

Generally, by increasing the retention time of polar compounds in the reversed phase column, you will get a better chance to separate the interfering compounds from the analytes.

On the other hand, increasing the pH of mobile phase will reduce the polarity of alkaline compounds, and may increase the retention time with a reversed phase column.

(ii) *Application of ion pairs*

In cases where the matrix is complex and very complex, the analytes often cannot be accurately measured. Extending the retention time of the

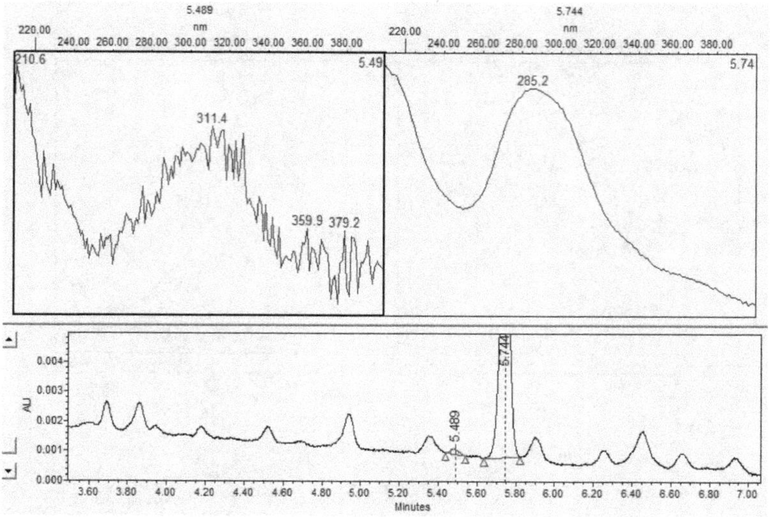

Figure 1.21: Chromatogram of folic acid, chromatography condition: C_{18} column, and mobile phase pH2.

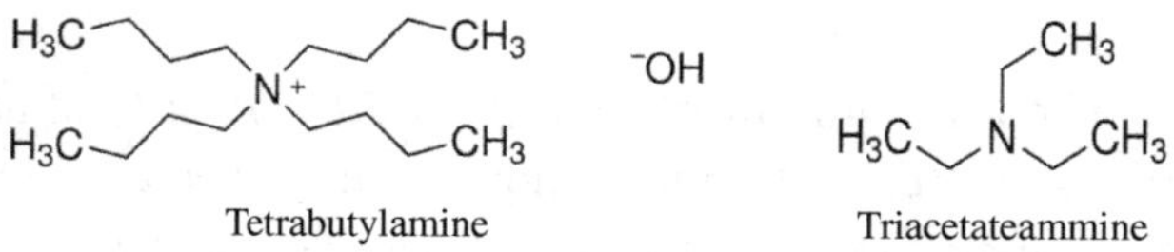

Figure 1.22: Molecules can be used as ion pair for acidic analytes.

analytes can help reduce the chance of interferes. To prolong the retention time of polar analytes, using an ion pairing technique is a very good choice.

In order to increase the retention time of polar analytes, add the opposite charged ions into the mobile phase, the analytes will attract the added ions and form a neutral ion pair, thus prolonging the analytes retention time in the reversed phase column.

If the analytes are negatively charged, add strong alkaline ions (such as tetraamine, triamine salts, see Figure 1.22) into the mobile phase. Usually, the longer carbon chain in the added alkaline ions, will result in longer retention times of the analytes. However, the bigger the molecule ions added, the more is the opportunity to damage the column and instruments.

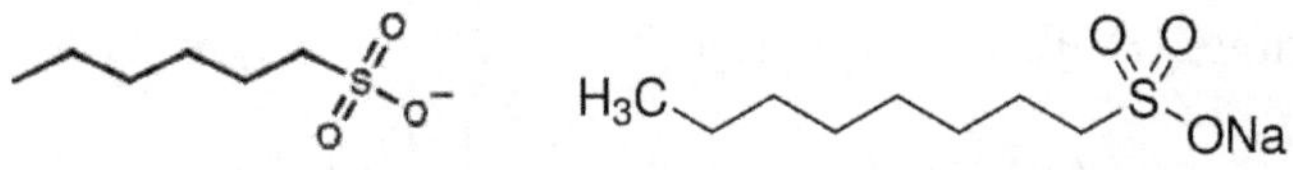

Figure 1.23: Molecules can be used as ion pair for alkaline analytes.

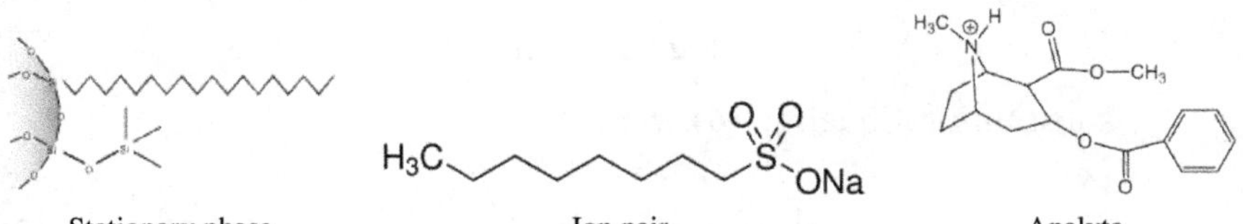

Figure 1.24: Schematic diagram of ion pair chromatogaphy.

On the opposite side, if the analytes are positively charged, a strong organic acid (Figure 1.23) can be added to the mobile phase. The positive analytes will attract the added acid ions to form neutral ion pairs and increase the retention time. Again, the bigger molecule acid added, the longer retention time will be. But the bigger the molecule acid added, the more is the opportunity to damage the column and instruments.

Figure 1.24 shows the mechanism of ion pair chromatography.

The pH of the ion pair mobile phase is also an important parameter.

The ion pair reagents are strong acidic or alkaline compounds; under normal pH conditions (pH 1–7) the polarity will not be changed much.

The analytes polarity may vary when the mobile phase pH changes. For example, to test acetic acid and formic acid with a reversed phase column, and the mobile phase containing tetrabutylamine salt, what should be the pH range of the mobile phase?

Following the formulas

$$Ka = \frac{[H+][Ac-]}{[HAc]} \tag{1}$$

$$[H+] = Ka\frac{[HAc]}{[Ac-]} \tag{2}$$

$$pH = -\log[H+] \tag{3}$$

Substitute [H+] from Equation (2)

$$p[H] = -\log Ka - \log\frac{[HAc]}{[Ac-]} \tag{4}$$

Due to

$$-\log Ka = pKa$$

By substituting Equation (4), we get

$$p[H] = pKa - \log\frac{[HAc]}{[Ac-]} \tag{5}$$

In order to properly use the ion pair method, the analytes should be dissociated as an anion. Here, it is assumed that when **dynamic equilibrium reaches,** 90% of analytes are dissociated.

$$\frac{[HAc]}{[Ac-]} \leq \frac{1}{10}$$

Then Equation (5) can be explained as,

$$pH = pKa + 1 \tag{6}$$

The *pKa* of acetic acid is 4.76. In order to let the ion pair method work properly and efficiently, the majority of acetic acid molecules should be dissociated, so the pH of mobile phase should not be less than *pKa* + 1 = 5.76.

pKa of formic acid is 3.75, the pH of mobile phase should not be less than 3.75 + 1 = 4.75.

If acetic acid and formic acid are tested simultaneously, the final pH of the mobile phase should not be less than 5.76.

If the analytes are alkaline compounds, then

$$Kb = \frac{[BH+][OH]}{[B]} \tag{7}$$

Here [*B*] is alkaline analyte molecule, [*BH*+] is protonated analyte.

$$[OH] = Kb\frac{[B]}{[BH+]} \tag{8}$$

$$p[OH] = -\log Kb - \frac{\log[B]}{[BH+]} \tag{9}$$

Since,

$$-\log Kb = pKb$$

So,

$$P[OH] = pKb - \log\frac{[B]}{[BH+]} \tag{10}$$

Again, assume most of the analyte molecules are protonated; the dynamic equilibrium reaches 90% of analytes when they are protonated.

$$\frac{[B]}{[BH+]} \leq \frac{1}{10}$$

$$p[OH] = pKb + 1 \tag{11}$$

Due to

$$pH = 14 - p[OH]$$

substitute Equation (11) for P[*OH*–], yield

$$pH = 14 - p[Kb] - 1 \tag{12}$$

because,

$$14 - pKb = pKa \tag{13}$$

So, Equation (13) also can be expressed as:

$$pH = pKa - 1 \tag{14}$$

For example, the *pKb* of aniline is known to be 9.13, and if sulfonate salt is used as an ion pair reagent, the pH of the mobile phase should not be greater than 14 – 9.13 – 1 = 3.87. If *pKa* value of the alkaline analyte is know, you can directly use Equation (14) to calculate the pH.

For bipolar compounds (e.g., amino acids, etc.), the adjustment of the pH should be determined according to the molecular isoelectric point. For example, cysteine isoelectric point is 5.05. It means at pH 5.05 the bipolar molecule is neutral, while the pH is less than 5.05, the molecule is positively charged; if pH higher than 5.05, the molecule will be negatively charged. If the sulfonate anion is used as an ion pair reagent, the pH should be adjusted to not higher than 5.05 – 1 = 4.05; if a strong alkaline is used as an ion pair reagent, the pH of mobile phase should be adjusted to not less than 5.05 + 1 = 6.05.

(iii) *Organic solvents in the mobile phase*

Table 1.1 compares the physical properties of commonly used organic solvents in liquid chromatography.

Based on Table 1.1, the viscosity of acetonitrile and the ultraviolet cut-off is ideal for using as mobile phases. Methanol, ethanol, isopropanol, hexane, chloroform, etc., are also commonly used as liquid chromatography mobile phase or mobile phase components.

Generally speaking, the stronger the non-polarity of the analytes in the reversed phase chromatography, the stronger the non-polarity of the mobile phase should be used to elute the analytes. However, using stronger non-polar solvents have an impact on the instrument and the column.

So, for very strong non-polar analytes, a less non-polarity column (such as C_8, C_4, etc., columns) can be used instead of C_{18} column, rather than using strong non-polar solvents.

Changing the percentage of organic solvents in the mobile phase can have different separation effects. Organic solvents in the mobile phase can also be added using a gradient to gradually increase the percentage to accelerate the elution of the analytes, thus reducing the peak width, and

Table 1.1: Physical properties of organic solvents commonly used in liquid chromatography.

Solvent	UV cut off	Viscosity
Acetonitrile	200nm	0.47
Methanol	240nm	0.69
Ethanol	240nm	1.36
Propanol	240	2.43

increasing the resolution. The principle of the operation is just like the gravity acceleration, where a basin of water falls from kilometers high with gravity acceleration divided into discontinuous water columns or droplets when it reaches the ground.

(iv) *Mobile phase in ion exchange chromatography*

Adjusting the mobile phase pH for a strong ion exchange chromatography, only considers the pH influence on analytes and ignores the influence on strong ions on the stationary phase. Increasing the polarity of the analytes will prolong the elution time, but if the polarity is too strong it will cause the analytes to be difficult to elute or even to be ineludible. Reducing the polarity of the analytes, will reduce the interaction force and shorten the elute time in strong ion exchange column. By changing the pH of mobile phase the polarity of analytes can be adjusted to cause a proper retention time.

For weak ion exchange chromatography, changing the mobile phase pH will affect both stationary phase and analytes. By reducing the pH of mobile phase, the weak cation exchange column will reduce the polarity, but may increase the polarity of analytes. Reducing the pH of mobile phase, will also increase the polarity of weak anion exchange stationary phase. It may, however cause the loss of polarity of analytes.

The strength of interaction force of weak ion exchange chromatography may vary with the change in pH. How to adjust the pH of the mobile phase to obtain the best chromatography effect depends on the analytes, sample matrix, composition of mobile phase and other factors. This needs to be explored in practice. However, the principle of adjustment of pH is extremely helpful for the development or adjustment of the testing method.

In addition, adding counter ions to the mobile phase can also regulate the peak retention time. In the strong cation exchange and strong anion exchange chromatography, the analytes are sometimes difficultly to elute, causing long retention time and wide peaks, or even not all the peaks are eluted. In order to control the retention time, we can intentionally add competitive ions with different strengths to the mobile phase. For example, in the anion exchange chromatography, we can add acetic acid ions to the mobile phase, occupy the active sites on the stationary phase, compete with the analyte anions, reduce the stationary phase partition coefficient of analytes ions to reduce the retention time. For cation exchange chromatography, ammonia or amine ions are often added to the mobile phase as competing ions.

The strength of the counter ions in the mobile phase depends on the structure and concentration of the ions.

Generally speaking, the higher the valence number is, the greater the radius of the ion is, thus the greater ion strength. The higher the ion concentration is, the greater the ion strength.

1.3 *Samples and standards solutions preparation*

There are different types of dietary supplements with different dosage forms, such as tablets, capsules, soft gels, solid powders, liquids, etc. It makes the sample preparation and extraction more difficult and complex. However, it does not matter what the dosage form is, the purpose of sample preparation is trying to completely extract and dissolve the analytes into the test solution. In general, if the analyte is water soluble, water can be used as a solvent to extract the analyte; if the analyte is oil-soluble, then use organic solvent extraction. But some adjustments are needed for some special samples.

(i) When testing the water-soluble components in soft gel or oil-based matrix, you cannot simply use water directly to extract the analytes, because water and oil are incompatible, the liquid–liquid extraction is inefficient and it is difficult to extract all the components under test into the water. Therefore, a small amount of dispersion solvent (miscible for both oil and water, could be methanol, acetonitrile, ethanol, etc.) should be mixed with the sample first, then water needs to be added to extract. The procedure is also called dispersion extraction. Dispersion extraction is much more efficient than liquid–liquid extraction, and can completely extract the analyte from the sample matrix.

(ii) When testing oil-soluble compounds in solid powders, they cannot be extracted directly by organic solvents, as many oil-soluble active compounds may be surrounded or coated in hydrophilic substances such as starch, cellulose, etc. Organic solvents are difficult to immerse in these hydrophilic substances, so it is difficult to extract all the oil soluble active compounds. These hydrophilic substances should be disintegrated with a small amount of warm water before the organic solvent extraction.

(iii) Some components in dietary supplement can react with each other, such as ferric ion can oxidize vitamin C. Also, metal ions can form chelate with some organic molecules, etc. All these reactions could affect the final test results. In order to protect the analytes that may be oxidized, during the sample preparation procedure add some reducing reagent, like sodium thiosulfate, vitamin C, or other reducing agents. In addition, in the protective reagent can also add some strong complex ligands such as EDTA to protect the analyte from being chelated.

(iv) Different extraction solvents can be used to reduce interferences. For example, vitamin B_{12} is generally extracted with water, but if the chromatogram is too messy, methanol or ethanol can be used instead, because B_{12} can be dissolved in either water or alcohol, but some interferants may be soluble only in water and not alcohol, offering a way to eliminate interferences.

(v) Some unstable compounds, such as carotenoids, can be degraded by oxygen. To extend the shelf life of the product, manufacturers will make these compounds as granulations, that is, using substances such as gelatin to coat these unstable ingredients into tiny beads to isolate them from the atmosphere. The produced materials are very stable. But these small beads must be broken down before extraction of the active ingredients or they will not be measured. Granulation is sometimes made using gelatin, and in the testing procedure bromelain must be used to break down the gelatin shell to expose the active ingredients and then use the appropriate solvent for extraction. Enzymatic digestions can usually be done in an hour at 37°C. But not all granulations are made by gelatin, some granulations are made by starch or denatured starch, wax, etc. The different kinds of granulation must have different break down and extraction methods. When testing these kind granulation products, request an extraction method from the manufacture first, then follow the method to prepare the test solution; otherwise, it will bring a lot of inconvenience to the test work.

(vi) Generally, the standard solution preparation should be the same as the sample solution preparation. However, with some unstable standard compounds, the purity should be determined before preparing the standard solution. For example, to measure the purity of lutein follow these steps: First the specified solvent is used to make a solution, measuring the UV absorption of the lutein solution, and using the extinction coefficient to calculate the concentration of the solution. Next, run HPLC with same UV wavelength as UV purity test, calculate the chromatography normalization purity. Finally, the purity measured by the ultraviolet spectrum is multiplied by the chromatography purity to obtain the real purity of the standard material.

In addition, some standards are very expensive and you cannot prepare new standard solutions every time you are testing. You can properly preserve the original standard solution for continuous use later. To ensure the stability of the original solution, a suitable stable compound can be added to the original solution as a reference. Run the liquid chromatography and record the peak area of the standard and the peak area of the reference. The ratio of the two peak areas is calculated. It can be used the next time if the peak area ratio remains unchanged, indicating that the original standard solution is stable. Stop using if the ratio of the areas is out of control, prepare a new standard solution is necessary.

1.4 *Introduction to the instrument*

(i) *High performance liquid chromatograph HPLC*

The high-performance liquid chromatograph is mainly composed of three components: injector, solvent compression pump and detector. The simplest way to deliver a sample is to manually inject it with a syringe. Modern instruments are generally computer controlled, have automatic samplers that have injection volumes from 1 to 100 μL. Different manufacturers have different injection techniques and corresponding devices. The repeatability and accuracy should be verified when installed.

The maximum pressure of the solvent compression pump of HPLC is generally 5,000–6,000 psi. There are two types of solvent compression pumps, high-pressure pumps and low-pressure pumps, where high and low pressures have a special definition. Low-pressure pump refers to the mobile phase solvent A, B, C, D mixed with different proportions and then compressed by a single compression pump to the column and detector. The high-pressure pump is solvent A and solvent B compressed through two individual pumps, after pumps the two solvents are mixed, it then goes to the column. The disadvantage of a low-pressure pump is that mixing of solvents will create bubbles that may accumulate into large bubbles that can cause unstable pressure and varying flow rates, affecting chromatography quality. In addition, the response time is slow when running on solvents gradients. So, the same gradient program in high-pressure and low-pressure HPLC coming out of the chromatography may not be exactly the same. The advantage is that it can make four different solvents mixture as mobile phase, and only one compression pump is required, to be more economical.

HPLC has a wide range of detectors, mainly ultraviolet/visible light (UV/Vis), fluorescence (FLR), refractive aberration (RI), evaporative light scattering (ELSD), mass spectrometry (MS or MS/MS), electrochemical (EC) and conductivity (CD). Only the most widely used UV/Vis and MS/MS are discussed here. ED and CD will be described in section of ion chromatography (IC).

Ultraviolet/visible light detector has two main categories: full-scan (PDA) detector and single wavelength (SWL) detector. PDA is a full-scan of each reading point (e.g., 200–500 nm), which means that each reading point can get a complete full-scan spectrum. The chromatographic peak spectrum of a pure compound should be consistent from start to finish and highly match with the spectrum of the standard. If the spectrum varies in the chromatography peak period or if it does not match the spectrum of standard, it is possible that the peak contains other compounds or are not at all the same compound as the standard.

Each reading point of the SWL only reads the adsorbed strength at a single wavelength. The purity of the chromatography peak is not possible to be identified. Therefore, it may result in an error in the final report. PDA is highly recommended for dietary supplement testing.

Mass spectrometry detectors are also highly recommended in mass/mass spectroscopy to increase selectivity, and avoid errors in detection. The Multiple Reaction Monitoring (MRM) model is the most widely used in qualitative and quantitative analyses. The molecular weight of the analyte is delivered to the instrument's software. Q1 focuses on this set molecular ion, any molecular ion that meets the set molecular weight will be sent by Q1 to Collision Cell to produce the corresponding fragments, which enters Q3 and accurately measures the mass and quantity. Different molecules of with same molecular weight do not produce exact the same fragments pattern after impact. In order to improve the selectivity, the three ion pairs were selected to compare with the standard.

Parent 1 > daughter ions 1,
parent 1 > daughter ions 2,
Parent 1 > daughter ions 3.

If the mass of the three fragments is the same as the standard, and the proportions are consistent in quantity, then it can be determined that the parent ion is the analyte ion. This, combined with HPLC retention time, further enhances certainty. The sum of the three ion pairs or the largest number of first set of ion pairs can be used for quantitative calculations. In the selection of ion pairs, one or two more ion pairs can be selected, in case the selected ion pair is disturbed.

MS/MS detector is very sensitive; the detection limit for B_{12} and biotin could reach to ppb level.

However, because the degree of ionization of the analyte molecules in different matrix backgrounds may be different, the repeatability may not be as good as UV/Vis detector. This may result in the data not being as accurate and precise as UV/Vis. Therefore, for high accuracy and precision quantitative testing is often better using UV/Vis detector, if possible.

Today, the advancement of high-resolution MS/MS spectrometer allows resolution to reach 6–7 digits after the decimal point. Such a high-resolution mass spectrometer is helpful for testing unknown compounds. For example, when a molecule monitored with molecular weight of 356.546734, there are very few possible molecules that fit this molecular weight. Combine the high-resolution isotopes and the fragment patterns to increase the certainty. Finally, a reference standard molecule (if available) can be used for final confirmation. The non-target testing has potential advantages, especially in food safety, new drug development, nutrition research, agriculture testing areas. In today's labs, most analytical tests are targeted tests, like melamine analysis, aflatoxins testing, certain listed pesticides screen, antibiotics screens, environment hazards tests, etc., all are testing targeted compounds. The limitation of the target testing is each test method only can test certain compounds. How can we check all harmful substances in the foods, such as pesticides, antibiotics, steroids, illegal drugs, adulterants, unproved colors, aflatoxins, etc., and even some unknown hazards? If we use existing methods to test the food safety, it will take a long time and result in many expenses, but still may probably miss some hazards and toxic compounds. As long as the compounds present in the sample, whether harmful or beneficial, high-resolution MS/MS spectrometer could identify and quantify, this will be an innovation in the testing industry.

The instruments are developing with time, the large data sets are going to be established with the internet, and the non-target test is becoming more and more practicable.

Now, the ion mobility spectrometer coupled LC/MS/MS is also used in the laboratory. Ion mobility spectrometer can separate ions with the same m/z value, but different stereo structures. Ions collide with buffer gas when they pass through the drift tube with same electric field, and through a series of different mechanisms, the ions with different stereo structures and sizes move differently in the drift tube to produce different drift times, thus playing a separation role. For example, different isomers, different molecular weight but same m/z value, same m/z value but different amino acid sequence peptides, sugar at different carbon of glycosides and so on, could be separated by ion mobility spectrometer.

(ii) *Ultra performance liquid chromatograph*

Ultra-Performance Liquid Chromatography (UPLC), also known as UHPLC, is the new generation of HPLC, developed in the last two decades. Its greatest advantage is speed, saving time and solvents.

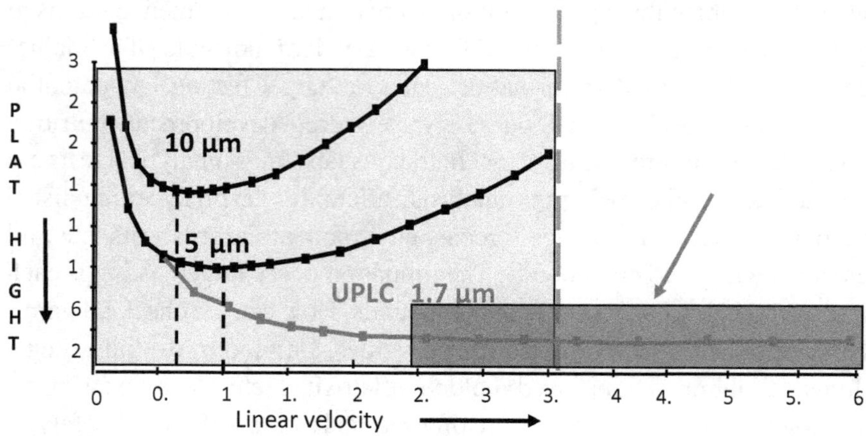

Figure 1.25: Van Deemter's curve.

Base on Van Deemter curve (see Figure 1.25), column efficiency is related to the mobile phase linear velocity. But if the particle size of carrier is small enough, we can keep the high efficiency even with fast linear velocity.

Base on the chromatography theory, the column efficiency (N) is inversely proportion to the partical size (dp) of carrier.

$$N \propto \frac{1}{dp}$$

The general HPLC carrier diameter is 5.0 μm, UPLC carrier diameter is 1.7 μm, compare the columns efficiency 5/1.7≈3.

So, the column efficiency of 5 cm long UPLC column equivalent 15 cm HPLC column.

Now let us compare the mobile phase linear velocity. Usually, 10 cm UPLC column flow rate is 0.6 ml/min, dead value is 0.2 ml; HPLC 25 cm column flow rate is 1.0 ml/min, dead value is 2.5 ml.

UPLC linear velocity = (0.6 ml/min) × (10 cm/0.2 ml) = 30 cm/min

HPLC linear velocity = (1.0 ml/min) × (25 cm/2.5 ml) = 10 cm/min

The linear velocity of UPLC is 3 times faster than HPLC. UPLC column efficiency is about 3 times higher than HPLC, and in order to get same column efficiency as HPLC, only 1/3 column length needed. So, with same column efficiency the UPLC is 3 × 3 = 9 times faster than HPLC.

See Figures 1.26 and 1.27.

The higher flow rate, smaller particle size of the carrier will create a high column back pressure. So UPLC need to solve two technical

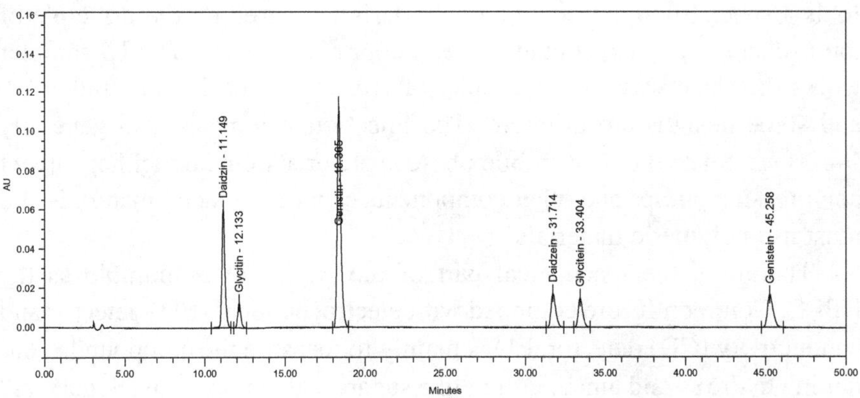

Figure 1.26: HPLC chromatogram with 25 cm column, 1.0 ml/min flow rate.

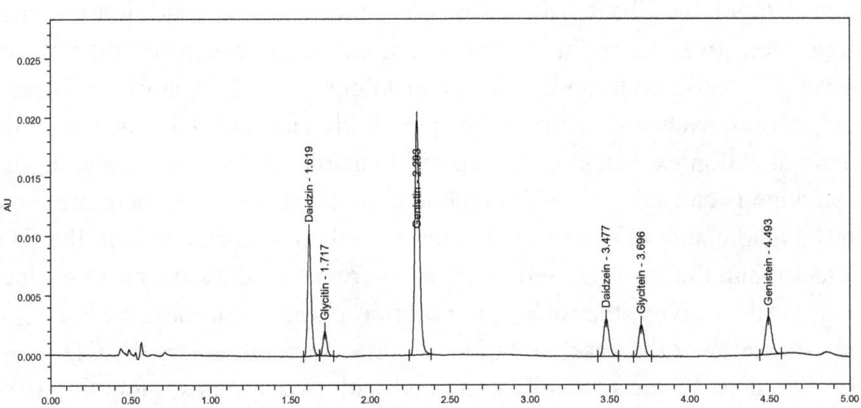

Figure 1.27: UPLC chromatogram with 10 cm column, 0.6 ml/min flow rate.

problems: (1) The carrier of the column can withstand high pressure (15,000 psi) and does not break and deform under high pressure conditions. (2) The instrument should be able to produce and withstand high pressure (15,000 psi) and not leak under high pressure conditions. At the end of the last century, the development of UPLC was successful, and now gradually became popular.

(iii) *Ion chromatograph (IC)*

IC is a special liquid chromatograph, designed based on the principle of ion exchange. IC also contains three major components. The IC sampler works the same way as the sampler of HPLC, except that the trademark and some designs are different. The injection volume is also generally 1–100 μL. Since the IC's mobile phase is either alkaline or acidic, solvent compression pumps and other components cannot use metal materials and must use polymeric materials.

Therefore, the mechanical part of the IC is not as durable as the HPLC. Common IC are equipped with electrochemical (ED) detector and conductivity (CD) detector. ED is mainly to measure the compounds containing hydroxy and amine group, like sugars and amino acids. Sugars and amino acids are negatively charged with a strong alkaline mobile phase. Therefore, sugars and amino acids can be separated with anion exchange chromatography. The sensitivity of ED under alkaline condition is quite high. Detection limits for sugars and amino acids can reach 50 ppb or lower. CD responds to both cations and anions. Therefore, anion exchange and cation exchange chromatography both can use CD as detector. General cation exchange is carried out in acidic mobile phase, and anion exchange is carried out under alkaline conditions. Because there are ions in the acidic and alkaline mobile phase, so there is a response in the CD detector and the baseline will be high. In order to reduce the baseline and increase sensitivity, the ions in the mobile phase are removed by a suppressor to lower the baseline before the mobile phase enters the CD.

Standard IC are generally equipped with two systems, including two compression pumps, corresponding to two sets of mobile phase devices and connected to ED and CD. Such a set of equipment can be used to test sugar, amino acids, anion and cation.

1.5 *Qualitative and quantitative testing of LC-ESI-MS/MS*

(i) *Qualitative test*

In order to improve the selectivity, avoid variation, HPLC or UPLC tandem mass spectrometer is used to authenticate the analyte molecule with the retention time of the chromatography and the m/z value of the mass spectrometry. However, in complex matrixes, there is a possibility that the same molecular weight compounds are mixed in one chromatographic peak. In this case LC/MS is limited in qualitative testing. Therefore, LC/MS/MS is recommended in dietary supplement testing. The MRM model usually is used for qualitative and quantitative testing. The molecular weight of the analyte is delivered to the instrument's software. Q1 focuses on this set molecular ion, and the m/z value of any ion that meets the set molecular ion is sent to Collision Cell by Q1 that produces the corresponding fragments, which enters Q3 and accurately measures the mass and quantity of the fragments. Different molecules with the same m/z value would not create an exact same fragment pattern. In order to improve the selectivity generally select the top three ion pairs for identification and quantitative analysis, i.e.,

Parent 1 > daughter ions 1,
Parent 1 > daughter ions 2,
Parent 1 > daughter ions 3.

The three ion pairs were selected to compare with the standard. If the mass of the three fragments is exactly same as that of the standard, and the quantitative proportions are consistent, then it can be determined that the parent molecule ion is the compound under measuring. This, combined with chromatography retention time, further enhances certainty. Additional one or two more ion pairs could be selected. In case the selected ion pairs interfered, the spare ion pairs can be used as a substitute.

(ii) *Quantitative testing*

The sum of or the largest one of the three ion pairs selected above can be used for quantitative calculations.

However, the ionization process (ESI) of mass spectrometers is easily interfered by the matrix (inhibited or enhanced, but in most cases, ionization is inhibited). Because the concentration of interferants in dietary supplement may greatly exceed the concentration of the analyte, energy may be absorbed by the interferants in the process of ionization and for this reason the analyte cannot be totally ionized or even completely not ionized. In contrast, the solvent standard solution is not affected by the matrix; the degree of ionization may be higher than the analyte in sample solution. Therefore, the actual test must determine the ionization degree of analyte in the sample matrix.

Quantitative analysis generally has two methods, one is the internal standard method, the other one is the external standard method, the following are discussions of the two methods.

(1) Internal standard method: The requirement of the internal standard compound is that the degree of ionization in the same chromatography condition should be same as or have a fixed proportion to the analyte, the physical and chemical properties of the internal standard should be similar to the compound to be measured to achieve fragmentation pattern consistency, and the internal standard compound is basically not present in the sample. To meet those requirements, only isotope molecules of the molecules to be tested are the ideal choice.

However, if the isotope internal standard in the sample matrix recovery rate is very low, then it cannot be used to calculate the result. For example, the recovery rate of the internal standard is only 20%, when the concentration of the internal standard and the analyte may be not proportional to the signal strength of MS/MS. For example, under certain condition of a matrix interference, the recovery rate of the internal standard is very low, in this case, if the peak area of the internal stand is 2,000, and the peak area of the analyte is only 1,000, it cannot be taken for granted that the concentration of the analyte is half of the concentration of the internal standard, because in this environment the signal of MS/MS and concentration may not be proportional. Therefore, in order to get an accurate result, one has to go through the following procedures.

Calculate the recovery of the internal standard.

First, prepare three different concentrations of solvent internal standard solutions[1] (no sample matrix), and inject it to the instrument system. Establish a standard work curve, at the same time check the linearity of the instrument. Prepare a sample solution,[2] and add a known amount of internal standard just before the injection. Calculate the recovery of the added internal standard in the sample solution:

$$Recovery = \frac{Peak\ area\ of\ internal\ standard\ measured}{theoretical\ peak\ area\ of\ added\ internal\ standard}$$

The theoretical peak area of added internal standard is calculated with standard working curve.

If the internal standard recovery is reasonable (e.g., 80%), use internal standard as reference to calculate the result.

$$Analyte\ (\%) = \frac{Aa \times C \times V \times 100\%}{Ai \times W}$$

Here

Aa = Peak area of analyte
Ai = Peak area of internal standard
C = Concentration of internal standard (mg/ml)
V = Total volume of sample solution (ml)
W = Sample weight (mg)

If the internal standard recovery exceeds the prescribed range, (such as 80–120%, the prescribed range of recovery is based on the test method, the matrix of the sample, the instrument used, etc., it should be with some level verification), the most efficient approach would then be to dilute the sample solution,[3] test sample solution[4] and the solvent internal standard solution[5] (if needed) to reach 3–5 times of instrument detection limit, and

---

[1] Sample solution*, sample solution without internal standard.
Test sample solution*, sample solution with internal standard.
Solvent standard solution*, standard solution without sample matrix.
[2] *Ibid.*
[3] Ibid.
[4] Ibid.
[5] Ibid.

then reinject into LC/MS/MS. If the internal standard recovery reaches the specified range, the result can be calculated by diluted solutions. If the recovery is still outside the acceptable range, there are two options:

Option one, after dilution make the peak area of the analyte and the peak area of the internal standard very close by adjusting the amount of internal standard spiked, and use the internal standard as reference to calculate the result.

Option two, the steps to establish an internal standard working curve with the sample matrix background are as follows: Prepare five sample solutions, and add different amounts of internal standard before injection, resulting in 0.05, 0.1, 0.5, 1.5 and 2 times as the internal standard in the test sample solution, together with the original test sample solution for a total of six points. The working curve of the quadratic function is established by the horizontal coordinate of the amount of spiked internal standard (or convert to concentrations), and the ordinate of the peak area of the internal standard (Figure 1.28). By entering the peak area of the analyte (not internal standard) in the test sample solution, the corresponding concentration can be found on the working curve, then calculate the result.

The above calculations assume that the ionization degree of the analyte molecule and the internal standard molecule is the same.

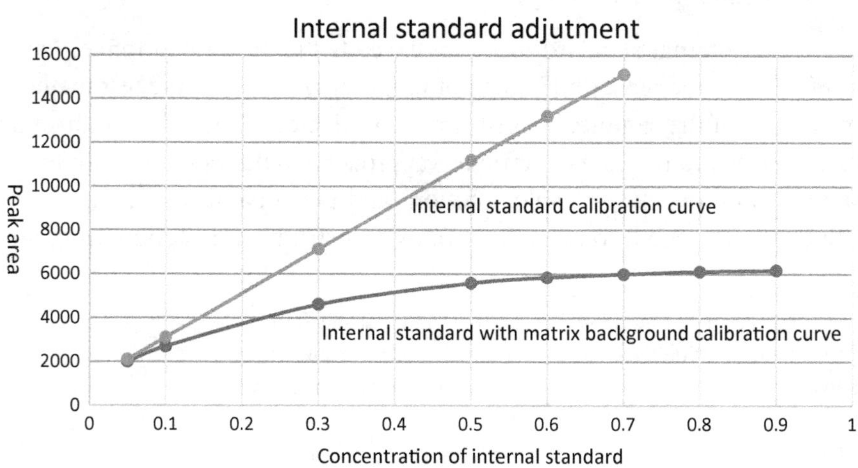

Figure 1.28: The blank calibration curve vs. matrix background calibration curve.

In addition, the deuterium (^{2}H) **or** (^{13}C) isotope internal standard may contain certain percentage of hydrogen (^{1}H) **or** (^{12}C) isotope. In this case, the actual concentrations of internal standard (^{2}H) **or** (^{12}C) solution should be used to calculate the result, and the calculated result should substrate the portion of hydrogen (^{1}H) **or** (^{12}C) isotope that comes from the internal standard. For example, the internal standard(^{2}H) isotope is only 90%, the other 10% is (^{1}H) isotope which is the analyte.

$$Analyte\ (\%) = \frac{C \times V \times 0.9}{W} \times 100\% \quad (R)$$

Here

C = Concentration of analyte in sample solution (mg/ml), obtained from the internal standard (with matrix) working curve

V = Total volume of sample solution (ml)

W = Sample weight (mg)

0.9 = (^{2}H) isotope purity

R = Calculated result

However, the aforementioned calculated result contains (^{1}H) isotope that comes from the internal standard. So, the calculated result should substrate this part of (^{1}H) isotope.

$$Final\ result = R - \frac{C \times V \times 0.1}{W} \times 100\%$$

Here

R = Above calculated result

C = Concentration of internal standard solution(mg/ml), obtained from the internal standard (with matrix) working curve

V = Total volume of sample solution (ml)

W = Sample weight of sample (mg)

0.1 = Percentage of (^{1}H) isotope impurity contained in the internal standard

In extreme cases, if the recovery of the internal standard is too low or there is no internal standard peak at all, the conditions of chromatography and mass spectrometry should be adjusted first, such as changing the chromatography columns, mobile phases, etc., so that the interferents could be separated. Also, different interfaces of MS/MS, for example, using APCI to replace ESI, and adjusting the mass spectrometry parameters, until the above procedures are implemented, can be tried.

If chromatography ion pair method is necessary, only volatile acids or alkalis can be used, such as trifluoroacetic acid, triethylamine, etc. When ion pair reagents are added to the mobile phase, the sensitivity of the mass spectrometer decreases significantly, making trace analysis impossible.

(2) External standard method: The isotope internal standard is more expensive, and some of isotope internal standards are not available. So, the external standard method is widely used.

Using the pure analyte as external standard, prepare different concentrations of external standard solutions, inject the different concentrations of standard solution into the LC/MS/MS system, create a working curve with the concentration as horizontal coordinates, signal strength (peak area) as vertical coordinates. Then inject the sample solution, get the corresponding peak area. The peak area is input into the working curve get the corresponding concentration.

However, the external standard method also has the problem of matrix interference. There is no matrix interference factor in the standard solution, so the ionization degree of the analyte in standard solution may be higher than the analyte in sample matrix solution. In order to have an accurate result follow the steps below to maximize the elimination of the interferes from the sample matrixes.

- Detection of spike recover.
- Separately take 1 ml of sample solution in to two vails, in one vail add know amount of standard. The two solutions are injected to LC/MS/MS separately.

The recovery of the added amount is calculated as follows:

$$Spike\,recovery = \frac{As - AO}{The\,theoretical\,area\,of\,the\,added\,standard} \times 100\%$$

Here

As = Peak area of spiked sample solution.
AO = Peak area of original sample solution.

The theoretical area of the added standard = Input the spiked amount (convert to concentration) to the working curve to get the corresponding peak area.

If the spike recovery is within the prescribed range, then the recovery is used to adjust the calculated result.

$$Actual\ result = \frac{Result\ calculated}{Spike\ recovery}$$

If the spike recovery is beyond the prescribed range (assuming 80–120%), the most efficient approach would then be to dilute the above sample and sample spiked solution, so that the concentration of analyte is 3–5 times of the instrument detection limit. Inject the diluted sample and sample spikred solution to LC/NS/MS separately, to calculate the spike recovery.

If the recovery is dropped in the prescribed range, the result calculated by diluted solutions can be adjusted by the recovery measured after dilution, to get an accurate result.

The prescribed range of recovery should be determined according to the sample matrix, different instruments, methods and other factors, and should be with some level vitrification.

If the sample solution cannot be diluted due to the instrument detection limit, or after dilution the spike recovery is still out of the range, then do the spike linear test. For example, in 0.995 ml sample solutions add 5 ul of 10 ppm standard stock solution; in 0.990 ml sample solution add 10 ul, in 0.985 ml sample solution add 15 ul, inject the three different concentration of spiked sample solutions and the no spike sample solution to LC-MS/MS. Then calculate the spike linearity as follows:

Point 1: Peak area of 5 ul spiked solution subtract peak area of no spike sample solution.
Point 2. Peak area of 10 ul spiked solution subtract peak area of no spike sample solution.
Point 3. Peak area of 15 ul spiked solution subtract peak area of no spike sample solution.

Then, input the above three points data,

Peak area from point 1, 5 ul
Peak area from point 2, 10 ul
Peak area from point 3, 15 ul

The amount of spiked as horizontal coordinate, and peak area as ordinate; calculate the linearity of spiked sample solutions.

If the linearity is good ($r^2 > 0.995$), we can still use the recovery to adjust the calculated results, although the recovery is out of the prescribed range.

But if the spike linearity is not good, the test method must be reset.

LC/MS/MS quantitative testing steps can be summarized as below.

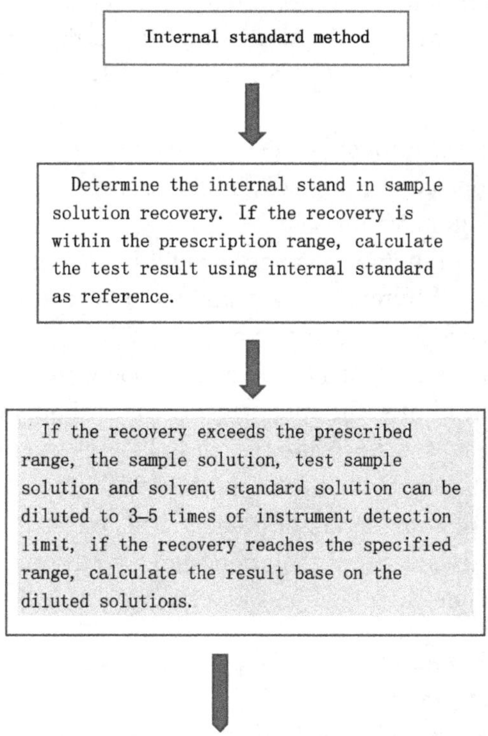

If the recovery is still beyond the acceptable range, but the peak area of analyte and internal standard are very close, calculate the result base on the diluted solutions.

↔

If the recovery is still beyond the acceptable range, or the sample solution cannot be diluted, a working curve of internal standard solutions with sample matrix should be established. Set the internal standard concentration as horizontal coordinates, peak area as the ordinate, and the working curve of the secondary function is established. By input the peak area of the analyte in the test sample solution, the corresponding concentration can be found on the working curve, calculate the result.

External standard method

↓

Prepare four different concentration external(analyte) standard solutions, Inject to the instrument, and create a work curve.

↓

Transfer 1 ml of sample solution to two individual injection vials separately, in one vial add know amount of analyte standard. Inject both sample and spiked sample solution to LC/MS/MS. Calculate the spike recovery. If recovery is within the prescription range, use recovery to adjust the calculated result.

↓

If the recovery exceeds the prescribed range, the sample solution and the spiked sample solution can be diluted to 3–5 times of instrument detection limit, reinject to LC/MS/MS, if the recovery reaches the specified range, calculate the result base on diluted solutions, the calculated result should be corrected by spike recovery which calculated after dilution.

↓

If the sample solution cannot be diluted or after dilution recovery is still out the prescription rang, then do the spike linearity test. For example, in the sample solution add 5ul, 10ul, 15ul of 10ppm standard solution, calculate the spike linearity. If the linearity is good, the calculated result can be adjusted by the spike recovery, though the spike recovery is out the prescription range.

Chapter 2

Vitamin and Related Nutrients Testing Methods

2.1 Testing Methods for Water-Soluble Vitamins

Water soluble vitamins include B_1, B_2, B_3, B_5, B_6, B_{12}, folic acid, biotin, and their derivatizations. There are two main forms of folic acid in dietary supplements: folic acid and methyl tetrahydrofolic acid. Methyl tetrahydrofolate is a metabolite of folic acid that can join the human biochemical system directly. Many dietary supplements now use methyl tetrahydrofolate instead of folic acid. There are also two types of B_3, one is a weak acidic niacin and the other is a weak alkaline niacinamide. B_{12} could be in the following four forms: cyanocobalamin, methyl cobalamin, hydroxy cobalamin and enzyme cobalamin. Mainly cyanocobalamin is used for dietary supplements, but now more and more dietary supplement products use methyl cobalamin instead of cyanocobalamin. The molecular structure of water-soluble vitamins are as follows:

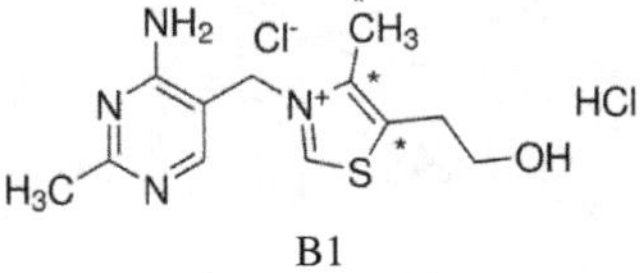

B1

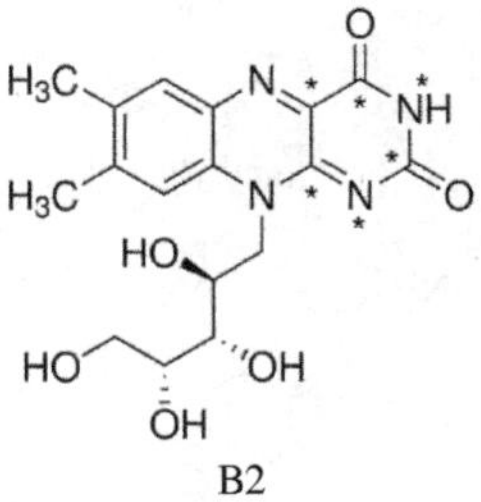

B2

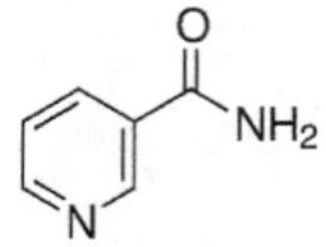

Niacinamide

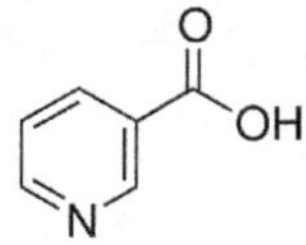

niacin

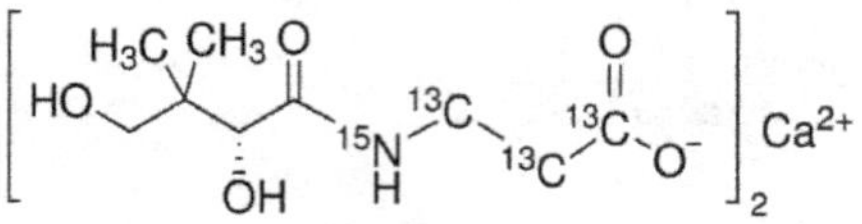

B5

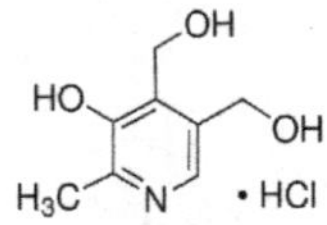

B6

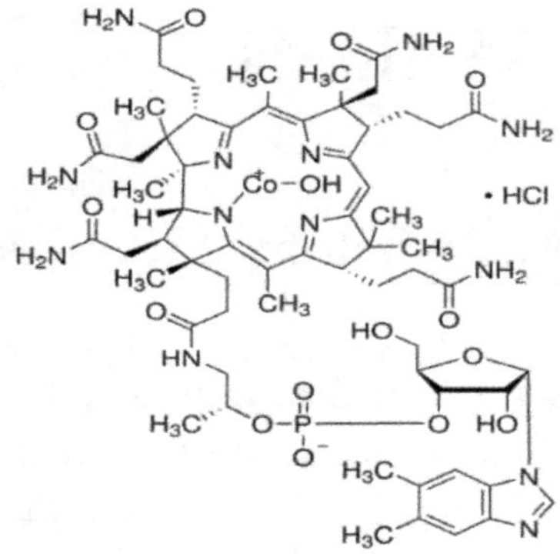

cynocobalamin

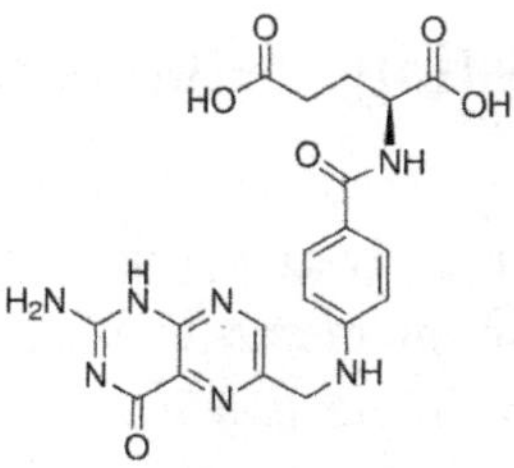

folic acid

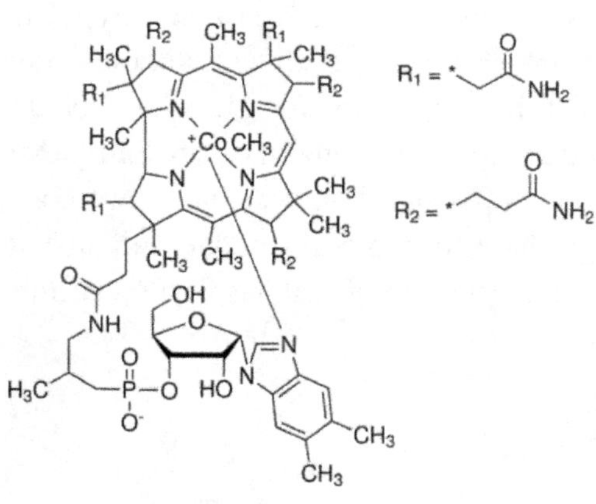

methylcobalamin

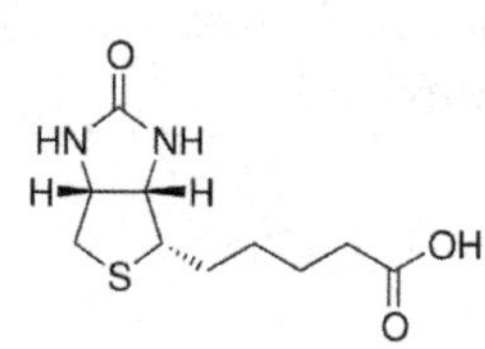

biotin

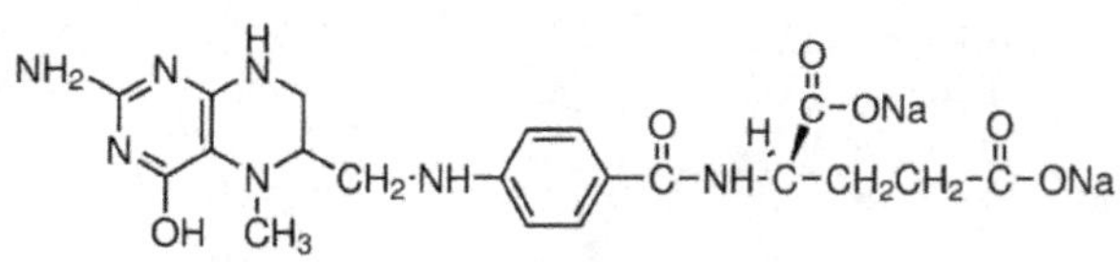

methyl tetrahydrofolic acid

2.1.1 *Water soluble vitamins test methods*

According to the molecular structure, most B vitamins are alkaline, except folic acid, B_5 and niacin which are acidic. If a C18 column is used to perform the chromatography, the resulting chromatogram is as Figure 2.1.

According to Figure 2.1, B_1 has almost no retention time, niacin, niacinamide and B_6 retention times are also very short. It is easy for these peaks to be disrupted in the analysis of actual samples.

If 10 millimole sodium hexamethyl sulfonate is added to the mobile phase as ion pair reagent, then the retention times can be extended (see Figure 2.2).

The retention times of the alkaline compounds after adding an ion pair reagent have been greatly prolonged, and the order of peak elution has been changed. Based on the chromatogram, the retention time and resolution are much better. The chromatographic interferences usually can be avoided if this step is used in the chromatography method. By lowering the pH of mobile phase, niacin and B_5 will have increased retention times, and have less chances of interferences.

An alternative method in some cases is using a phenyl column to replace C18 column. As shown in Figure 2.3, the retention time of niacin, niacinamide and pyridoxine were extended. Relatively, B_5 and biotin,

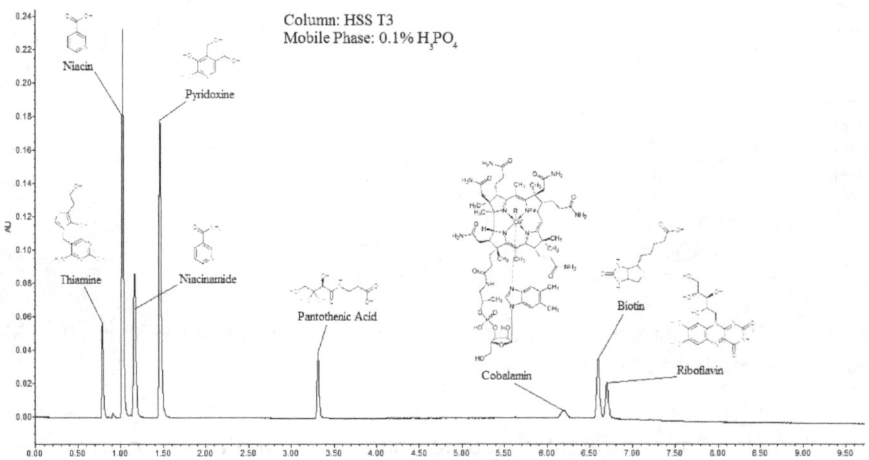

Figure 2.1: Chromatogram of water-soluble vitamins with C18 column.

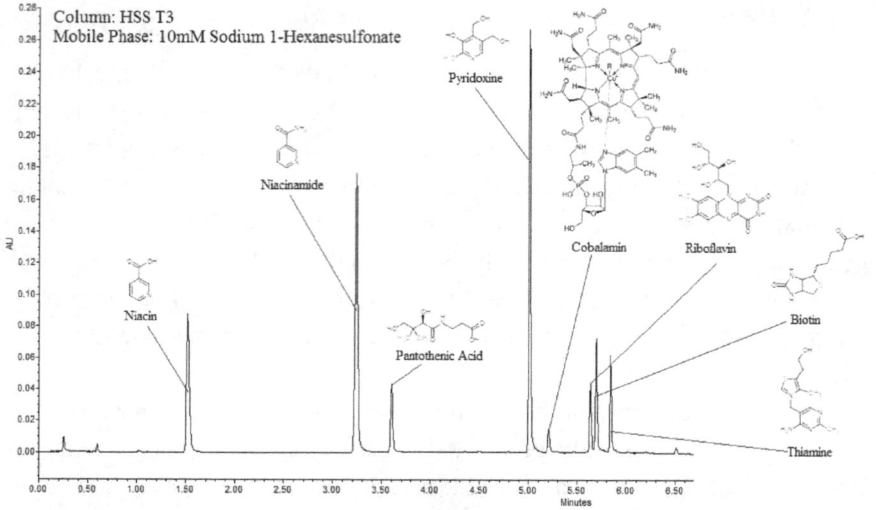

Figure 2.2: Chromatogram of water-soluble vitamins with C18 column, 10 mM sodium hexansulfonate in mobile phase.

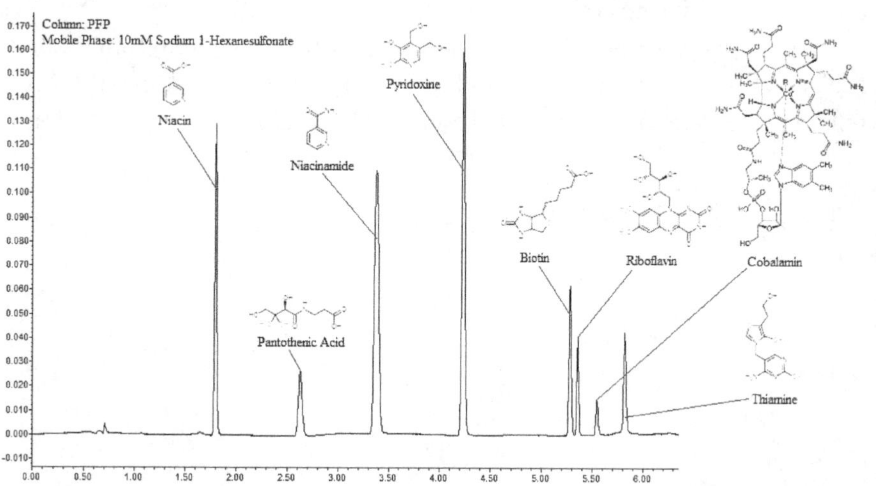

Figure 2.3: Chromatogram of water-soluble vitamins with phenyl column, 10 mM sodium hexansulfonate in mobile phase.

which do not have conjugated double bonds in the molecule, the retention times, were reduced, and the elution orders were reversed with niacinamide and riboflavin.

When the polarity of interferant is similar to the analyte, using a C18 column may not separate them, then the phenyl columns could be considered, especially when the UV spectrum of the interferant differs greatly from the UV spectrum of the analyte. Comparing Figures 2.2 and 2.3, we can see that the absolute retention time of some compounds (e.g., B_6) were shorter, this is because the dispersion force of the phenyl column is not as strong as a C18 column, but if a compound has a similar polarity as to B_6 but no conjugate double bond, it will retain much less than B_6.

(i) *Test procedures*

Preparation solutions

Solution A (sample preparation solvent) — To 950 ml Nano pure water add 50 ml acetonitrile and 2 ml phosphoric acid, shake and mix well. The solvent can be used for three months.

Solvent B (mobile phase A) — Add 10 mM sodium hexansulfonate to 1,000 ml nano pure water, sonicate for 10 min. Use potassium phosphate monobasic and phosphoric acid to adjust pH to 3.0, mix well, and filter through a 0.2 μm membrane. It will be stable for one month.

Solvent C (Mobile phase B) — Acetonitril

Standard solutions preparation: Folic acid can only be dissolved in an alkaline solution, B_2 can only be dissolved in hot water, B_{12} and biotin are generally in the sample at microgram level, so above standards should be prepared in a stock solution first.

B_2 stock solution — Accurately weight about 10 mg of B_2 standard, transfer it to a 50 ml volumetric flask, add about 30 ml nano pure water, put in 80°C water bath, until the solution becomes clear, cool to room temperature, add nano pure water to mark, shake and mix well.

Folic acid stock solution — Accurately weight about 10 mg folic acid standard, transfer it to a 100 ml volumetric flack, add about 60 ml pH 11 sodium hydroxyl solution, shake, until completely dissolved, add same solvent to mark, mix well.

B_{12} and biotin stock solution — Accurately weight about 10 mg B_{12} and 10 mg biotin standards, transfer to a 100 ml volumetric flask, add about 60 ml of solvent A, sonicate until both standards are completely dissolved, cool to room temperature, add solvent A to mark, mix well.

Standard solution — Accurately weight about 10 mg B_1, B_6, niacin and niacinamide, 30mg B_5, transfer to a 100 ml volumetric flask, add about 60 ml solvent A, keep in water bath sonicate for 3 min. Then transfer 20 ml B_2 stock solution, 5 ml folic acid stock solution and 2 ml B_{12} and biotin stock solution to the aforementioned 100 ml volumetric flask, shake, cool to room temperature. Add solvent A to mark, mix well. Make further dilution with solvent A, if necessary.

Suggested concentration of standard solution, B_1, B_2, B_6, B_5, niacin and niacinamide is 10 ppm; Folic acid, B_{12} and biotin 1 ppm.

Sample solutions preparation

Solid or powder samples — Weigh 20 tablets or capsules, and calculate the average weigh per tablet or capsule. Take at least 20 g of samples, grind to fine powder, weigh an amount of sample powder to bring the vitamins content close to the standard solution, transfer to a 100 ml volumetric flask. Add 20 ml of warm water (about 50°C), let it stand for 15 min with frequent shaking, then add 40 ml of solvent A. Cover with a cap and shake for 15 min. If needed, using water bath, sonicate for 5–10 min, cool to room temperature, add solvent A to mark, and mix well. Filter or centrifuge the sample solution, the resulting clear solution is ready for injection.

Liquid or soft gel samples — Cut open the soft gel to get the average content weight per soft gel, take certain amount of the sample into a 100 ml volumetric flask so that the vitamin content is close to that of the standard solution. Add about 10–15 ml of methanol, shake or sonicate in a water bath for 5 min, and then slowly add 50 ml of solution A, side-by-side shake, or sonicate. Finally, fill solution A to mark, and mix well. Filter through a 0.4 μm filter paper, or centrifuge for 5–10 min. Place the clear solution in an injection vial, and prepare for injection.

If testing ingredients include B_2, the sample preparation should be carried out under 80°C.

If folic acid is found in the sample, the sample preparation should be separated with other vitamins, and process with a pH 11 solvent.

(ii) *Chromatography conditions*

HPLC condition

Column: Phenomenex Prodigy 5 um 4.6 × 250 mm
Injection volume: 20 μl
UV wavelength: B_1,245 nm; B_2,268 nm; niacin and niacinamide, 261 nm; B_5,211 nm; B_6,291 nm; B_{12},360 nm; folic acid,280 nm; biotin, 210 nm.
Mobile phase A: Solvent B
Mobile phase B: Solvent C
Flow rate: 1.1 ml/min
Column temperature: Room temperature

Mobile phase gradient

Time (min)	A%	B%
0	85	15
1.0	85	15
1.0–9.0	65	35
9.00–11.0	65	35
11.00–14.0	20	80
14.00–16.0	20	80
16.00–16.5	85	15
20.0	85	15 End

UPLC condition

Column: Water Acquity UPLC HSS Ts C18, 1.8 um, 2.1 × 150 mm
Injection volume: 1 ul
UV wave length: B_1,245 nm; B_2,268 nm; niacin and niacinamide, 261 nm; B_5,210 nm; B_6,291 nm; B_{12},360 nm; folic acid, 280 nm; biotin, 210 nm
Mobile phase A: Solvent B
Mobile phase B: Solvent C
Flow rate: 0.4 ml/min
Column temperature: 45°C

Mobile phase gradient:

Time (min)	A%	B%
0	97	3
0–1.0	97	3
1.0–3.0	90	10
3.0–7.0	64	36
7.0–7.8	64	36
7.8–8.2	97	3
10	97	3 End

Result calculation

$$Analyte(mg)\ per\ unite = \frac{Aa \times Wstd \times Vsam \times UW}{As \times Wsam \times Vstd}$$

or

$$Analyte\ (\%) = \frac{Aa \times Wstd \times Vsam \times 100\%}{As \times Wsam \times Vstd}$$

Aa = Peak area of analyte in sample solution
As = Peak area of analyte in standard solution
$Wstd$ = Weight of standard (mg)
$Wsam$ = Weight of sample (mg)
$Vsam$ = Total volume of sample solution (ml)
$Vstd$ = Total volume of standard solution (ml)
UW = Unit weight (mg)

Adjustment of liquid chromatography conditions

As mentioned early, due to different formulations, different matrices and different dosage forms one may encounter some unexpected interferences in chromatography. To eliminate these interferences adjusting some of the liquid chromatography conditions may be helpful.

Eliminating interferences for acidic vitamins: The water-soluble vitamins niacin, pantothenic acid and folic acid are acidic compounds that reduce the pH of mobile phase, and will reduce the polarity and extend the retention time. However, the interfering compounds may not be acidic compounds, and the retention times would not be changed, thus they may be separated from the acidic vitamins. When the pH is less than 2, niacin will become a positive ion, so that can attract the ion pair molecule in the mobile phase to form neutral ion pair, and can further extend the retention time.

(2) Eliminate interference for other vitamins: Thiamin (B_1), pyridoxine (B_6), niacinaminde (B_3) and cyanocobalamin (B_{12}) are alkaline compounds. The following adjustments can be made when the chromatography shows interferences.

(a) Adjust the mobile phase gradient — If the gradient rate is too fast, sometimes different compounds could be co-eluted. So, by reducing the gradient rate before the analyte peak is eluted, sometimes the interferences can be separated. It should be noted that the effect of the change of mobile phase on the peak is a lagging effect.
(b) Substitute a phenyl column — Because the alkaline vitamins contain low-energy π electrons they can interact with phenyl column to form $\pi - \pi$ interaction force beside the dispersion force, but the interfering molecule may not contain low-energy π electrons so it may be separated.
(c) Adjusting the wavelength of the detector — Select the wavelength with minimal or no interference from the chromatography peak spectrum. For example, when testing B_2, if there is interference at 268 nm, then choose 373 nm or 446 nm at which there may be no interference. For quantitative analysis, the sample and standard must be measured at the same wavelength.
(d) Using larger molecule ion pair reagents — Such as adding octanesulfonate to the mobile phase instead of hexansulfonate, to extend the retention time of the analyte further.

2.1.2 *B_{12} and Biotin LC-MS/MS test method*

Usually in the formulation of dietary supplement products, B_{12}, biotin and folic acid are at microgram levels. In order to reduce the concentration of interferences and other components in the matrix, the final concentrations of B_{12}, biotin and folic acid in sample solution are often in the ppb range.

The UV/Vis detector has difficulty identifying and quantitating them at that concentration, so it is recommended to use an MS/MS detector. Modern MS/MS quantitation limits can reach ppb levels for all the aforementioned three compounds.

(i) *Test procedures (B_{12} and biotin)*

Preparation of three standard solutions with different concentrations.

Number of standards	B_{12} (ppb)	Biotin (ppb)
1	5	5
2	25	25
3	125	125

The aforesaid standard concentration can be adjusted according to the specific situation in the laboratory.

First, inject three different concentrations of standard solutions, establish working curves for each analyte, the linear R^2 of each working curve should be greater than 0.995.

Preparation of sample solution — Following Section 2.1.1(i) "sample solution preparation", make a dilution to match the concentration of the standard solution.

Preparation of spiked sample solution — If the estimated concentration of analyte is 50 ppb, add 5 ul of 10 ppm stock standard solution to 995 ul sample solution, shake well.

Inject sample solution and spiked sample solution to LC/MS/MS separately, calculate the spike recovery.

$$Spike\,recovery = \frac{(Ass - As) \times 100\%}{theoretical\ area\ of\ the\ added\ standard}$$

Here

Ass = Peak area of spiked sample solution.

As = Peak area of sample solution.

The theoretical area of the added standard = Input the spiked amount (convert to concentration) to the standard working curve, get corresponding peak area.

UPLC condition

Column: Water Acquity UPLC HSS Ts C18, 1.8 um, 2.1 × 150 mm
Injection volume: 1 ul
Mobile Phase A: 0.1% formic acid in nano pure water
Mobile Phase B: 0.1% formic acid in acetonitrile
Flow rate: 0.4 ml/min
Column temperature: 45°C

Gradient:

Time (min)	A%	B%
0	95	5
0–3.2	80	20
3.2–4.0	70	30
4.0–5.2	70	30
5.2–5.5	95	5
5.5–8.0	95	5 End

MS/MS parameters:

To accurately identify and quantify the analytes, three ion pairs were selected for each parent ion (see Chapter 1, Section 1.1.5).

Biotin: m/z of the parent ion is +245.1, pick three daughter ions as follows:

Ion pair one: 245.13 → 97.06
Ion pair two: 245.13 → 123.01
Ion pair three: 245.13 → 166.38

The chromatography peak of biotin must contain these three ion pairs, and the proportion of the three ion pairs should be close to the standard. Add the three ion pairs (Total Ion Count, TIC) or the primary ion pair can be used to calculate result.

B_{12}: The m/z of the parent ion is +678.52 (1357.04/2^+).
Ion pair one: 678.52 → 147.25
Ion pair two: 678.52 → 359.25
Ion pair three: 678.52 → 456.91

The selected ion pairs may differ for different instruments.

The following MS/MS parameters are from Waters UPLC-MS/MS TQS instrument.

Biotin

Type	MRM
Ion Mode	ES+
Inter Channel Delay(sec.)	−1.000
InterScan Time (sec.)	−1.000
Span (Da)	0
Start Time(min)	2.0
End Time(min)	4.5

Ch	Prnt(Da)	Dau(Da)	Dwell(s)	Cone(V)	Coll(eV)	Delay(s)	Compound	Formula
1	245.13	97.06	0.025	28.00	24.00	−1.000	Biotin	244.1
2	245.13	123.01	0.025	28.00	26.00	−1.000	Biotin	244.1
3	245.13	166.38	0.025	28.00	20.00	−1.000	Biotin	244.1

B_{12}

Type	MRM
Ion Mode	ES+
Inter Channel Delay (sec)	−1.000
InterScan Time (sec)	−1.000
Span (Da)	0
Start Time (min)	**4.6**
End Time (min)	**6.3**

Ch	Prnt(Da)	Dau(Da)	Dwell(s)	Cone(V)	Coll(eV)	Delay(s)	Compound	Formula
1	678.52	147.21	0.05	28.00	16.00	−1.000	B12	677.3
2	678.52	359.25	0.05	28.00	16.00	−1.000	B12	677.3
3	678.52	456.91	0.05	28.00	16.00	−1.000	B12	677.3

Result calculation

Follow Chapter 1, Section 1.1.5 “Qualitative and quantitative testing of LC-MS/MS”.

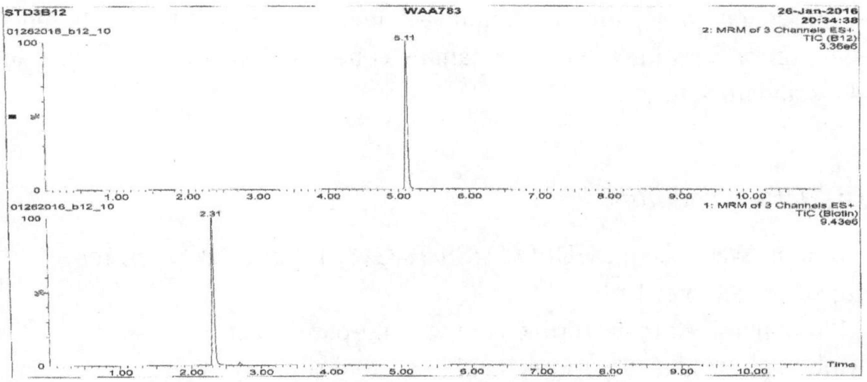

Figure 2.4: TIC chromatogram of biotin and B_{12}.

2.1.3 *Conducting LC-MS/MS to analyze trace water soluble vitamins*

In food (such as fruit, fruit juice, etc.) the water-soluble vitamins content is quite low it could be determined by LC-MS/MS. MS/MS is sensitive to all water-soluble vitamins.

(i) *Test procedure*

Preparation of standard solution — Same as above Section 2.1.1 (i) "Preparation of standard solution", but the suggested concentrations of standard solution are as follows.

Vitamin	STD 1 (ppb)	STD 2 (ppb)	STD 3 (ppb)	STD 4 (ppb)
B_1	5	10	20	40
B_2	5	10	20	40
B_5	5	10	20	40
B_6	5	10	20	40
Niacin	5	10	20	40
Niacinamide	5	10	20	40
Folic acid	2	4	8	16
B_{12}	2	4	8	16
Biotin	2	4	8	16

Preparation of sample solution — Same as Section 2.1.1 (i) "Sample solution preparation", but the vitamins concentration should be close to the standard solution.

(ii) *UPLC condition*

Column: Water Acquity UPLC HSS Ts C18, 1.8 um, 2.1 × 150 mm
Injection volume: 1 ul
Mobile phase A: 0.1% formic acid in nano-pure water
Mobile phase B: 0.1% formic acid in acetonitrile
Flow rate: 0.4 ml/min
Column temperature: 45°C

Gradient:

Time (min)	**A%**	**B%**
0	95	5
0–3.5	85	15
3.5–7.5	60	40
7.5–8.0	60	40
8.0–8.5	95	5
8.5–12.0	95	5 End

The following MS/MS parameters are from Waters UPLC-MS/MS TQS instruments.

Niacinamide:

Type	**MRM**
Ion Mode	ES+
Inter Channel Delay (sec)	–1.000
InterScan Time (sec)	–1.000
Span (Da)	0
Start Time (min)	2.4
End Time (min)	3.0

Ch	Prnt(Da)	Dau(Da)	Dwell(s)	Cone(V)	Coll(eV)	Delay(s)	Compound	Formula
1	122.97	53.03	0.025	2.00	20.00	–1.000	Niacinam.	122.0
2	122.97	95.97	0.025	2.00	14.00	–1.000	Niacinam.	122.0

For niacinamide only two ion pairs can be found.

Niacin:

Type	MRM
Ion Mode	ES+
Inter Channel Delay (sec)	–1.000
InterScan Time (sec)	–1.000
Span (Da)	0
Start Time (min)	1.0
End Time (min)	2.2

Ch	Prnt(Da)	Dau(Da)	Dwell(s)	Cone(V)	Coll(eV)	Delay(s)	Compound	Molecule
1	123.97	53.03	0.025	36.00	20.00	–1.000	Niacin	123.0
2	123.97	80.55	0.025	36.00	16.00	–1.000	Niacin	123.0
3	123.97	95.98	0.025	36.00	14.00	–1.000	Niacin	123.0

B_6:

Type	MRM
Ion Mode	ES+
Inter Channel Delay (sec)	–1.000
InterScan Time (sec)	–1.000
Span (Da)	0
Start Time (min)	2.3
End Time (min)	2.85

Ch	Prnt(Da)	Dau(Da)	Dwell(s)	Cone(V)	Coll(eV)	Delay(s)	Compound	Molecule
1	170.10	76.70	0.025	2.0	28.00	–1.000	B6	169.0
2	170.10	77.09	0.025	2.0	28.00	–1.000	B6	169.0
3	170.10	134.07	0.025	2.0	18.00	–1.000	B6	169.0

B_5:

Type	MRM
Ion Mode	ES+
Inter Channel Delay (sec)	–1.000
InterScan Time (sec)	–1.000
Span (Da)	0
Start Time (min)	2.3
End Time (min)	2.85

Ch	Prnt(Da)	Dau(Da)	Dwell(s)	Cone(V)	Coll(eV)	Delay(s)	Compound	Molecule
1	220.07	90.13	0.025	2.00	10.00	–1.000	B5	219.1
2	220.07	184.16	0.025	2.00	10.00	–1.000	B5	219.1
3	220.07	202.17	0.025	2.00	8.00	–1.000	B5	219.1

B_1:

Type	MRM
Ion Mode	ES+
Inter Channel Delay (sec)	–1.000
InterScan Time (sec)	–1.000
Span (Da)	0
Start Time (min)	2.5
End Time (min)	3.6

Ch	Prnt(Da)	Dau(Da)	Dwell(s)	Cone(V)	Coll(eV)	Delay(s)	Compound	Molecule
1	265.10	80.98	0.025	2.00	28.00	–1.000	B1	264.2
2	265.10	122.08	0.025	2.00	12.00	–1.000	B1	264.2
3	265.10	144.05	0.025	2.00	10.00	–1.000	B1	264.2

B_2:

Type	MRM
Ion Mode	ES+
Inter Channel Delay (sec)	–1.000
InterScan Time (sec)	–1.000
Span (Da)	0
Start Time (min)	6.0
End Time (min)	8.0

Ch	Prnt(Da)	Dau(Da)	Dwell(s)	Cone(V)	Coll(eV)	Delay(s)	Compound	Molecule
1	377.18	172.12	0.025	2.00	36.00	–1.000	B2	376.15
2	377.18	198.06	0.025	2.00	34.00	–1.000	B2	376.15
3	377.18	243.11	0.025	2.00	20.00	–1.000	B2	376.15

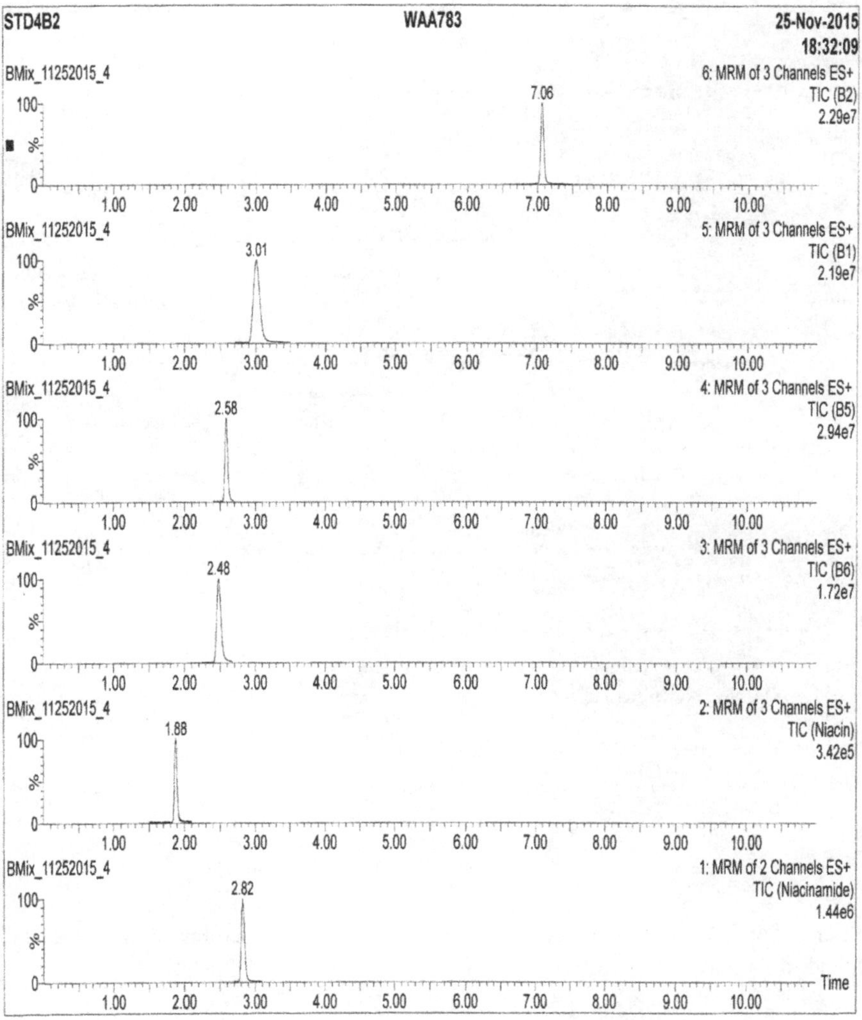

Figure 2.5: LC-MS/MS TIC chromatograms of water-soluble vitamins.

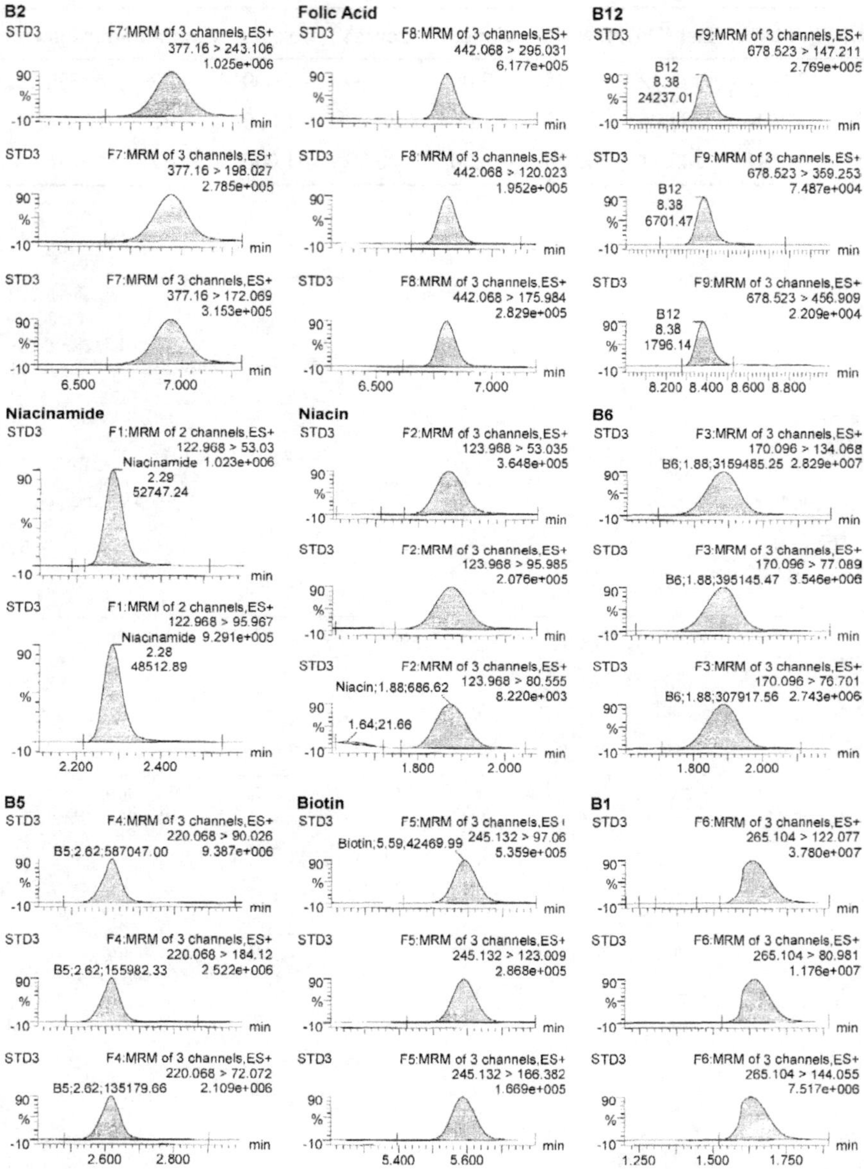

Figure 2.6: Water-soluble vitamins LC-MS/MS ion pairs spectrum; niacinamide only found two ion pairs.

(iii) *Results and calculation*

The result calculation is carried out in accordance with the steps found in Chapter 1, Section 1.1.5 "Qualitative and quantitative testing of LC-MS/MS".

2.1.4 *Testing method for methylcobalamin*

Methylcobalamin (methyl B_{12}) is a different form of vitamin B_{12} (Cyanocobalamin). Nowadays in many products cyanocobalamin is replaced by methylcobalamin.

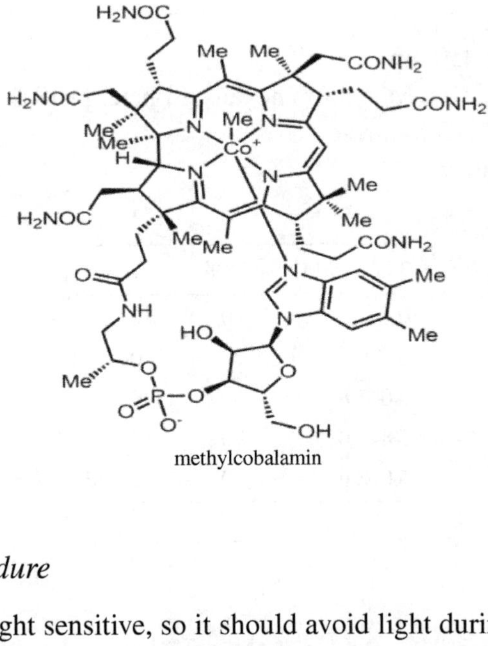

methylcobalamin

(i) *Test procedure*

Methyl B_{12} is light sensitive, so it should avoid light during analysis.

Solvent A (for sample preparation) — Add 50 ml of acetonitrile in 950 ml of nano-pure water, and 2 ml of phosphoric acid, shake and mix well. The shelf life is three months.

Preparation of standard solution — Accurately weight about 10 mg of methyl B_{12} standard, transfer to 100 ml light protection volumetric flask, add 60 ml solvent A, vortex a few minutes until all of the standard is dissolved. Add solvent A to mark, shake well. Use solvent A to dilute the solution until it is about 1 ppm.

Preparation of the sample solution — Take a certain amount of ground sample containing about 0.1 mg of methyl B_{12}, transfer it to a 100 ml light protection volumetric flask, add 60 ml solvent A, shake for 15 min, then sonicate for 5 min, cool to room temperature, add solvent A to mark, shake well and centrifuge for 5 min, and finally take the upper-level clear solution for injection.

(ii) *UPLC conditions*

Column: Acquity UPLC HSS T3 1.8 μm, 2.1 × 100 mm
Flow rate: 0.4 ml/min
Injection volume: 2 μl
UV wavelength: 350 nm
Mobile Phase A: 10 mM sodium hexansulfonate, pH 3.0
Mobile Phase B: Acetonitrile
Column temperature: 45°C

Gradient:

Time (min)	A%	B%
0	90	10
0–5.0	60	40
5.0–5.8	60	40
5.8–6.0	90	10
6.0–8.0	90	10 End

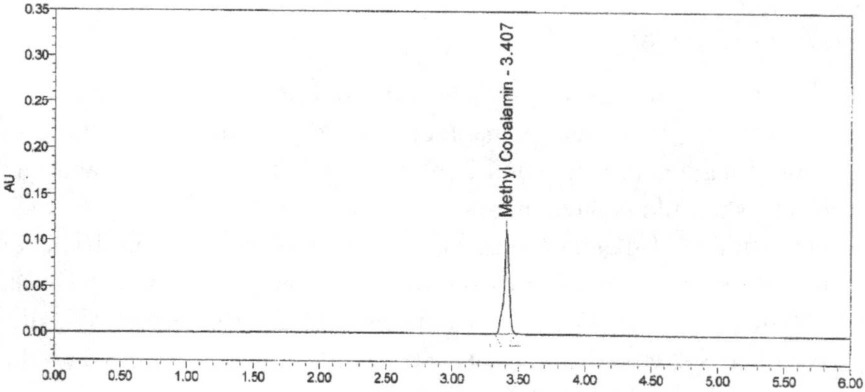

Figure 2.7: Chromatogram of methylcobalamin.

(iii) *Results calculation*

$$Methylcobalamin\ (\mu g/unit) = \frac{Aa \times Wstd \times Vsam \times UW}{As \times Wsam \times Vstd}$$

or

$$Methylcobalamin\ (\mu g/g) = \frac{Aa \times Wstd \times Vsam}{As \times Wsam \times Vstd}$$

Aa = Peak area of sample
As = Peak area of analyte
Wstd = Weight of standard (μg)
Wsam = Weight of sample (g)
Vsam = Total volume of sample solution (ml)
Vstd = Total volume of standard solution (ml)
UW = Unit weight (g)

2.1.5 *5-Methyltetrahydrofolate test method*

5-methyltetrahydrofolic acid (5-MTHF) is a metabolite of folic acid that can directly enter the biochemical system of the human body. So, the trend now is using 5-methyltetrahydrofolic acid to replace folic acid.

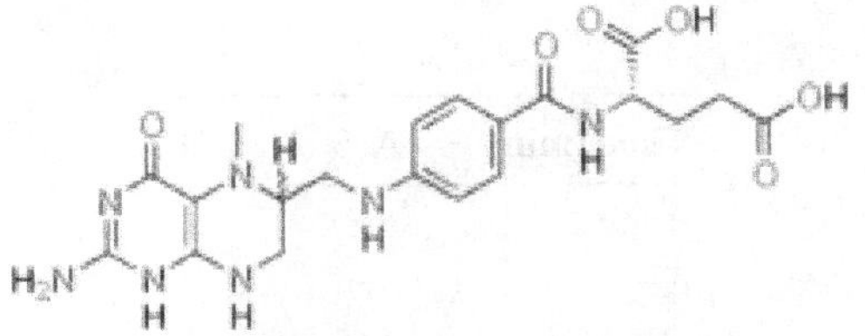

5-methyltetrahydrofolic acid

(i) *Test procedure*

5-methyltetrahydroyfolic acid is soluble in an alkaline solution, but under alkaline conditions 5-methyltetraoxyfolic acid is not stable. This method uses 0.1 N hydrochloric acid to prepare the standard and sample solutions.

Preparation of standard solution — Accurately weigh about 10 mg 5-methyltetrahydrofolic acid standard, transfer it to 100 ml volumetric flask, add 60 ml 0.1 N hydrochloric acid solution, sonicate until the standard completely dissolved. Cool to room temperature, fill the 0.1 N hydrochloric acid solution to the mark, shake and mix well. Dilute to about 1 ppm with a 0.1 N hydrochloric acid solution.

Preparation of sample solution — Take certain amount of ground sample powder or liquid sample containing about 0.1 mg 5-methyltetrahydrofolic acid, transfer to a 100 ml volumetric flask. Add 60 ml of 0.1 N hydrochloric acid solution, shake for 15 min, then sonicate for 5 min, after cooling fill 0.1 N hydrochloric acid solution to the 100 ml mark, shake and mix well. Centrifuge for 5 min, the upper-level clear solution is ready for injection.

(ii) *UPLC conditions*

Column: Acquity UPLC HSS T3, 1.8 μm, 2.1 × 100 mm
Flow rate: 0.4 ml/min
Injection volume: 1 μl
UV wavelength: 292 nm
Mobile Phase A: 0.1% phosphoric acid in water
Mobile Phase B: Acetonitrile
Column temperature: 45°C

Gradient:

Time (min)	A%	B%
0	98	2
0–5.0	92	8
5.0–5.8	92	8
5.8–6.0	98	2
6.0–6.8	98	2

(iii) *Results calculation*

$$5-MTHF\ (\mu g/unit)=\frac{Aa\times Wstd\times Vsam\times UW}{As\times Wsam\times Vstd}$$

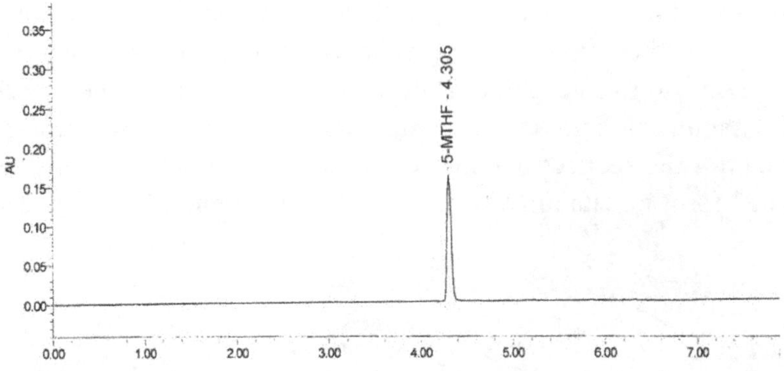

Figure 2.8: UPLC chromatogram of 5-methyltetrahydrofolic acid.

or

$$5-MTHF\ (\mu g/g) = \frac{Aa \times Wstd \times Vsam}{As \times Wsam \times Vstd}$$

Aa = Peak area of sample
As = Peak area of analyte
$Wstd$ = Weight of standard (μg)
$Wsam$ = Weight of sample (g)
$Vsam$ = Total volume of sample solution (ml)
$Vstd$ = Total volume of standard solution (ml)
UW = Unit weight (g)

2.1.6 *Determination of ascorbic acid (Vitamin C) by HPLC and UPLC*

Vitamin C in a dietary supplement may exist in two forms, one is reduced vitamin C (L-ascorbic acid), and the other is oxidized vitamin C (dehydro-L-ascorbic acid). The bioactivities of these two forms of vitamin C are the same. So, when testing vitamin C, you should measure the sum of the two forms. There are two test methods, the first one is using chromatography to separate the two forms of vitamin C, and then using individual external standards to calculate the oxidized state and reduced state vitamin C, then adding up the total vitamin C content. Another method is by first using a reducing reagent, Tris (2-carboxyethyl) Phosphine Hydrochloride to reduce the oxidized state vitamin C to reduced state vitamin C, then using chromatography to quantify the reduced vitamin C as total vitamin C with only using reduced form of vitamin C as standard. This method is introduced as follows.

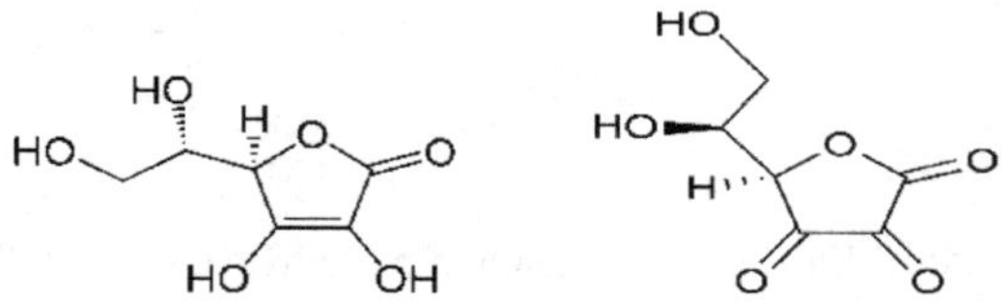

Ascorbic acid   Dehydroascorbic acid

(i) *Test procedure*

Preparation of standard solutions — Accurately weigh about 20 mg of vitamin C (reduced) standard, transfer it to 50 ml of volumetric flask, add about 30 ml of 0.01% of phosphoric acid, 5% acetonitrile in water, sonicate until all of the standard dissolved. Cool to room temperature, add same solvent to 50 ml, shake and mix well. Dilute 20 times with the same solvent.

Preparation of sample solutions — Weigh a certain amount of ground sample containing about 20 mg of vitamin C, transfer to a 50 ml volumetric flask, add about 30 ml of 0.1% phosphoric acid and 5% acetonitrile water solution, shake with wrist action shaker for 5 min, then sonicate for 10 min, cool to room temperature, add same solution to 50 ml, shake and mix well. Take 3 ml of sample solution to 5 ml of centrifuge tube, centrifuge for 5 min. Take the upper-level clear solution to dilute 20 times with the same solvent.

Reduction reaction — Take 0.6 ml of each standard solution, sample solution and blank solution (only the 0.01% phosphoric acid and 5% acetonitrile water solution) into 2 ml injection vails individually, add 0.6 ml of 10 mg/ml Tris (2-carboxyethyl) Phosphine Hydrochloride water solution to each injection vails, vortex for 1 min, and keep at room temperature for 10 min. It is ready for injection.

(ii) *Chromatography condition*

UPLC condition

Column: Acquity HSS Ts C18, 0.18 um, 2.1 × 150 mm
Flow rate: 0.4 ml/min
Column temperature: 45ºC
Mobile phase: 10 mM Tetrabutylammonium Hydrogen Sulfate (TBAB) water solution, pH 5.5.
Run time: 6 min

HPLC condition

Column: Phenomenex Prodigy 5 um, 4.6 × 250 mm
Flow rate: 1.0 ml/min
Column temperature: Room temperature
Mobile phase A: 10 mM Tetrabutylammonium Hydrogen Sulfate, pH 5.5
Mobile phase B: Acetonitrile
Mobile phase A: Mobile phase B = 97:3
Run time: 10 min

Result calculation

$$VC\ (mg/unit) = \frac{Aa \times Wstd \times Vsam \times UW}{As \times Wsam \times Vstd}$$

or

$$VC\ (\%) = \frac{Aa \times Wstd \times Vsam \times 100\%}{As \times Wsam \times Vstd}$$

Aa = Peak area of sample
As = Peak area of analyte
Wstd = Weight of standard (mg)
Wsam = Weight of sample (mg)
Vsam = Total volume of sample solution (ml)
Vstd = Total volume of standard solution (ml)
UW = Unit weight (mg)

2.2 Testing Methods for Oil-Soluble Vitamins

Oil-soluble vitamins include vitamin A (vitamin A, vitamin A acetate, vitamin A palmitate), vitamin E (vitamin E, vitamin E acetate, vitamin E succinate), vitamin D_2, vitamin D_3, precursor of vitamin D_3, vitamin K_1, vitamin K_2 (MK4, MK7), vitamin K_3. Β-carotene has the same bioactivity as vitamin A. In dietary supplements manufacturers often use Β-carotene as an alternative to vitamin A. Due to the large molecular weight of Β-carotene, long retention time, and inclusion of different isomers, it is recommended to test it separately from other oil-soluble vitamins. See "Β-carotene test method".

Vitamin D_3 may contain a small amount of vitamin D_3 precursor (1,25-Dihydroxycalciferol). The precursor of vitamin D_3 is an intermediate in the synthesis of D_3 progress, and now considered as part of D_3, should also be included when testing total D_3.

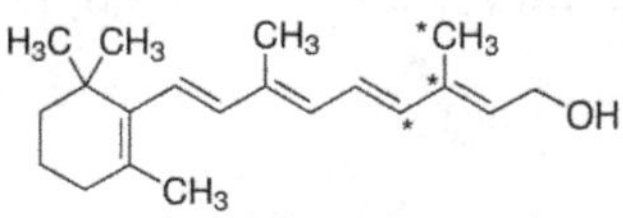

vitamin A

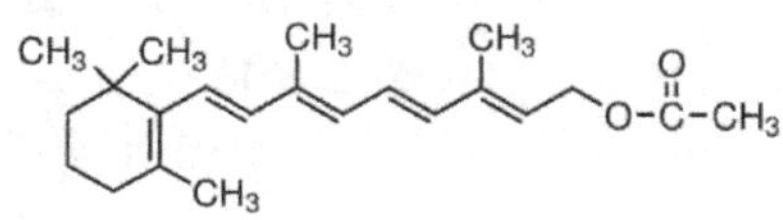

vitamin A Acetate

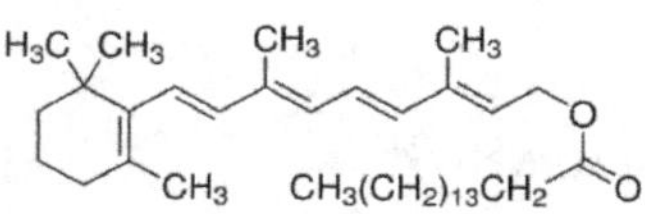

vitamin A Palmitate

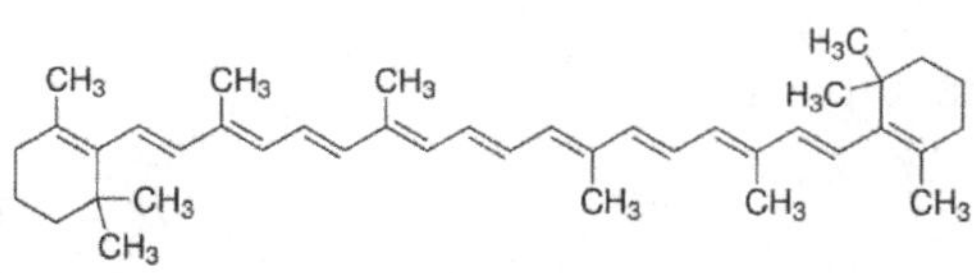

β-Carotene

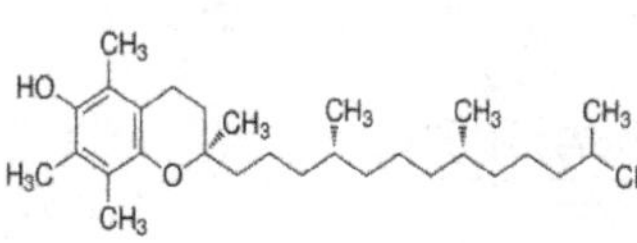

vitamin E

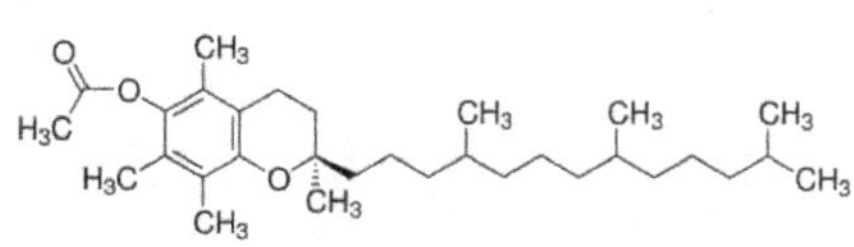

vitamin E Acetate

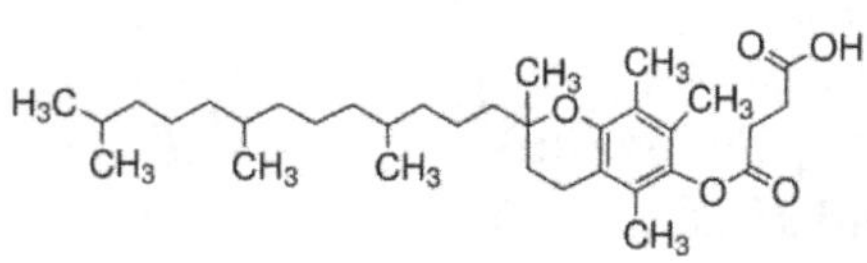

Vitamin E Succinate

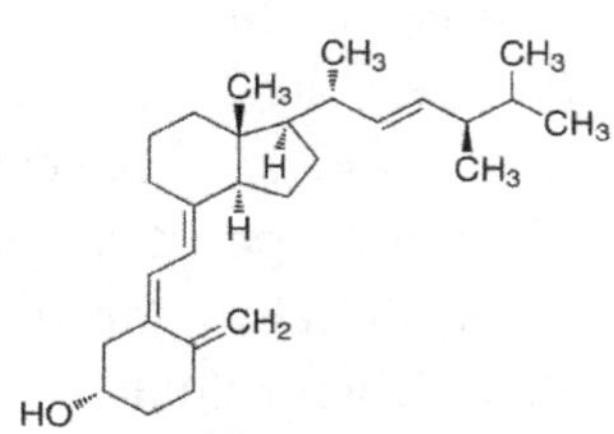

Vitamin D_2

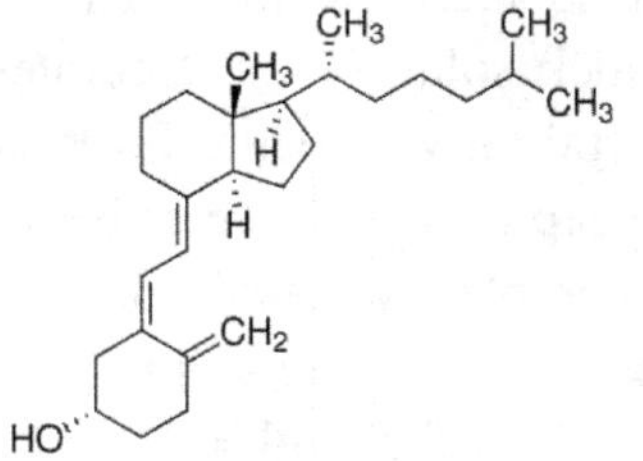

vitamin D_3

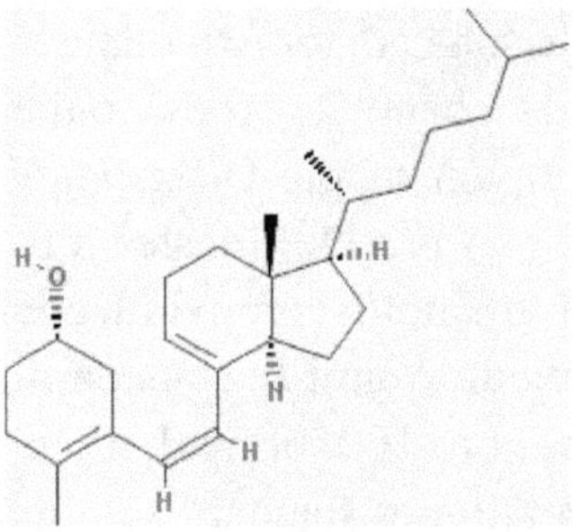

pre-vitamin D_3

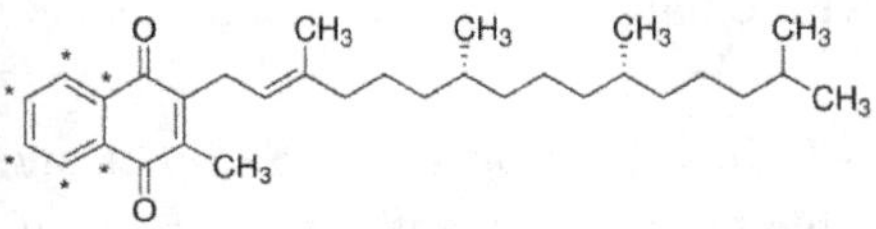

vitamin K_1

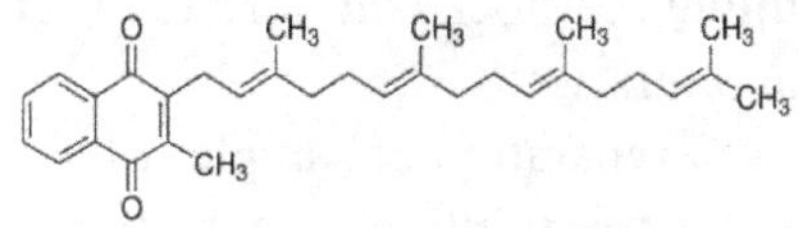

vitamin K_2 (MK4)

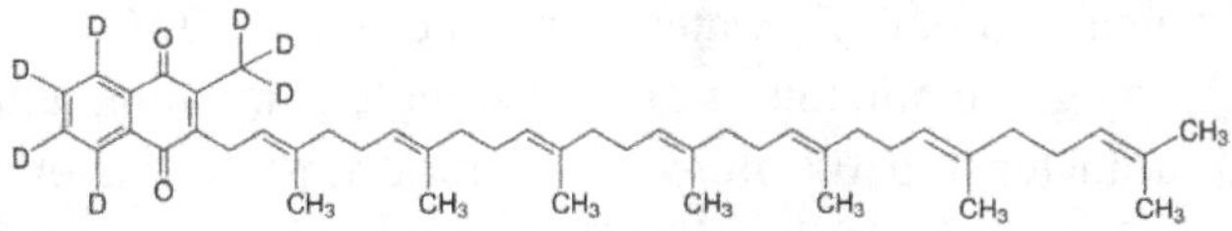

Vitamin K_2 (MK-7)

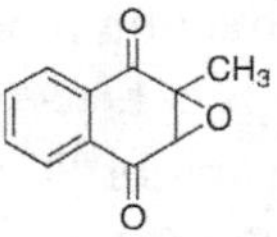

Vitamin K_3

From the aforementioned molecular structures it can be seen that all oil-soluble vitamins are relatively non-polar compounds, and with C18 columns we can get a long retention time, and the compounds are relatively easy to separate.

2.2.1 *Vitamin D_2, D_3 and D_3 precursor test method*

Vitamin D_3 may contain a small amount of vitamin D_3 precursors (1,25-Dihydroxycalciferol, pre-D_3). Vitamin D_2, D_3 and pre-D_3 have a relatively close molecular structure, so it is difficult to separate, but if the gradient is well regulated, the three compounds can be completely separated.

(i) *Test procedure*

Preparation of D_2 and D_3 standard stock solution — Accurately weigh about 10 mg of each vitamin D_2 and D_3 standards, transfer it to a 100 ml volumetric flask, add about 60 ml of 1:1 ethanol/isopropyl alcohol, put in 70ºC water bath, sonicate for few minutes, until all standards are dissolved. After cooling add ethanol/isopropyl to the mark, shake and mix well.

Preparation of pre-D_3 standard stock solution — Accurately weigh about 5 mg of pre-D_3, transfer it to a 100 ml volumetric flask, add about 60 ml 1:1 ethanol/isopropyl alcohol, keep in a 70°C water bath, sonicate for few minutes until the standard is completely dissolved. Fill with the same solvent to 100 ml mark after it is cooled, shake and mix well.

Preparation of standard solution — Transfer 1 ml of D_2 and D_3 stock solution, 0.5 ml of pre-D_3 stock solution to a 100 ml volumetric flask, dilute the stock solutions to 100 ml with ethanol/isopropyl alcohol, shake and mix well.

Preparation of sample solution — Follow Section 1.1.3 "Samples and standards solutions preparation" in Chapter 1. To effectively extract oil-soluble vitamins from the sample, it is recommended that the entire extraction process be carried out in a water bath condition of 70°C.

First, accurately weigh an amount of ground sample containing about 0.1 mg of D_2 or D_3, transfer to a 100 ml of volumetric flask, mix sample with a 20 ml of DMSO, soak for 15 min in a 70°C water bath, sonicate for 5 min, then add 50 ml 1:1 ethanol/isopropyl alcohol, sonicate for 10 min at 70°C with frequent shake, after cooling add 1:1 ethanol/isopropyl alcohol to mark, shake and mix well. After centrifuging (12,000 rpm) for 5 min, take the clear solution for injection.

If the sample is a fatty liquid, just add 60 ml 1:1 ethanol/isopropyl alcohol, sonicate for 10 min under 70°C, after cooling fill same solution to mark, shake well, centrifuge (12,000 rpm), take the clear solution for injection.

The conditions for sample preparation should be adjusted as necessary according to the specific sample and the analytes. In some cases, powdered samples can be extracted directly using organic solvents, without involving water.

(ii) *Chromatography conditions*

HPLC chromatography conditions

Column: Phenomenex Synergi 5 μm 4.6 × 250 mm 100A
Injection volume: 20 ul

Mobile phase A: Methanol
Mobile phase B: Ethanol
Flow rate: 1.0 ml/min
Column temperature: Room temperature
UV wavelength: 269 nm

Gradient:

Time (min)	A%	B%
0	35	65
0–1.0	35	65
1.0–15.0	0	100
15.0–18.0	0	100
18.0–18.5	35	65
25.0	35	65 结束

UPLC chromatography conditions

Column: Acquity UPLC® BEH C18 1.7 μm, 2.1 × 150 mm
Injection volume: 2 ul
UV wavelength: 269 nm
Mobile phase A: 0.1% phosphoric acid water solution
Mobile phase B: 0.1% Phosphoric acid in acetonitrile
Flow rate: 0.5 ml/min
Column temperature: 55°C

Gradient:

Time (min)	A%	B%
0	15	85
0–7.0	0	100
7.0–8.8	0	100
8.8–9.0	15	85
9.0–12.0	15	85

Result and calculation (for both HPLC and UPLC methods)

$$Dvitamin\ (\mu g/unit) = \frac{Aa \times Wstd \times Vsam \times UW}{As \times Wsam \times Vstd}$$

or

$$Dvitamin\ (\mu g/g) = \frac{Aa \times Wstd \times Vsam}{As \times Wsam \times Vstd}$$

Aa = Peak area of corresponding VD in sample solution
As = Peak area of corresponding VD in standard solution
Wstd = Weight of standard (μg)
Wsam = Weight of sample (g)
Vsam = Total volume of sample solution (ml)
Vstd = Total volume of standard solution (ml)
UW = Unit weight (g)

2.2.2 *Vitamin A test method*

Vitamin A has three different forms: vitamin A, vitamin A acetate and vitamin A palmitate. The molecules of the three forms of vitamin A contain different number of carbons, so they can easily be separated by reversed phase chromatography.

The standards of all three forms of vitamin A are available from Sigma-Aldrich and other suppliers. The test process does not need hydrolysis of the sample to determine the total vitamin A. You can use the three forms vitamin A standards to individually quantify the content of each form of vitamin A. By avoiding the hydrolysis procedure, you can save time and may get more accurate results. The more the steps in the sample preparation, the more the chances of errors. For example, different sample matrixes may have different hydrolysis recoveries, and this also may introduce more human errors.

(i) *Test procedure*

Preparation of standard solution — Accurately weigh about 5 mg of each vitamin A, vitamin A acetate and vitamin A palmitate. Transfer it to a 100 ml volumetric flask, add about 60 ml 1:1 ethanol/isopropyl alcohol, put in 70°C water bath, sonicate for few minutes, until all standards are dissolved. After cooling, fill 1:1 ethanol/isopropyl alcohol to the mark, shake and mix well, the standard solution is ready for injection.

Preparation of sample solution — Follow Section 1.1.3 in the previous chapter for sample preparation. To effectively extract oil-soluble vitamins from the sample, it is recommended that the entire extraction process be carried out in a water bath condition of 70°C.

Accurately weigh a certain amount of sample containing about 5 mg of vitamin A, or vitamin A acetate, or vitamin A palmitate, transfer to a 100 ml of volumetric flask, mix sample with 20 ml DMSO, soak for 15 min in a 70°C water bath, sonicate for 5 min, 50 ml 1:1 ethanol/isopropyl alcohol, sonicate for 10 min at 70°C with frequent shaking, after cooling add 1:1 ethanol/isopropyl alcohol to mark, shake and mix well. After centrifuging (12,000 rpm), take the clear solution for injection.

If the sample is fatty liquid, just add 60 ml 1:1 ethanol/isopropyl alcohol, sonicate for 10 min under 70°C, after cooling fill the same solution to mark, shake well, after centrifuging for 5 min (12,000 rpm). Take the clear solution for injection.

The conditions for sample preparation may be adjusted as necessary according to the specific sample and the analytes. In some cases, the powdered sample can be extracted using organic solvents directly, without water being used.

(ii) *Chromatography conditions*

HPLC conditions

Column: Phenomenex Synergi 5 μm 4.6 × 250 mm 100A
Injection volume: 20 ul
Mobile phase A: Methanol
Mobile phase B: Ethanol
Flow rate: 1.0 ml/min
Column temperature: Room temperature
UV wavelength: 326 nm

Gradient:

Time (min)	A%	B%
0	35	65
0–1.0	35	65
1.0–15.0	0	100
15.0–18.0	0	100
18.0–18.5	35	65
25.0	35	65 End

UPLC conditions

Column: Acquity UPLC® BEH Phenyl 1.7 μm, 2.1 × 150 mm
Injection volume: 1 ul
UV wavelength: 326 nm
Mobile phase A: 0.1% phosphoric acid water solution
Mobile phase B: 0.1% Phosphoric acid in acetonitrile
Flow rate: 0.5 ml/min
Column temperature: 55°C

Gradient:

Time (min)	A%	B%
0	15	85
0–7.0	0	100
7.0–8.0	0	100
8.0–8.3	15	85
8.3–11.0	15	85 End

Result and calculation

$$Individual\,vitamin\,A(mg/unit) = \frac{Aa \times Wstd \times Vsam \times UW}{As \times Wsam \times Vstd}$$

or

$$Individual\,vitamin\,A\ (\%) = \frac{Aa \times Wstd \times Vsam \times 100\%}{As \times Wsam \times Vstd}$$

Aa = Peak area of corresponding vitamin A in sample solution
As = Peak area of corresponding vitamin A in standard solution
Wstd = Weight of standard (mg)
Wsam = Weight of sample (mg)
Vsam = Total volume of sample solution (ml)
Vstd = Total volume of standard solution (ml)
UW = Unit weight (mg)

2.2.3 *Vitamin E test method*

Like vitamin A, there are three forms of vitamin E (vitamin E, vitamin E acetate and vitamin E succinate) that may be found in dietary supplements. The reference standards of all three vitamin E forms are available, so the total vitamin E determination can be carried out by quantifying each individual vitamin E form, instead of quantifying total vitamin E after hydrolysis.

In addition, from the molecular structure of vitamin E it can be seen that there are three chair centers in vitamin E molecule, so they should have up to (2^3) eight enantiomers. Natural vitamin E is only RRR form, called d-vitamin E, and synthetic vitamin E contains all eight enantiomers such as RSR, SSR, RRS etc., called dl-vitamin E. The bioactivity of d-vitamin E is higher than dl-vitamin E. To accurately measure the bioactivity (IU) of the sample, the d or dl form of vitamin E should be identified.

Pure Vitamin E raw materials can be identified by specific rotation measurement; however, once vitamin E is mixed with other ingredients in the dietary supplement finished products, specific rotation method is not applicable. In order to identify natural or synthetic vitamin E in the finished products, Waters research scientist successfully separated some Vitamin E enantiomers by carbon dioxide supercritical chromatography (see Figure 2.9). Although carbon dioxide supercritical chromatography cannot separate each enantiomer completely, it is enough to identify the natural or synthetic vitamin E. Natural vitamin E is entirely in RRR form enantiomer, and should exhibit a single peak. Synthetic vitamin E is a combination of all enantiomers, and it should exhibit multiple peaks.

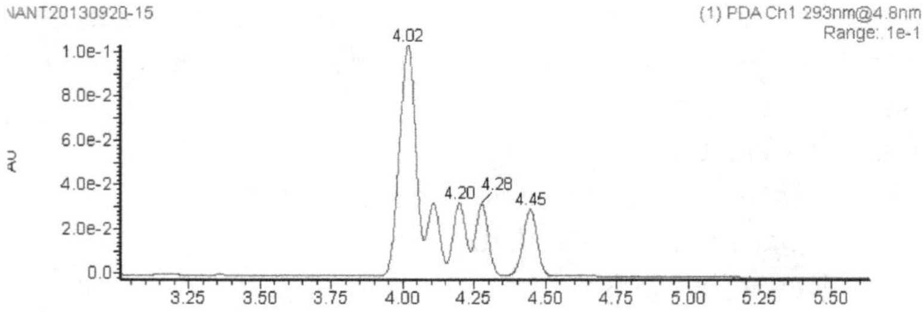

Figure 2.9: Carbon dioxide supercritical chromatogram for vitamin E enantiomers.

The following chromatography method cannot identify d or dl forms of vitamin E.

(i) *Test procedure*

Preparation of standard solution — Accurately weigh about 10 mg of each vitamin E, vitamin E acetate and vitamin E succinate standards, transfer it to a 100 ml volumetric flask, add about 60 ml of ethanol, put in 70ºC water bath, sonicate for few minutes, until all standards are dissolved. After the solution is cooled, fill ethanol to the mark, shake and mix well, the standard solution is ready for injection.

Preparation of sample solution — The sample preparation for vitamin E can follow Section 1.1.3 of Chapter 1. To effectively extract oil-soluble vitamins from the sample, it is recommended that the entire extraction process be carried out in a water bath condition of 70ºC.

Accurately weigh a certain amount of the ground sample containing about 10 mg of vitamin E, or vitamin E acetate, or vitamin E succinate, transfer it to a 100 ml of volumetric flask, mix the sample with 20 ml of DMSO, let it stand for 15 min in a 70ºC water bath, sonicate for 5 min, then add 60 ml 1:1 ethanol/isopropyl alcohol and sonicate for another 10 min under 70ºC water bath with frequent shaking. After cooling add 1:1 ethanol/isopropyl alcohol to mark, shake and mix well. After centrifuging (12,000 rpm), take the clear solution for injection.

If the sample is fatty liquid, just add 60 ml 1:1 ethanol/isopropyl alcohol, sonicate for 10 min under 70ºC, after cooling fill the same solution to mark, shake well. After centrifuging (12,000 rpm), take the clear solution for injection.

The conditions for sample preparation may be adjusted as necessary according to the specific sample and the analytes. In some cases, the powdered samples can be extracted with organic solvents directly, without water being involved.

(ii) *Chromatography conditions*

HPLC condition

Column: Phenomenex Synergi 5 μm 4.6 × 250 mm 100A
Injection volume: 20 ul
Mobile phase A: Methanol
Mobile phase B: Ethanol
Flow rate: 1.0 ml/min
Column temperature: Room temperature
UV wavelength: 269 nm, 285 nm, 295 nm

Gradient:

Time (min)	**A%**	**B%**
0	35	65
0–1.0	35	65
1.0–15.0	0	100
15.0–18.0	0	100
18.0–18.5	35	65
25.0	35	65 End

UPLC conditions

Column: Acquity UPLC® BEH Phenyl 1.7 μm, 2.1 × 150 mm
Injection volume: 2 ul
UV wavelength: 269 nm, 285 nm, 295 nm
Mobile phase A: 0.1% phosphoric acid water solution
Mobile phase B: 0.1% Phosphoric acid in acetonitrile
Flow rate: 0.4 ml/min
Column temperature: 45°C

Gradient:

Time (min)	A%	B%
0	35	65
0–6.0	10	90
6.0–6.5	10	90
6.5–6.8	0	100
6.8–8.0	0	100
8.0–8.3	35	65
8.3–10.0	35	65

Results and calculation

$$Vitamin\,E\,(mg/unit) = \frac{Aa \times Wstd \times Vsam \times UW}{As \times Wsam \times Vstd}$$

or

$$Vitamin\,E\ (\%) = \frac{Aa \times Wstd \times Vsam \times 100\%}{As \times Wsam \times Vstd}$$

Aa = Peak area of corresponding vitamin E in sample solution
As = Peak area of corresponding vitamin E in standard solution
Wstd = Weight of standard (mg)
Wsam = Weight of sample (mg)
Vsam = Total volume of sample solution (ml)
Vstd = Total volume of standard solution (ml)
UW = Unit weight (mg)

Total content of vitamin E is the sum of the content of each individual vitamin E form.

2.2.4 *Vitamin K_1, K_2(MK-4 and MK-7), K_3 test method*

Vitamins K_1, K_2 (MK4 and MK7), K_3 are easily separated due to molecular differences. However, K_1 and K_2 have trans and cis isomers, and cis K_1, K_2 are considered to be inactive, so it is necessary to separate the trans and cis K_1, K_2. Both C18 and phenyl columns can be used to separate the isomers.

In dietary supplements, the vitamin K content is at low levels. The concentration of standard solution should be around 1 ppm or less.

Vitamin K_2 (including MK-4 and MK-7) are not stable, the actual purity of standards should be calibrated following Section 1.1.3 in Chapter 1.

(i) *Test procedure*

Preparation of standard solution — Accurately weigh about 5 mg of each K_1, K_2 (MK-4 and MK-7) and K_3, transfer it to a 50 ml volumetric flask, add about 30 ml 1:1 ethanol/isopropyl alcohol. Keep in a 70ºC water bath and sonicate for a few minutes until all the standards are dissolved. Add the same solvent to 50 ml volume, shake and mix well. Transfer 1 ml of the above standard stock solution to a 100 ml volumetric flask, add 1:1 ethanol/isopropyl alcohol to mark, then shake and mix well. The standard solution is ready for injection.

Preparation of sample solution — For sample solution preparation follow Section 1.1.3 in the previous chapter. To effectively extract oil-soluble vitamins from the sample, it is recommended that the entire extraction process be carried out in a water bath at of 70ºC.

Accurately weigh a certain amount of ground sample containing about 0.1 mg of vitamin K_1, or K_2, or K_3, transfer it to a 100 ml of volumetric flask, mix sample with 20 ml DMSO, soak for 15 min in a 70°C water bath, sonicate for 5 min, then add 50 ml 1:1 ethanol/isopropyl alcohol, sonicate for another 10 min under 70ºC water bath with frequent shaking, cool the flask to room temperature, add 1:1 ethanol/isopropyl alcohol to the volume, shake and mix well. After centrifuging for 5 min (12,000 rpm), take the clear solution for injection.

If the sample is fatty liquid, just add 60 ml 1:1 ethanol/isopropyl alcohol, sonicate for 10 min under 70ºC, after cooling fill same solvent to mark and shake well. After centrifuging for 5 min (12,000 rpm), take the clear solution for injection.

The conditions for sample preparation may be adjusted as necessary according to the specific sample and the analytes. In some cases, the powdered samples can be extracted with organic solvents directly, without water being used.

(ii) *Chromatography condition*

HPLC conditions

Column: Phenomenex Synergi 5 μm 4.6 × 250 mm 100 A
Injection volume: 20 ul
Mobile phase A: Methanol
Mobile phase B: Ethanol
Flow rate: 1.0 ml/min
Column temperature: Room temperature
UV wavelength: 269 nm

Gradient:

Time (min)	A%	B%
0	35	65
0–1.0	35	65
1.0–15.0	0	100
15.0–18.0	0	100
18.0–18.5	35	65
25.0	35	65 End

UPLC conditions

Column: Acquity UPLC® BEH Phenyl 1.7 μm, 2.1 × 150 mm
Injection volume: 2 ul
UV wavelength: 269 nm
Mobile phase A: 0.1% phosphoric acid water solution
Mobile phase B: 0.1% Phosphoric acid in acetonitrile
Flow rate: 0.5 ml/min
Column temperature: 55°C

Gradient:

Time (min)	A%	B%
0	20	80
6.0	0	100
6.0–9.5	0	100
9.5–10.0	20	80
10.0–12.0	20	80

Result and calculation

$$\textit{Individual vitamin K content}(\mu g/unit) = \frac{Aa \times Wstd \times Vsam \times UW}{As \times Wsam \times Vstd}$$

or

$$\textit{Individual vitamin K content}(\mu g/g) = \frac{Aa \times Wstd \times Vsam}{As \times Wsam \times Vstd}$$

Aa = Peak area of corresponding vitamin K in sample solution
As = Peak area of corresponding vitamin K in standard solution
$Wstd$ = Weight of corresponding standard (μg)
$Wsam$ = Weight of sample (g)
$Vsam$ = Total volume of sample solution (ml)
$Vstd$ = Total volume of standard solution (ml)
UW = Unit weight (g)

2.2.5 *Adjustment of liquid chromatography conditions*

Oil-soluble vitamins are non-polar compounds and they have a longer retention time in reverse phase chromatography. With different products, the interferences may be different, and the chromatography conditions may need to be adjusted. The following are suggestions for adjustments.

(1) Adjust gradients — The gradient setting is dependent on the analyte and matrix composition. In order to separate different components in the different formulas and matrices, a change to the gradient settings may be required. Reducing the gradient rate will not always get better separation; this adjustment should be based on experience.
(2) Using different columns and mobile phases — If C18 columns cannot separate the interferant, a different type of column can be required (such as phenyl, C30, etc.). Changes to the mobile phases can also be useful. For example, if C18 column with acetonitrile mobile phase cannot separate the interferant, a phenyl column with methanol mobile phase may be able to affect the required separation.

(3) Adjust the wavelength of the UV/Vis detector — Select a wavelength with minimal or no interferences based on the UV spectrum.
(4) Dilute the sample solution — Dilute the concentration of the sample solution as much as possible to reduce the concentration of the interferences.
(5) Select detector — Select a detector to avoid matrix interfere, for example, use MS/MS detector to replace the UV/visible detector, etc.

2.2.6 *LC-MS/MS methods for vitamin D and K tests*

Dietary supplement products generally contain vitamin D and K levels in the microgram concentration. In order to reduce the challenges of matrix and compound interferences, the analyte concentration in the sample solution should be as low as possible. It is important to use a very sensitive detector. Usually, the sensitivity of LC-MS/MS is around 100 times superior to LC-UV. Also, LC-MS/MS has better selectivity.

(i) *Test procedure*

Preparation of standard solution — Accurately weigh about 5 mg of vitamin D_2, D_3, pre D_3, K_1, K_2 (MK4, MK7) and K_3 standards as needed, transfer it to a 100 ml volumetric flask, add about 60 ml of 1:1 ethanol/isopropyl alcohol, put in 70°C water bath, sonicate for few minutes until all standards are dissolved. Cool the sample flask to room temperature, fill 1:1 ethanol/isopropyl to the mark, shake and mix well. Transfer 1.0 ml of the above standard stock solution to a 100 ml volumetric flask, dilute to volume with ethanol/isopropyl alcohol, shake and mix well. Make further dilutions with the same solvent to get 200 ppb, 40 ppb and 8 ppb standard solutions for each analyte. Use these three standard solutions to establish a working curve for each analyte.

Preparation of sample solution — For the sample solution preparation follow Section 1.1.3 in the previous chapter. In order to effectively extract oil-soluble vitamins from the sample, it is recommended that the entire extraction process be carried out in a water bath at of 70°C.

Accurately weigh a certain amount of powdered sample containing about 5 μg of any K_1, K_2, K_3, D_3, D_2 and pre D_3, transfer it to a 100 ml volumetric flask, mix sample with 10 ml of DMSO (70ºC), soak for 15 min in a 70°C water bath, sonicate for 5 min, then add 60 ml isopropyl alcohol, sonicate for 10 min under 70ºC water bath with frequent shaking, cool the flask to room temperature, add 1:1 ethanol/isopropyl alcohol to the volume, shake and mix well. After centrifuging for 5 min (12,000 rpm), take the clear solution for injection.

If the sample is fatty liquid, just add 60 ml 1:1 ethanol/isopropyl alcohol, sonicate for 10 min under 70ºC, after cooling fill same solution to mark and shake well. After centrifuging for 5 min (12,000 rpm), take the clear solution for injection.

The conditions for sample preparation may be adjusted as necessary according to the specific sample and the analytes being measured. In some cases, powdered samples can just use organic solvents to extract the analytes directly, without using water.

(ii) *UPLC condition*

Column: Acquity UPLC® BEH Phenyl 1.7 μm, 2.1 × 150 mm
Flow rate: 0.5 ml/min
Injection volume: 2 ul
Column temperature: 55°C
Mobile phase A: 10mM formic acid in nano pure water
Mobile phase B: 10mM formic acid in acetonitrile

Gradient:

Time (min)	**A%**	**B%**
0	15	85
0–6.0	0	100
6.0–9.5	0	100
9.5–9.8	15	85
9.8–12	15	85 End

MS/MS parameter: (From Waters UPLC-MS/BMS TQS)

D_2:

Type	MRM
Ion Mode	ES+
Inter Channel Delay (sec)	–1.000
InterScan Time (sec)	–1.000
Span (Da)	0
Start Time (min)	2.0
End Time (min)	7.0

Ch	Prnt(Da)	Dau(Da)	Dwell(s)	Cone(V)	Coll(eV)	Delay(s)	Compound	Formula
1	397.31	67.06	0.05	22.00	20.00	–1.000	D2	396.3
2	397.31	81.10	0.05	22.00	24.00	–1.000	D2	396.3
3	397.31	95.08	0.05	22.00	24.00	–1.000	D2	396.3

K_2(MK-4):

Type	MRM
Ion Mode	ES+
Inter Channel Delay (sec)	–1.000
InterScan Time (sec)	–1.000
Span (Da)	0
Start Time (min)	5.0
End Time (min)	6.1

Ch	Prnt(Da)	Dau(Da)	Dwell(s)	Cone(V)	Coll(eV)	Delay(s)	Compound	Formula
1	445.20	81.06	0.025	26.00	28.00	–1.000	MK-4	444.3
2	445.20	95.10	0.025	26.00	30.00	–1.000	MK-4	444.3
3	445.20	187.05	0.025	26.00	16.00	–1.000	MK-4	444.3

K_1:

Type	MRM
Ion Mode	ES+
Inter Channel Delay (sec)	–1.000
InterScan Time (sec)	–1.000
Span (Da)	0
Start Time (min)	6.0
End Time (min)	6.9

Ch	Prnt(Da)	Dau(Da)	Dwell(s)	Cone(V)	Coll(eV)	Delay(s)	Compound	Formula
1	451.33	128.15	0.05	42.00	66.00	–1.000	K1	450.3
2	451.33	187.09	0.05	42.00	24.00	–1.000	K1	450.3
3	451.33	225.43	0.05	42.00	16.00	–1.000	K1	450.3

D_3:

Type	MRM
Ion Mode	ES+
Inter Channel Delay (sec)	–1.000
InterScan Time (sec)	–1.000
Span (Da)	0
Start Time (min)	2.0
End Time (min)	7.0

Ch	Prnt(Da)	Dau(Da)	Dwell(s)	Cone(V)	Coll(eV)	Delay(s)	Compound	Formula
1	385.33	81.11	0.05	22.00	26.00	–1.000	D3	384.3
2	385.33	107.15	0.05	22.00	24.00	–1.000	D3	384.3
3	385.33	259.27	0.05	22.00	14.00	–1.000	D3	384.3

K_2(MK-7):

Type	MRM
Ion Mode	ES+
Inter Channel Delay (sec)	–1.000
InterScan Time (sec)	–1.000
Span (Da)	0
Start Time (min)	7.2
End Time (min)	9.0

Ch	Prnt(Da)	Dau(Da)	Dwell(s)	Cone(V)	Coll(eV)	Delay(s)	Compound	Formula
1	649.47	81.04	0.08	50.00	42.00	–1.000	MK-7	648.5
2	649.47	95.09	0.08	50.00	42.00	–1.000	MK-7	648.5
3	649.47	187.09	0.08	50.00	30.00	–1.000	MK-7	648.5

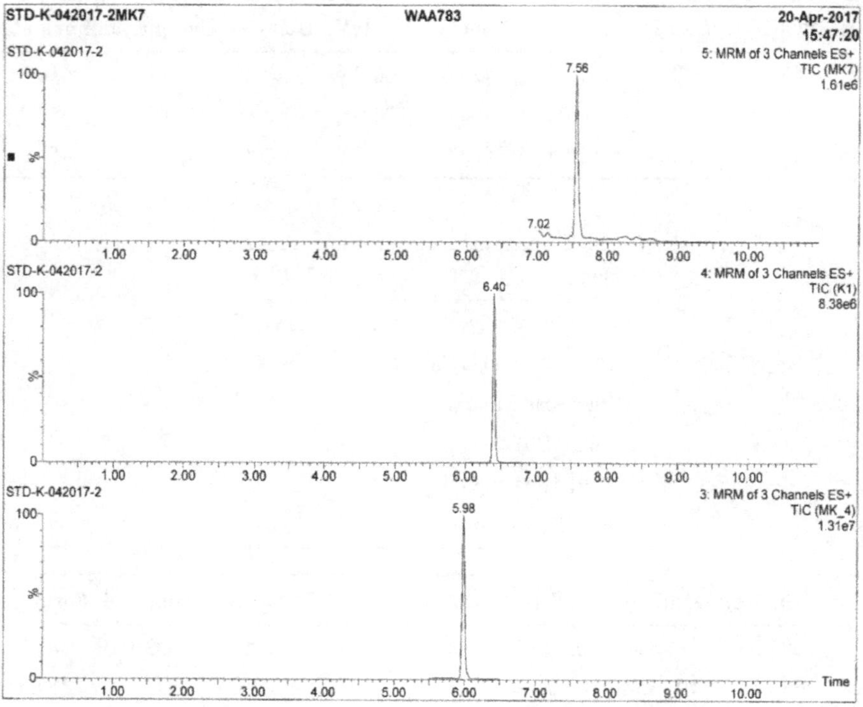

Figure 2.10: Vitamin K_1, MK-4 and MK-7 TIC chromatogram.

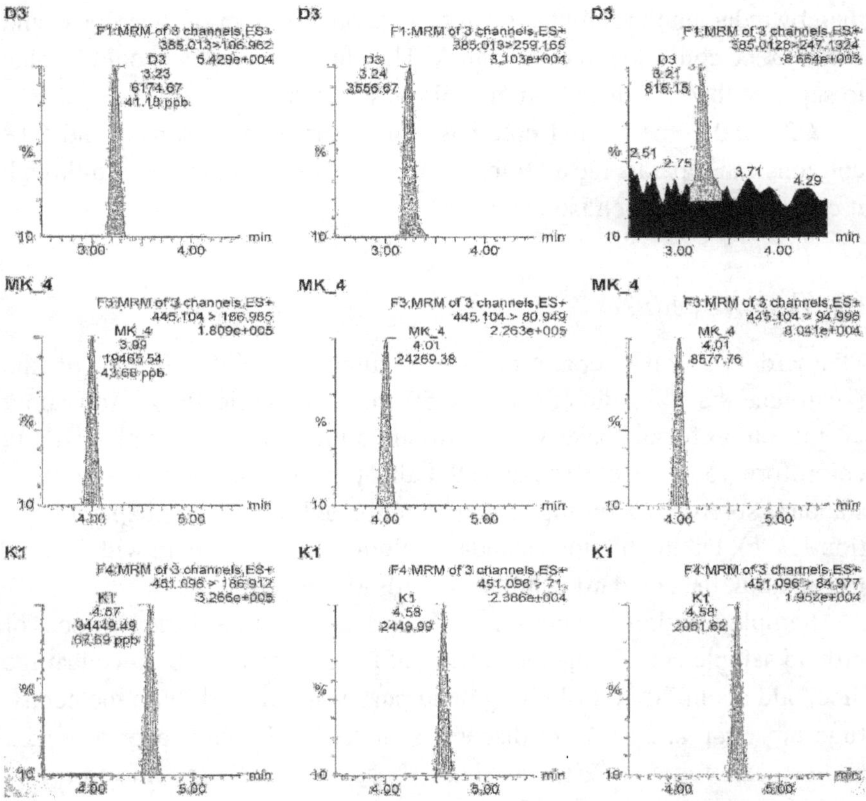

Figure 2.11: D_3, MK-4 and K_1 ion pairs spectrum.

(iii) *Result calculation*

Follow Chapter 1, Section 1.1.5 "Qualitative and quantitative testing of LC-MS/MS".

2.3 Tests for *β*-carotene

β-carotene can be converted to vitamin A in the human body. The all trans *β*-carotene is the most commonly found form, plus 9-cis, 11-cis, 13-cis and 15-cis *β*-carotenes. The all-trans *β*-carotene is the most bioactive isomer but it can be converted into cis *β*-carotene under exposure to sun light and heat, thereby reducing the activity. α-carotene, another isomer of β-carotene, and it cannot be converted into vitamin A. The chromatography should be able to separate these isomers from the all trans β-carotene.

C30 and some phenyl columns can separate each isomer, and C18 columns can separate the all trans β-carotene from other isomers, although it cannot separate each isomer.

(i) *Test procedure*

Standard solution preparation — Accurately weigh 20 mg of the β-carotene standard directly into a 50 mL volumetric flask. Add about 20 mL chloroform, shake well to dissolve the standard completely, add chloroform to 50 ml, and shake well. Label the concentration of β-carotene standard solution according to actual calibrated purity see chapter1, section 1.3 (e). Dilute the stock standard solution to about 2 ppm with isopropyl alcohol, the standard solution is ready for injection.

Sample solution preparation — Accurately weigh a certain amount of ground sample containing about 1 mg of β-carotene in a 50 ml centrifuge tube, add about 20 ml of boiling nano pure water directly into the centrifuge tube, cap and shake to disperse sample. Put into a beaker or a rack and sonicate for about 20 min. Shake occasionally during sonication.

Quantitatively transfer 20 mL chloroform into the tube. Cap immediately and tightly, wrap with aluminum foil, and shake vigorously for 30 min.

Centrifuge for 5 min. Use the Pasture pipette to collect the bottom layer (chloroform layer) into a syringe and filter through 0.45 μm Gelman Acrodisk (discard the first few drops). Transfer 1 ml of the clear solution to a 25 ml volumetric flask, dilute to volume with isopropyl alcohol, shake well, the solution is ready for injection.

If the sample is fatty liquid, transfer to a 50 ml volumatric flask, add chloroform to volume, sonicate for 10 min under 70°C. Centrifuge for 5 min (12,000 rpm), transfer 1 ml of clear chloroform to 10 ml volumetric flask dilute to volume with isopropyl alcohol. The sample solution is ready for injection.

If the β-carotene raw material is microencapsulated, follow the extraction procedure provided by the manufacturer.

The conditions for sample preparation may be adjusted as necessary according to the specific sample and analytes.

(ii) *Charomatography condition*

(1) *HPLC condition*

Column: Phenomenex Synergi 5 um, 4.6 × 250 mm
Flow rate: 1 ml/min
injection volume: 20 ul
Column temperature: Room temperature
Mobile phase A: Methyl alcohol
Mobile phase B: Ethanol
UV wavelength: 450 nm

Gradient:

Time (min)	A%	B%
0	20	80
0–10.0	0	100
10.0–18.0	0	100
18.0–18.5	20	80
25.0	20	80 end

(2) *UPLC condition*

Column: Waters Acquit BEH Phenyl 1.7 um, 2.1 × 150 mm
Flow rate: 0.5 ml/min
Injection volume: 2 ul
mobile phase: Acetonitrile
UV wavelength: 450 nm
Column temperature: 45°C
Run time: 12 min

In addition, for some specific testing a C30 columns method may be needed. This method has a relatively longer run time. An injection may take 1 h. The following method comes from the system 2 method used in the validation of the AOAC beta-carotene test method.

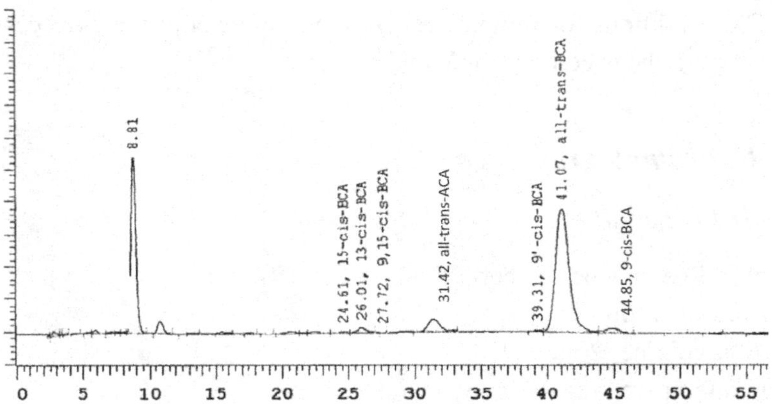

Figure 2.12: C30 chromatogram of β-carotene sample. BCA is β-carotene, ACA is α-carotene.
15-sic-BCA 24.61 min
13-cis-BCA 26.01 min
9,15-cis-BCA 27.72 min
all-trans-ACA 31.42 min
9'-cis-BCA 39.31 min
All-trans-BCA 41.07 min
9-cis-BCA 44.85 min

Column: YMC-Pck C30, 5 μm, 4.6 × 250 mm
Injection volume: 20 ul
Column temperature: 30°C
Mobile phase A: 900 ml methanol + 20 mg Vitamin C + 100 ml MTBE
Mobile phase B: Methyl tert-butyl ether (MTBE)
UV wavelength: 445 nm

Gradient:

Time (min)	A%	B%	Flow rate (ml/min)
0	100	0	0.9
0–57	100	0	0.9
57–59	0	100	0.9
59–60	0	100	2.0
60–62	0	100	2.0
62–63	100	0	0.9
63–68	100	0	0.9

(iii) *Result calculation*

$$\beta-carotene\ content\ (\%) = \frac{Aa \times Wstd \times Vsam \times 100\%}{As \times Wsam \times Vstd}$$

Aa = Peak area of β-carotene in sample solution
As = Peak area of β-carotene in standard solution
Wstd = Weight of β-carotene standard (mg)
Wsam = Weight of sample (mg)
Vsam = Total volume of sample solution (ml)
Vstd = Total volume of standard solution (ml)

1 mg of β-carotene = 1667 IU

2.4 Oil Soluble Vitamin Activity Factors

1 mg synthetic vitamin E acetate = 1 IU
1 mg natural vitamin E acetate = 1.39 IU
1 mg synthetic vitamin E succinate = 0.89 IU
1 mg natural vitamin E succinate = 1.21 IU
1 mg synthetic vitamin E = 1.10 IU
1 mg natural vitamin E = 1.49 IU
1 mg vitamin A = 3333 IU
1 mg vitamin A acetate = 2941 IU
1 mg vitamin A palmitate = 1818 IU
1 mg β-carotene = 1667 IU
1 mg vitamin D (D2或D3) = 40000 IU
1 ug vitamin D(D2或D3) = 40 IU

2.5 Tests for Total Tocopherols and Tocotrienols

Total tocopherols are composed of: α-tocopherol, β-tocopherol, γ-tocopherol and δ-tocopherol. α-Tocopherol is also known as vitamin E. The raw material of vitamin E often contains small amounts of β, γ and δ-tocopherols. C18 columns can separate α-tocopherol from other tocopherols, though β and γ are impossible to separate because they are isomers.

Tocotrienols are similar as tocopherols but contain three double bonds on the straight carbon chain. Similar to tocopherols, C18 column can be used to separate α-tocotrienol from β, γ and δ tocotrienols, but not β and γ because they are isomers.

People have used normal phase chromatography column to successfully separate all the eight compounds. Some phenyl column also can be used to separate all the above eight compounds. The following is a separate method from Phenomenex.

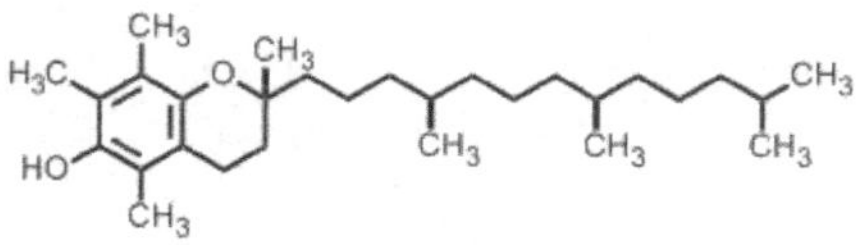

alpha-Tocopherol
"Vitamin E"

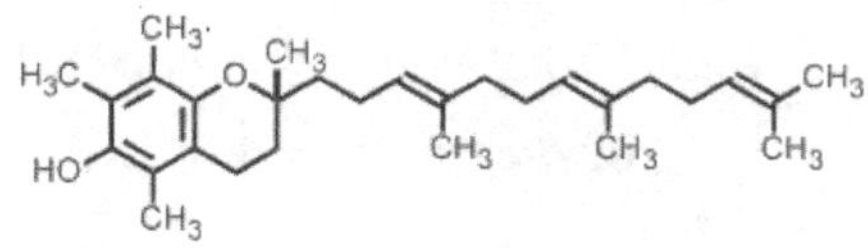

alpha-Tocotrienol

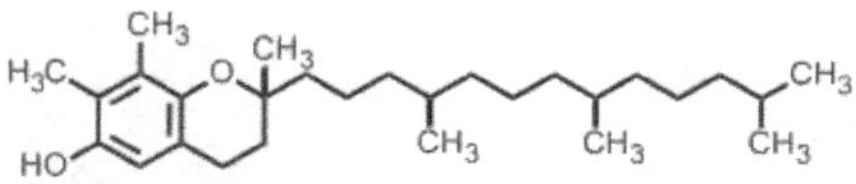

gamma-Tocopherol

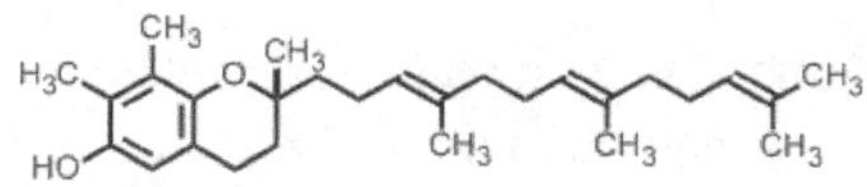

gamma-Tocotrienol

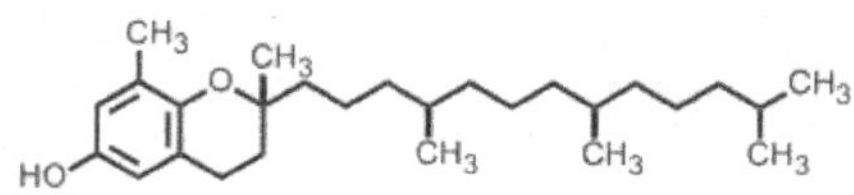

delta-Tocopherol

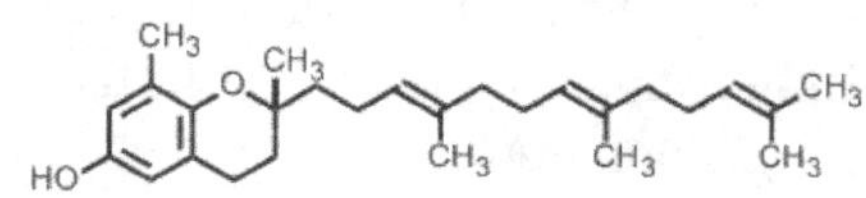

delta-Tocotrienol

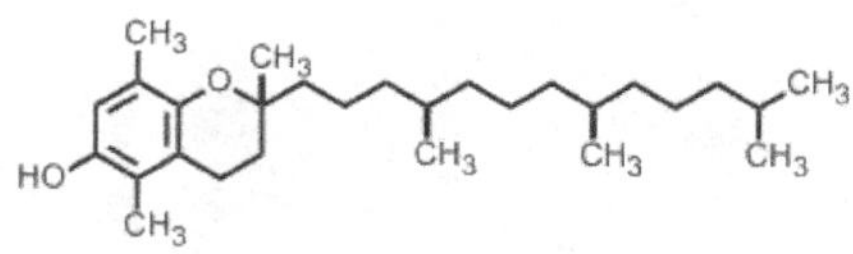

beta-Tocopherol

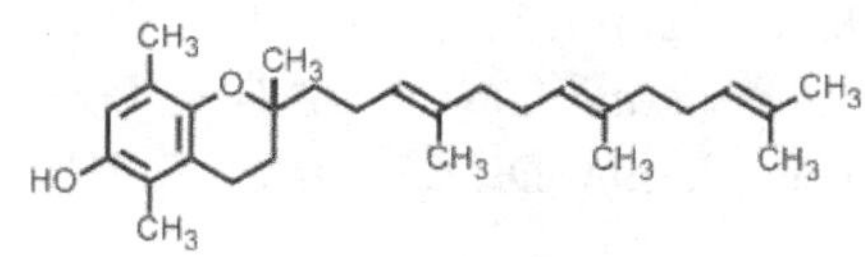

beta-Tocotrienol

(i) *Test procedure*

Standard solution preparation — Accurately weigh about 20 mg of each tocopherol and tocotrienol, transfer it to a 100 ml volumetric flask, add 60 ml IPA (isopropyl alcohol) to dissolve the standards, then add ethanol

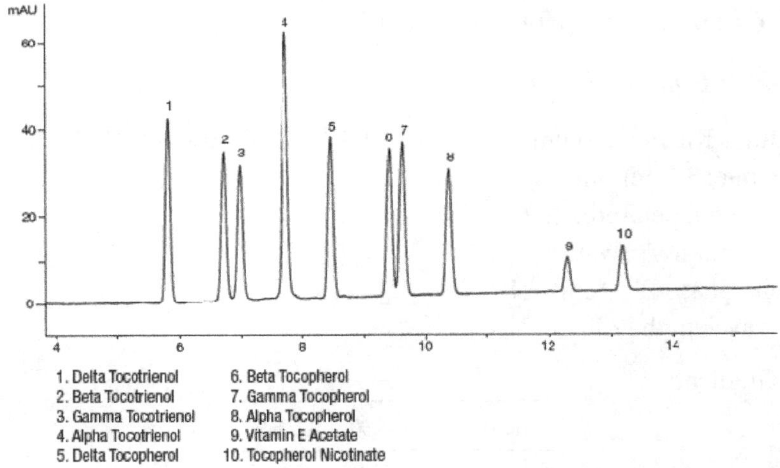

Figure 2.13: Chromatogram from Phenomenex Kinetex 2.6 um F5 Core-Shell column instruction manual.

to mark, shake and mix well. Use ethanol to dilute 10 times. The diluted standard solution is ready for injection.

Prepare sample solution — Accurately weigh an amount of sample that contains about 2 mg of any tocopherols or tocotrienols, transfer it to a 100 ml volumetric flask. If the sample is solid powder, first mix sample with a small amount (no more than 10 ml) of hot water (70°C). Place this in a 70°C water bath for 15 min, sonicate for 5 min, then add about 60 ml isopropyl alcohol. Sonicate for another 10 min in the 70°C water bath with frequent shaking, cool to room temperature, add isopropyl alcohol to the 100 ml volumetric flask, shake and mix well. Filter or centrifuge the sample solution. The clear solution is ready for injection.

If the sample is fatty liquid, add 60 ml isopropyl alcohol in the sample flask, shake and sonicate for 10 min. Cool to room temperature, add isopropyl alcohol to the 100 ml, shake and mix well. Filter or centrifuge th samplesolution, and the clear solution is ready to injection.

The conditions for sample preparation may be adjusted as necessary according to the specific sample and the analytes. In some cases, the powdered sample of the analytes can be extracted directly with organic solvents.

(ii) *Chromatography condition*

(1) *HPLC method*

Column: Kinetex 2.6 um, F5 core-shell 4.6 × 150 mm, 00F-4723-EO
Flow rate: 1.2 ml/min
Column temperature: 42°C
Mobile phase A: Water
Mobile phase B: Methanol
UV wavelength: 290 nm

Gradient:

Time (min)	A%	B%
0	15	85
1.0–15.0	0	100
17.0–18.0	15	85
23.0	15	85 End

(iii) *Result and calculation*

$$Tocotrienol/tocopherol(mg/unit) = \frac{Aa \times Wstd \times Vsam \times UW}{As \times Wsam \times Vstd}$$

or

$$Tocotrienol/tocopherol\ (\%) = \frac{Aa \times Wstd \times Vsam \times 100\%}{As \times Wsam \times Vstd}$$

Aa = Peak area of sample solution
As = Peak area of standard solution
Wstd = Weight of standard (mg)
Wsam = Weight of sample (mg)
Vsam = Total volume of sample solution (ml)
Vstd = Total volume of standard solution (ml)
UW = Unit weight (mg/unit)

Sum of the calculated individual items to get total tocopherols or total tocotrienols.

2.6 Tests of Carotenoids

There are many kinds of carotenoids in nature. The following carotenoids are commonly used in dietary supplements, Beta-carotene, lycopene, lutein/zeaxanthin and astaxanthin.

Preparation of carotenoids sample solution: Carotenoid compounds are unstable, they are easily decomposed or isomerized in the natural environment and have a short shelf life. To stabilize the compounds and extend the shelf life, industry uses a micro-encapsulation technique to isolate them from the atmosphere and to extend the shelf life. So, it is important to make sure that the beadlets are broken, and the active ingredients are completely extracted to the test solution during sample preparation. Otherwise, you will get very low test results due to poor recovery. The beadlets are generally opened using an enzymatic digestion, and then extracted with organic solvents. The methods to open the microencapsulated particles and to extract the active ingredients may vary depending on the granulation process and the raw materials used. To effectively extract the compounds of interest, it is important to obtain the correct extraction method. Usually, the manufacturers can provide a specific extraction method that should be used to break the encapsulation for their specific products.

Preparation of carotenoid standard solution: Accurately weigh an amount of carotenoid standard in a volumetric flask, add the corresponding solvent to dissolve the standard, and fill to the volume. Measure the UV absorption at the corresponding wavelength. The concentration of the solution is calculated by the UV extinction coefficient, and the UV purity of the standard is calculated. Use the same solution to run the chromatography with same UV wavelength, using the normalization method to calculate chromatographic purity. The exact purity of the standard is obtained by multiplying the UV purity by the chromatography purity. Because the standard is unstable, the purity of the standard must be recalibrated before each test, to obtain accurate and reliable results. Finally, dilute the solution to about 2 ppm with ethanol, and it is ready for injection. The entire test procedure should avoid exposure to light and heat.

The beta-carotene test method has been described previously, and it is not repeated here.

2.6.1 *Testing of lycopene*

Natural lycopene contains 11 conjugate double bonds with all-trans form.

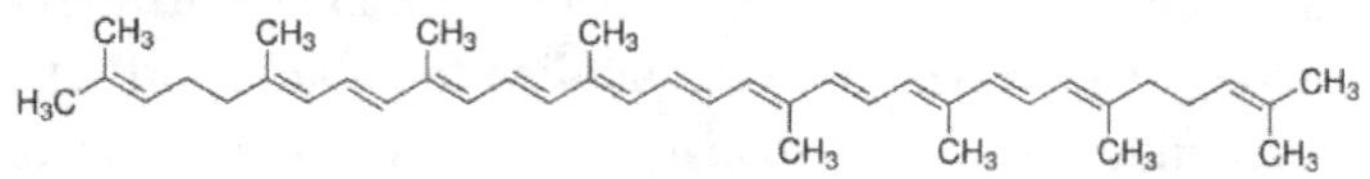

lycopene

(i) *Test procedure*

Lycopene is also an unstable compound, so the preparation of the standard solutions should be carried out following the preparation procedures described previously.

If lycopene in the sample is micro-encapsulated, the sample is first extracted according to the extraction method provided by the manufacturer.

Preparation of the standard solution: Accurately weigh 5 mg of a lycopene standard directly into a 25 ml volumetric flask. Add 10 mL chloroform, shake well to dissolve the standard completely, add chloroform to mark, and shake well. Transfer 1 ml stock standard to a 100 ml volumetric flask, add 60 ml isopropyl alcohol, mix well, add isopropyl alcohol to 100 ml, and shake well. The purity of standard should be calibrated following the procedure described earlier see chapter1, section 1.3 (e).

Preparation of sample solution: (1) Accurately weigh a certain amount of ground powdered sample that contains about 0.1 mg of lycopene into a 50 ml centrifuge tube. (2) Add about 15 mL of hot nano pure water directly into the centrifuge tube, cap and shake to disperse the sample. Put it into a beaker or a rack and sonicate for about 20 min. Shake occasionally during sonicating. (3) Quantitatively transfer 20 mL chloroform into each tube. Cap immediately and tightly, wrap with aluminum foil, and shake vigorously by hand to mix evenly. Then shake with a wrist action shaker at highest intensity for 30 min. (4) Centrifuge the solutions for 5 min. Use the Pasteur pipette to collect the bottom layer (chloroform layer) into the syringes and filter through 0.45 μm Gelman Acrodisk into a glass tube (discard the first few drops). Transfer 0.5 ml of the filtered sample solution into an HPLC injection vail, quantitatively pipette 0.5 ml isopropyl alcohol to the vail, and vortex for 1 min. This solution can be injected to the HPLC system.

If the sample is fatty liquid, just weight a certain amount of sample containing 0.1 mg lycopene into a 50 ml volumetric flask, add 20 ml chloroform, sonicate for 5 min, add isopropyl alcohol to mark, mix well and centrifuge for 5 min. The resulting clear solution is ready for injection.

If the lycopene raw material in the sample is micro-encapsulated, the sample must first be extracted according to the extraction method provided by the manufacturer.

(ii) *UPLC conditions*

Column: Acquity UPLC® BEH C18, 1.7μm, 2.1 × 150 mm
Flow rate: 0.5 mL/min
Injection volume: 2.0 ul
Column temperature: 45°C
UV wavelength: 472 nm
Mobile Phase A: Deionized water
Mobile Phase B: Acetonitrile

Gradient:

Time (min)	**A%**	**B%**
0	8	92
0–6.0	0	100
6.0–8.0	0	100
8.0–8.3	8	92
11.0	8	92 End

(iii) *Result calculation*

$$Lycopene\ (mg/unit) = \frac{Aa \times Wstd \times Vsam \times Purity \times UW}{As \times Wsam \times Vstd}$$

or

$$Lycopene\ (\%) = \frac{Aa \times Wstd \times Vsam \times Purity \times 100\%}{As \times Wsam \times Vstd}$$

Aa = Peak area of sample solution
As = Peak area of standard solution
Wstd = Weight of standard (mg)
Wsam = Weight of sample (mg)
Vsam = Total volume of sample solution (ml)
Vstd = Total volume of standard solution (ml)
UW = Unit weight (mg/unit)
Purity = standard purity

6.2.2 *Tests of lutein and zeaxanthin*

Lutein and zeaxanthin are naturally co-existing compounds.

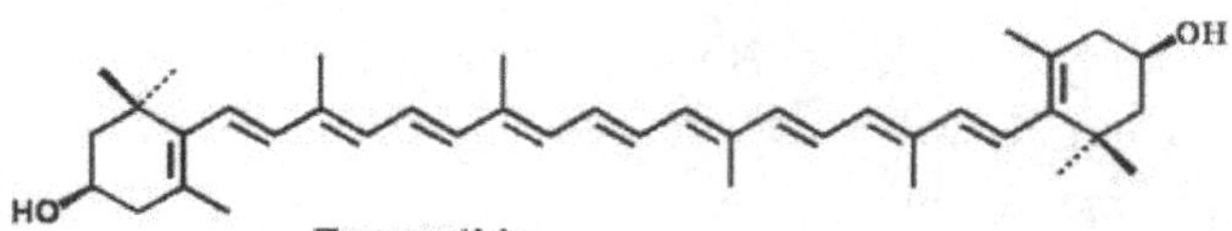

Zeaxanthin

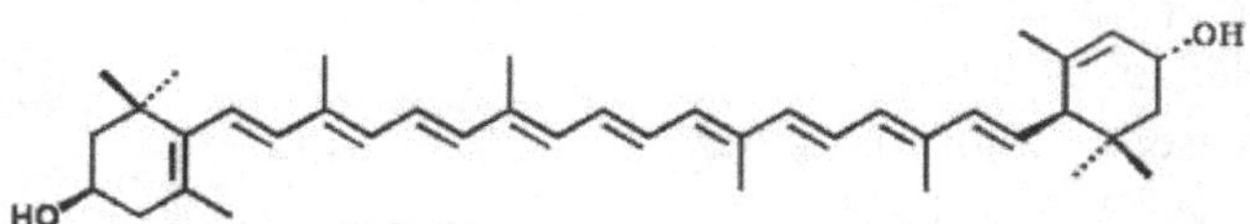

Lutein

(i) *Test procedure*

Lutein and zeaxanthin can be separated using a C30 or phenyl column. The preparation of samples and standard solutions should be carried out according to the previous descriptions.

If the lutein and zeaxanthin in the sample are micro-encapsulated, the sample must first be extracted according to the extraction method provided by the manufacturer.

Standard solution preparation — Accurately weigh 20 mg of lutein/zeaxanthin suspension standard directly into a 50 mL volumetric flask. Add about 20 mL chloroform, shake well to dissolve the standard completely, add chloroform to 50 ml, and shake well. Label the concentration of lutein/zeaxanthin standard solution according to calibrated actual purity see chapter1, section 1.3 (e). Dilute the stock standard solution to about 2 ppm with isopropyl alcohol, the solution is ready for injection.

Sample solution preparation — Accurately weigh a certain amount of ground sample that contains about 1 mg of lutein/zeaxanthin in a 50 ml centrifuge tube, add about 15 ml of boiling nano pure water directly into the centrifuge tube, cap and shake to disperse sample. Put it into a beaker or a rack and sonicate for about 20 min. Shake occasionally during sonicating.

Quantitatively transfer 20 mL of chloroform into the tube. Cap immediately and tightly, wrap with aluminum foil, and shake vigorously for 30 min with a wrist action shaker.

Centrifuge for 5 min. Use the Pasture pipette to collect the bottom layer (chloroform layer) into the syringes and filter through 0.45 μm Gelman Acrodisk (discard the first few drops). Transfer 1 ml of the clear solution to a 25 ml volumetric flask, dilute to volume with isopropyl alcohol and shake well. This solution is ready for injection.

If the sample is fatty liquid, just weight certain amount of sample contains 0.1 mg lutein/zeaxanthin in a 50 ml volumetric flask, add 20 ml chloroform, sonicate for 5 min, add isopropyl alcohol to mark, mix well and centrifuge for 5 min. The resulting clear solution is ready for injection.

If the lutein/zeaxanthin in the sample are micro-encapsulated, the sample must first be extracted according to the extraction method provided by the manufacturer.

(ii) *UPLC conditions*

Column: Aquity BEH Phenyl, 1.7 um, 2.1 × 150 mm
mobile phase A: 0.1% phosphoric acid in water
Mobile phase B: 0.1% phosphoric acid in acetonitrile
Flow rate: 0.50 ml/min
Column temperature: 45°C
UV wavelength: 475 nm
Injection volume: 2 ul

Gradient:

Time (min)	A%	B%
0	20	80
0–6.0	0	100
6.0–7.5	0	100
7.5–8.0	20	80
8.0–10.0	20	80

(iii) *Results and calculations*

The calculation can either be carried out by total peak area of lutein and zeaxanthin in sample solution vs. total peak area in standard solution, getting a total content of lutein and zeaxanthin in the sample; or by individually calculating the content of lutein and zeaxanthin.

$$Lutein/zeaxanthin\ (mg/unit) = \frac{Aa \times Wstd \times Vsam \times Purity \times UW}{As \times Wsam \times Vstd}$$

or

$$Lutein/zeaxanthin\ (\%) = \frac{Aa \times Wstd \times Vsam \times Purity \times 100\%}{As \times Wsam \times Vstd}$$

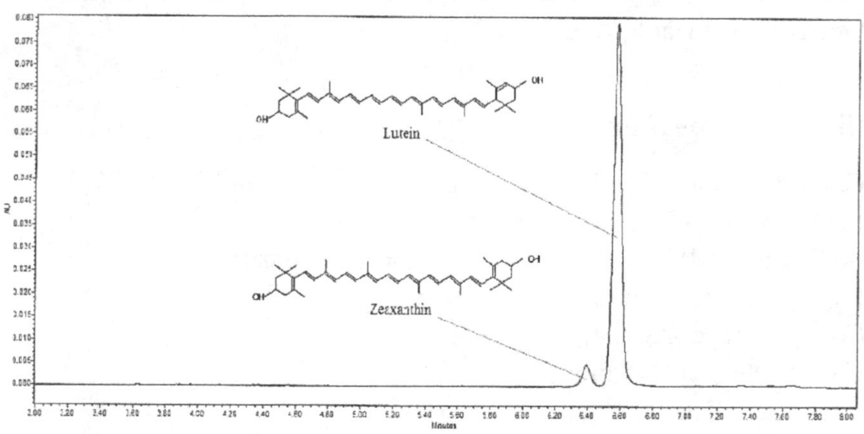

Figure 2.14: Chromatogram of lutein and zeaxanthin.

Aa = Peak area of sample solution
As = Peak area of standard solution
Wstd = Weight of standard (mg)
Wsam = Weight of sample (mg)
Vsam = Total volume of sample solution (ml)
Vstd = Total volume of standard solution (ml)
UW = Unit weight (mg/unit)
Purity = standard purity

2.6.3 *Testing for astaxanthin*

Natural astaxanthin is often present in the form of a variety fatty acid esters. Quantitative analysis with a chromatography method does generally not quantify of each individual fatty acid esters. This is because there are many possible fatty acid esters, and the corresponding individual standards are not easy to find.

Cholesterol esterase is used to digest astaxanthin esters in organic solvents yielding free astaxanthin and fatty acids. Then after digestion, a chromatography method is used to quantify the total free astaxanthin.

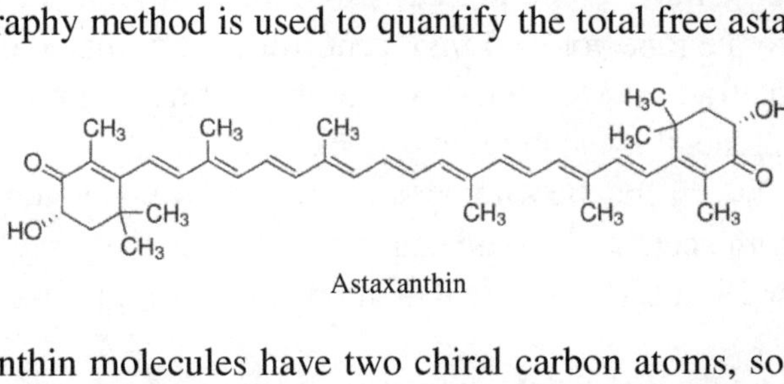

Astaxanthin

Astaxanthin molecules have two chiral carbon atoms, so there could be four different enantiomers. Because the proportion of enantiomers are varied with the sources of the raw materials, and there is no knowledge about the difference of the bioactivity for the enantiomers, this method will not separate the enantiomers during the test. The final result will be the total of the enantiomers.

(i) *Testing process*

Cholesterol esterase solution preparation — Dissolve an accurately weighed quantity of cholesterol esterase in 50 mM tris hydrochloride buffer (pH 7.0), having a known concentration of 4 units per ml.

Preparation of standard solution — Accurately weigh about 5 mg of an astaxanthin standard into a 200 ml volumetric flask, add about 100 ml acetone to dissolve the standard, then fill acetone to mark, and shake and mix well. The standard solution is ready for injection. The standard solution must be prepared on the same day of test. The purity of the standard can be determined according to the previously described procedure.

Sample solution preparation:

(1) If the sample is liquid, warm the sample in a pre-heated water bath at 50–60°C for 30 min, and shake very well for 10 min intervals.
(2) Accurately weight certain an amount of liquid or ground solid sample containing about 35 mg of free astaxanthin in a 10 mL glass tube and add approximately 5 mL of acetone, vortex for 5 min, then centrifuge for 5 min.
(3) Pipette the clear sample solution from the glass tube into a 100 mL volumetric flask. Rinse the tube with more acetone to recover all remaining orange color. For each additional rinse, add 5 mL of acetone into the tube vortex 5 min, centrifuge for 5 min, and pipette the clear solution into the flask. Make up the final volume to 100 mL with acetone, this is the sample stock.
(4) Pipette 2.0 mL of the sample stock into a 20 mL volumetric flask, dilute with acetone to volume and mix. This is the assay solution A.
(5) Transfer 2.0 mL of the assay solution A to a 10 mL glass centrifuge tube.
(6) Set block heater at 37°C, add 3.0 mL of cholesterol esterase solution to the glass centrifuge tube, and mix by gentle inversion.
(7) Allow to react at 37°C for 45 min. Gently/slowly invert every 10 min.
(8) Add 1 g of sodium sulfate dehydrate and 2 mL of petroleum ether, vortex for 30 sec, and centrifuge at 5,000 rpm for 5 min.
(9) Transfer the petroleum ether layer to a 10 mL-glass centrifuge tube containing 1g of sodium sulfate anhydrate. Repeat step 8 once, combine the petroleum ether.

(10) Evaporate the petroleum ether under nitrogen gas stream at room temperature. Then add 3 mL of acetone, sonicate to dissolve the residual, and centrifuge at 10,000 rpm for 5 min. The clear solution is the assay sample solution B and it can be usd for HPLC injection.
Note: If astaxanthin in the sample is micro-encapsulated, follow the extraction method provide by manufactures.

(ii) *UPLC conditions*

Column: Acquity BEH Phenyl, 1.7 um, 2.1 × 150 mm
Mobile phase A: Nano pure water
Mobile phase B: Methanol
Flow rate: 0.50 ml/min
Column temperature: 45°C
UV wavelength: 475
Injection volume: 1 ul

Gradient:

Time (min)	**A%**	**B%**
0	35	65
0–6	0	100
6.0–16.5	0	100
16.5–16.9	35	65
20	35	65 End

If there is any other peak after astaxanthin peak in the chromatogram with the same UV spectrum as astaxanthin should be astaxanthin esters peaks, it means the sample did not digest completely, the sample should be re-digested by cholesterol esterase with a longer reaction time.

(iii) *Result calculation*

$$Astaxanthin\ (mg/unit) = \frac{Aa \times Wstd \times Vsam \times Purity \times UW}{As \times Wsam \times Vstd}$$

or

$$Astaxanthin\ (\%) = \frac{Aa \times Wstd \times Vsam \times Purity \times 100\%}{As \times Wsam \times Vstd}$$

Aa = Peak area of sample solution
As = Peak area of standard solution
Wstd = Weight of standard (mg)
Wsam = Weight of sample (mg)
Vsam = Total volume of sample solution (ml)
Vstd = Total volume of standard solution (ml)
UW = Unit weight (mg/unit)
Purity = standard purity

Chapter 3

Sugar, Oligosaccharide and Poly-Saccharide Test Methods

3.1 Testing Methods for Monosaccharides and Disaccharides

The test methods for sugars include the determination of monosaccharides and disaccharides. This is accomplished mainly with GC methods, or HPLC and IC methods. The IC method is described here.

The sugars' pKa are all within 12–13, so under the strong alkaline condition they are dissociated and negatively charged, can be separated, and quantified by anion exchange chromatography with an EC detector.

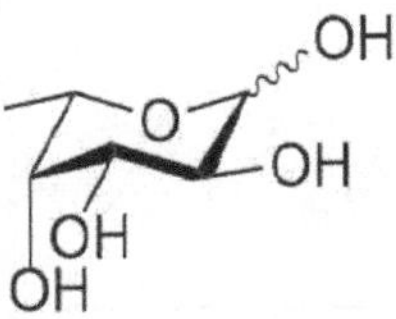

Fucose

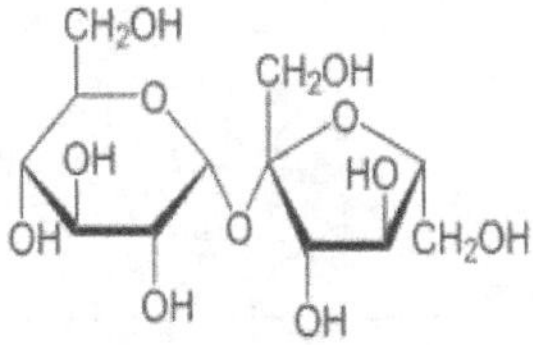

Sucrose

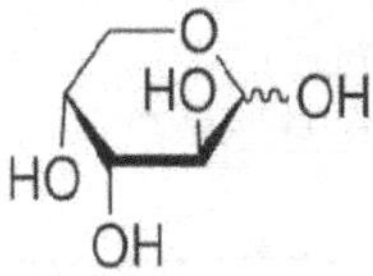

Arabinose

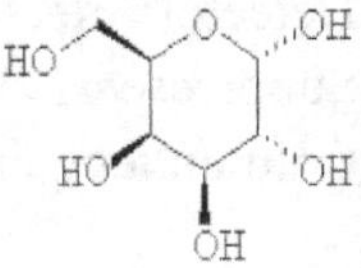

Galactose

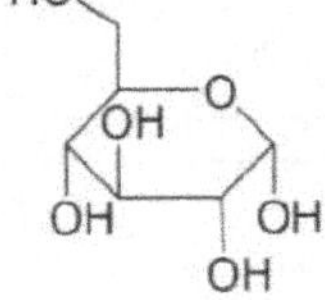

Glucose

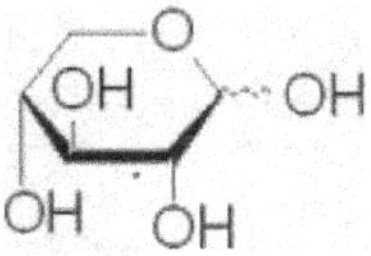

Xylose

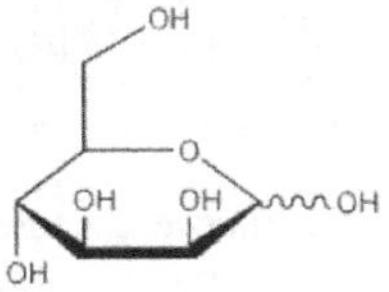

Mannose

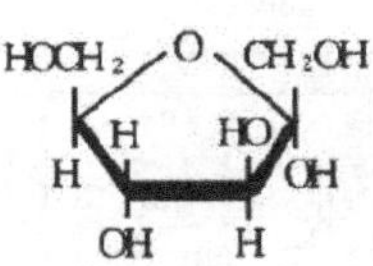

Fructose

(i) *Test procedure*

Preparation of standard solution — Accurately weigh about 20 mg of the following standards: fucose, sucrose, arabinose, galactose, glucose, xylose, mannose and fructose. Transfer these to a 100 ml volume flask. Add 60 ml of water, sonicate until the standards are completely dissolved, add water to the mark and shake well. Further dilute with water to about 10 ppm per sugar standard, and shake well. This solution is ready for injection (see Figure 3.1).

Preparation of sample solution — Accurately weigh a certain amount of ground sample containing about 20 mg of any of the aforementioned sugars, transfer to 100 ml of volumetric flask, add 60 ml of water, sonicate 10 min, cool to room temperature, fill water to mark and shake well. Centrifuge (12,000 rpm) for 5 min, take the clear solution to dilute with water to reach about 10 ppm per sugar. Shake and mix these solutions well. The sample solution is ready for injection.

(ii) *IC conditions*

Column: Dionex CarboPac SA10, 4 × 250 mm, 4 μm
Flow rate: 1.5 ml/min
Injection volume: 10 μL
Eluent: 12 mM potassium hydroxy
Detector: Electrochemistry
Suppresser: Not need
Column temperature: 35°C

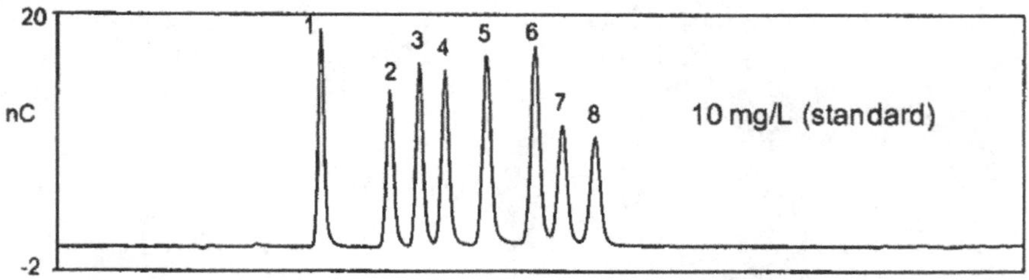

Figure 3.1: IC chromatogram 1. fucose, 2.sucrose, 3. arabinose, 4. galactose, 5. glucose, 6. xylose, 7. mannose, 8. fructose (chromatogram comes from Dionex/Thermo Science CarboPac SA10 instruction manual).

(iii) *Result calculation*

$$Individual\ sugar\ content\ (mg/unit) = \frac{Aa \times Wstd \times Vsam \times UW}{As \times Wsam \times Vstd}$$

or

$$Individual\ sugar\ content\ (\%) = \frac{Aa \times Wstd \times Vsam \times 100\%}{As \times Wsam \times Vstd}$$

where

Aa = Peak area of sample solution
As = Peak area of standard solution
Wstd = Weight of standard (mg)
Wsam = Weight of sample (mg)
Vsam = Total volume of sample solution (ml)
Vstd = Total volume of standard solution (ml)
UW = Unit weight (mg/unit)

3.2 Testing Methods for Oligosaccharides

Oligosaccharides generally contain 3–10 monosaccharides, such as xylo-oligosaccharide, Raffinose and oligogalactose (Galacto-oligosaccharide), etc. Oligosaccharides have demonstrated health benefits, including improvements in blood sugars and lipids, digestive health benefits, and beneficial changes to immune markers. They are used widely in dietary supplements, food and beverages. Determination of oligosaccharides involves two tests: identification and quantification tests.

Compare sample chromatograms with standard chromatograms, in order to check the retention times of each peak, and to see if it matches with the standard, as well as if the proportions of each peak are similar.

Acidic hydrolysis of the oligosaccharides during testing will produce free monosaccharides. Then you can quantify each monosaccharide by IC, the sum of each monosaccharide is the content of oligosaccharides being tested.

3.2.1 *Test of xylo-oligosaccharide*

(i) *Test procedure*

Sample solution A — Accurately weigh about 200 mg of xylo-oligosaccharide sample or reference standard, transfer to 50 ml of volumetric flask, add about 30 ml of water, sonicate for 10 min, cool to room temperature, then add water to the mark. Shake and mix this well, centrifuge (12,000 rpm) for 5 min, take the clear solution to dilute 50 times with deionization water. Shake and mix this well. Label it as "sample solution A".

Sample solution B — Accurately weigh the sample containing approximately 200 mg of xylo-oligosaccharide or reference standard, transfer to a 50 ml volumetric flask, and add 20 ml of 1 M hydrochloric acid solution. After shaking put this in a boiling water bath for 2.5 h (150 min), and shake every 15 min. After cooling, fill with deionized water to mark, shake and mix well, and centrifuge (12, 000 rpm) for 5 min. Dilute the clear solution 500 times with deionization water, shake and mix well, and label it "sample solution B". This solution is ready for injection.

Preparation of sugar standards solution — Accurately weigh about 30 mg of xylose and 5 mg of glucose, transfer to a 100 ml volumetric flask, add 60 ml water, then sonicate until all of the standards are dissolved. Add deionized water to the mark, then shake and mix well. Pipette 4, 2, 1 and 0.5 ml of the aforementioned clear solution to different 100 ml volumetric flask separately, add deionization water to mark, and shake well. The working curve of xylose and glucose can be created with these four standard solutions.

The hydroxyl group of sugar can be dissociated in an alkaline solution to form anions. Oligosaccharides contain more hydroxy groups than mono and disaccharides, so they should have more interaction with an anion exchange column. It will be difficult to elute these using same IC conditions as mono and disaccharides. To elute the oligosaccharides molecules, this method adds acetate anion as counter ions to the mobile phase. By adding counter ions, the oligosaccharide molecules will be "pushed out" (see "The application of mobile phases" in Chapter 1); thus, can get a full IC chromatogram pattern of oligosaccharides.

(ii) *Identification test*

IC conditions (for identification test)

Column: Thermo Scientific/Dionex Carbonpack PA1 4 × 250 mm
Column temperature: 35°C
Flow rate: 1.2 ml/min
Eluent: 100 mM potassium hydroxyl (50%) and 100 mM potassium acetate (50%) mixture.

Equilibrate the column with the eluent for 1 h, then inject 20 microliters of sample solution A into the chromatography system, and allow a run time of 30 min. Calculate the proportion of each of the peaks. Compare the sample chromatogram pattern with an industry reference standard. If the retention time of each peak, and the proportion of the peak areas are consistent with the standard product, it can be verified that the sample under test is the same substance as reference standard (see Figure 3.2).

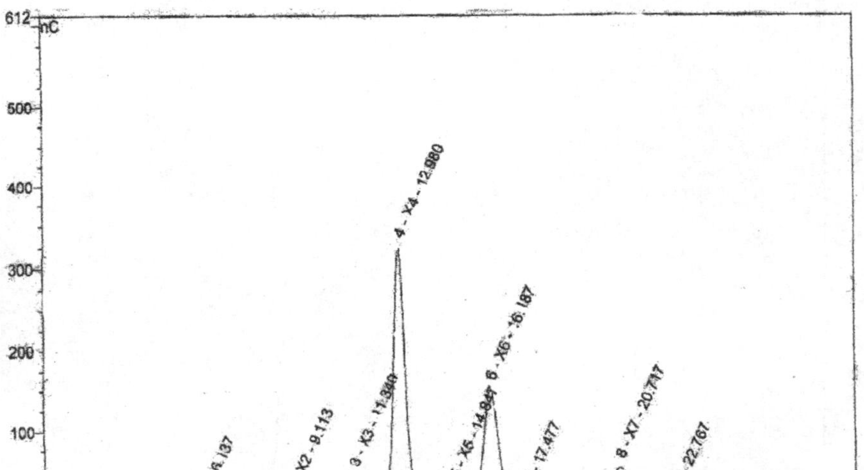

Figure 3.2: IC chromatogram of xylo-oligosaccharide.

(iii) *Quantitative test*

IC condition (quantitative test)

Column: Thermo Scientific/Dionex Carbonpack PA1 4 × 250 mm
Column temperature: 35°C
Flow rate: 1.2 ml/min
Eluent: 10 mM potassium hydroxide

Equilibrium the column with the eluent for 1 h, then inject 20 microliters of sample solution A into the chromatography system. Then calculate the pre-existing free xylose and grouse contents if existing.

Inject 20 microliters of sample solution B to IC system, calculate the total content of xylose and grouse after hydrolysis (see Figures 3.3 and 3.4).

(iv) *Results calculation*

Staring with total content of xylose and glucose that was measured after hydrolysis, subtract the content of pre-exiting xylose and glucose, and this

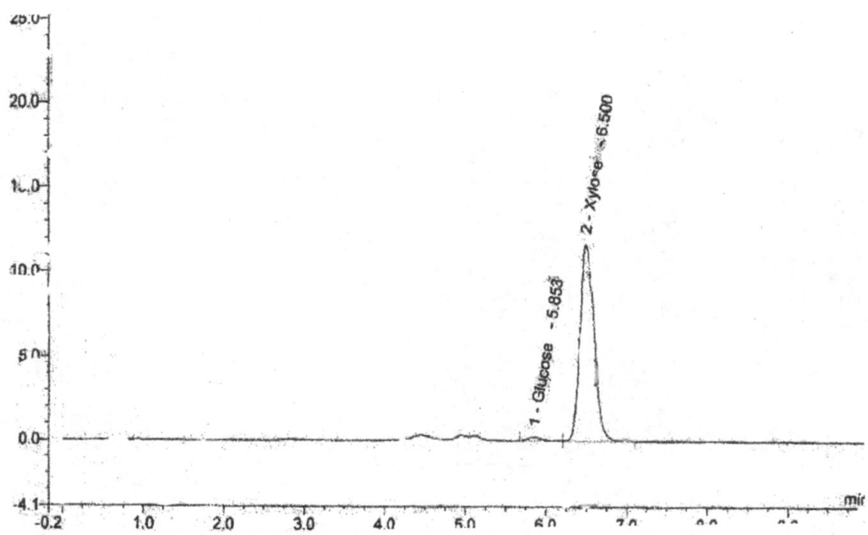

Figure 3.3: Chromatogram of total glucose and xylose of hydrolyzed xylo-oligosaccharide.

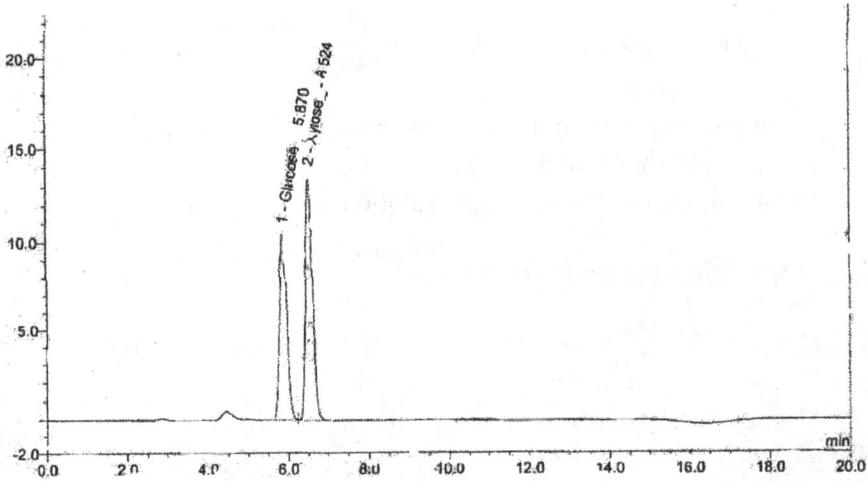

Figure 3.4: IC chromatogram of glucose and xylose standards.

is the content of glucose and xylose from xylo-oligosaccharide in the sample.

The total amount of xylose and glucose produced by hydrolysis of xylo-oligosaccharide may exceed 100%. This is because the monosaccharides produced after hydrolysis contain additional water molecules, introduced by hydrolysis. For example, disaccharides will bring in one additional water molecule, after the hydrolysis; trisaccharides will bring in two additional water molecules; tetra saccharide will produce three additional water molecules. . . . However, the absolute amount measured is unimportant. The relative quantity determined by comparing it with the industry standards is more valuable.

(v) *Quantitative calculations*

$$Pre-exiting\,glucose\% = \frac{Csam \times Vsam \times 100\%}{Wsam}, \text{ Glu B}$$

Csam = Concentration of glucose before hydrolysis (mg/ml)
Wsam = Weight of sample (mg)
Vsam = Total volume of sample solution (ml)

$$Pre-exiting\,xylose\% = \frac{Csam \times Vsam \times 100\%}{Wsam}, \text{Xyl B}$$

Csam = Concentration of xylose before hydrolysis (mg/ml)
Wsam = Weight of sample (mg)
Vsam = Total volume of sample solution (ml)

$$Total\,glucose\,after\,hydro\% = \frac{C'sam \times V'sam \times 100\%}{W'sam}, \text{Glu A}$$

C′sam = Concentration of total glucose after hydrolysis (mg/ml)
W′sam = Weight of sample (mg)
V′sam = Total volume of hydrolyzed sample solution (ml)

$$Total\,xylose\,after\,hydro\% = \frac{C'sam \times V'sam \times 100\%}{W'sam}, \text{Xyl A}$$

C′sam = Concentration of total xylose after hydrolysis (mg/ml)
W′sam = Weight of sample (mg)
V′sam = Total volume of hydrolyzed sample solution (ml)

$$Xylo-oligosaccharide\ \% = (XylA - XylB) + (Glu\,A - Glu\,B)$$

Xyl A = xylose content after hydrolysis
Xyl B = xylose content before hydrolysis
Glu A = glucose content after hydrolysis
Glu B = glucose content before hydrolysis

Compare the xylo–oligo content of sample with xylo–oligo content of reference standard to obtain a relative percentage which can be used to evaluate the quality of sample.

$$Relative\,percentage(\%) = \frac{xylo-oligo\,content\,of\,sample \times 100\%}{xylo-oligo\,content\,of\,reference\,standard}$$

Other oligosaccharide can be tested by the same principle.

3.3 Test for Polysaccharides and Related Compounds

There are many kinds of polysaccharides: chondroitin sulfate (CS) and hyaluronic acid (HA) are the most popular and important polysaccharides used in dietary supplement industry. Here, we will describe the test methods for chondroitin sulfate and HA.

3.3.1 *Chondroitin sulfate test method*

Quantitative analysis of CS in raw materials and dietary supplements has been extremely challenging owing to the wide molecular weight variation of CS polymers, its poor UV absorbance and strongly ionic nature. Other related Glycosaminoglycans (GAGs) (such as dermatan sulfate, HA, heparin, heparin sulfate and keratin sulfate) may be present as impurities or adulterants in CS materials, and thus, any analytical methodology designed to quantify CS must be selective for CS in the presence of these other GAGs and other possible interferences or even adulterants. There are several CS test methods used by the dietary supplement industry now.

Carbazole method: CS is treated with sulfuric acid and heated to hydrolyze the CS to hexuronic acid and hexosamine. Carbazole is then added that reacts with the hexuronic acid to form a colored compound that can be measured by colorimetry. Although relatively easy to use and rugged, the method is non-specific; any other compounds containing hexuronic acid moieties, such as glycosaminoglycans, will react with the carbazole to give a positive response.

Cetyl pyridnium (CPC) titration method: This method widely used by industry to test CS. CPC is a positively charged organic cation, and can attract negative anions in solution and form a precipitate. By measuring the solvent turbidity it is possible to quantify the CS in the sample. The problem with this method is CPC not only can attract CS but also any other anions in the solution to form a precipitate if the anion molecule weight is large enough. There are lots of possible anions in the sample solution, like other GAGs, proteins and even surfactants. Some adulterants materials can pass the CPC test, but they are not CS at all.

Size exclusion chromatography method: Because CS is a polymeric species, size-exclusion chromatography (SEC) can be used to separate it from small molecules often found in dietary supplements. Its lack of a chromophore; however, necessitates use of either short-wavelength UV detection (<210 nm) or refractive index detection. In addition, SEC cannot distinguish between CS and other polymers of similar size; therefore, its selectivity is not good.

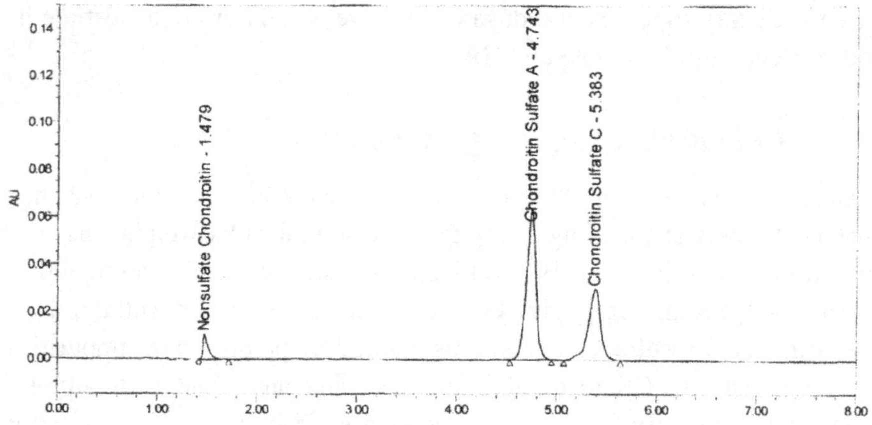

Figure 3.5: UPLC chromatogram of sample solution.

A method to quantify CS in raw materials and dietary supplements has been developed and validated. The CS is first selectively hydrolyzed by chondroitinase ACII enzyme yeld un-, mono-, di- and trisulfated unsaturated disaccharides with a conjugated double-bond feature UV absorption at 232 nm, can be monitored by UV PDA detector (see Figure 3.5). The resulting disaccharides are then quantified by ion-pairing liquid chromatography with ultraviolet detection. The amounts of the individual disaccharides are summed to yield the total amount of CS in the material.

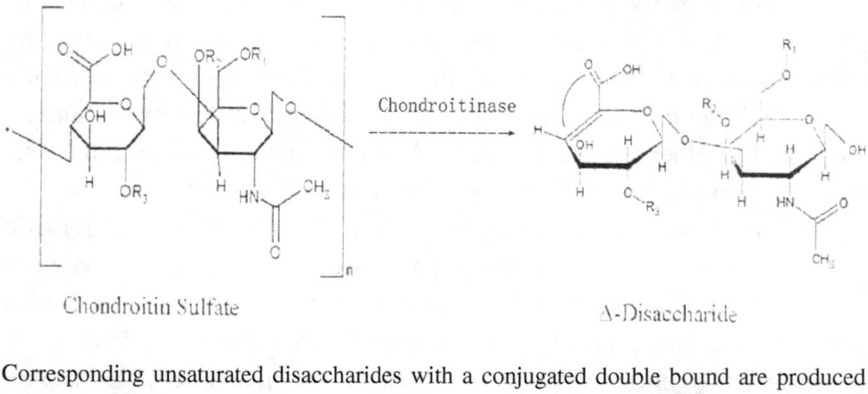

Corresponding unsaturated disaccharides with a conjugated double bound are produced after hydrolysis.

Table 3.1: Enzymatic hydrolysis of CS producing unsaturated disaccharides.

Abbreviation	**R**	**R_2**	**R_3**
ΔDi-0S	H	H	H
ΔDi-4S	H	SO_3	H
ΔDi-6S	SO_3	H	H
ΔDi-di(2,6)S	SO_3	H	SO_3
ΔDi-di(4,6)S	SO_3	SO_3	H
ΔDi-tri(2,4,6)S	SO_3	SO_3	SO_3

CS A after hydrolysis yield unsaturated disaccharide-4-sulfate, ΔDi-4S; CS C yield unsaturated disacchride-6-sulfate, ΔDi-6S; non-sulfate chondroitin yield disaccharide-0-sulfate, ΔDi-0S; CS D yield chondroitin 2,6 disulfate, ΔDi-di(2,6)S; CS E yield chondroitin 4,6 disulfate, ΔDi-di(2,6)S; chondroitin tri-sulfate yield chondroitin 2,4,6 trisulfate, ΔDi-tri(2,4,6)S (see Table 3.1).

Reagents and standard

Tris-(hydroxymethyl) aminomethane (Sigma# T-1503)
Sodium acetate, Anhydrous (Sigma# S-8750)
Acetic acid, Glacial (Sigma# A-0808)
Sodium chloride (any source of reagent grade)
Bovine serum albumin (Sigma Cat#A-4378)
Chondroitinase AC II Arthro (Seikagaku Bio Business Corporation)
Chondroitin sulfate (USP reference material)
Tetrabutylammonium hydrogen sulfate (aka TBAB)
Nanopure water

Preparation of solutions

(1) 0.13 M HCl — Carefully add 1.1 mL concentrated HCL to 99 mL water and mix well.
(2) Enriched tris buffer — Dissolve 3 g of tris (hydroxymethyl) aminomethane, 2.4 g of sodium acetate, 1.46 g of sodium chloride and 50

mg of crystalline bovine serum albumin in 100 mL of 0.13N HCl. The pH should be 8.0. Store this solution in refrigerator.

(3) Chondroitinase ACII solution — Dissolve 10 units of the enzyme in 1.0 mL of nano pure water. Store this solution in < 0°C.

(4) CS (USP) standard solution — Accurately weigh about 200 mg into a 50 mL volumetric flask and dissolve in nano pure water. Store in refrigerator.

(5) Sample solution — Accurately weigh about 500 mg of CS raw material into a 100 mL volumetric flask. If sample is not entirely chondroitin, then increase sample size according to claimed amount to be equivalent to 500 mg raw materials. Add about 60 mL nano pure water and sonicate for 15 min. Dilute to volume with nano pure water. Filter through a 0.2 μm membrane.

(6) Internal mark solution preparation — Accurately weigh about 50 mg a-Ketoglutaric acid into a 50 ml volumetric flask. Add about 10 mL water and sonicate until the standard is completely dissolved (about 2 min). Dilute to volume with water and mix well.

(7) Mobile phase A — Weigh 340 mg of tetrabutylammonium hydrogen sulfate, transfer it to a 1,000 ml volumetric flask, add 500 ml nano pure water, sonicate until all dissolved. Use phosphoric acid and potassium phosphate monobasic to adjust pH to 3.5, add nano water to 1,000 ml, shake and mix well, filter through a 0.2 μm membrane.

(8) Mobile phase B — Acetonitrile

Enzymatic hydrolysis of standards and samples

Pipette 20 μl TRIS buffer solution, 20 μl enzyme solution and 20 μl standard or sample solution into a 2 mL HPLC injection vial with a 200 μl insert, for the blank add 20 μl water instead of sample solution, mix well. Place the vial in a 37°C dry bath for 3 h. Allow it to cool to room temperature. Transfer the solution into an LC injection vial. Rinse the 200 μl insert with exactly 100 μl water twice, and quantitatively transfer this into the LC vial. Add 100 μl of internal standard solution to the standard solution only. Dilute to 1.00 mL by adding 640 μl mobile phase A to the standard

LC vial. Mix well. For sample solution, dilute to 1.00 mL by adding 740 μl mobile phase A to the LC vial. Mix well.

HPLC conditions

Column: Phenomenex Prodigy 4.6 × 250 mm 5 μm
Flow rate: 1.0 mL/min
UV Detection: 232 nm
Injection: 20 μL
Mobile phase A: 88%
Mobile phase B: 12%
Column temperature: Room temperature

UPLC conditions

Column: Waters Acquity UPLC® HSS T3 1.8 μm, 2.1 × 150 mm
Column temperature: 45°C
Flow rate: 0.45 ml/min
Injection: 2 μL
Detection: 232 nm
Mobile phase A: 85%
Mobile phase B: 15%

CS from terrestrial animals mainly contains three kinds of chondroitin sulfates: CS A, CS C and non-sulfate chondroitin, and the content of CS A is greater than CS C.

Currently, the U.S. Pharmacopeia (USP) test method is limited to CS source from terrestrial animals. In fact, marine animals also contain significant qualities of CS. An example is shark cartilage which contains a high content of CS. There are many marine CSs in the dietary supplement market. The marine CSs contain not only CS A, CS C and non-sulfate chondroitin but also CS D, CS E and trisulfate chondroitin. The content of CS C is greater than CS A.

If the peak area ratio of CS A vs. CS C in chromatogram is less than 1.5, the sample may contain the marine source CSs. In this case, it is

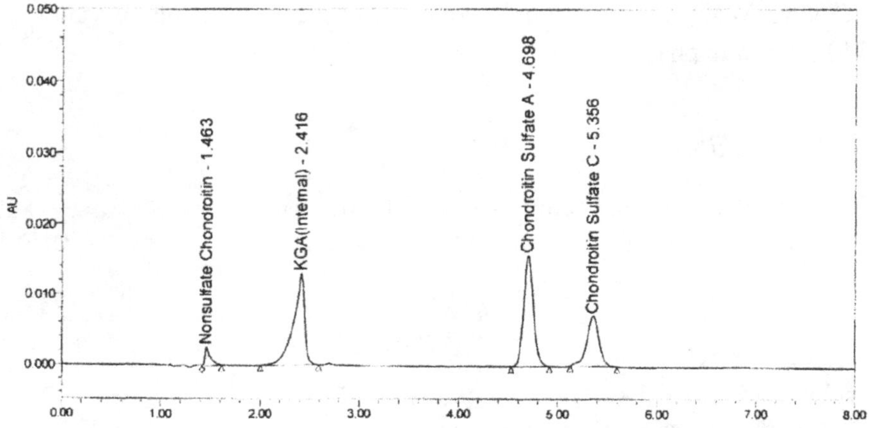

Figure 3.6: UPLC chromatogram of standard solution with internal marker. Approximate retention times: ADi-0S (1.5 min), internal standard (2.4 min), ADi-4S (4.7 min) and ADi-6S (5.4 min).

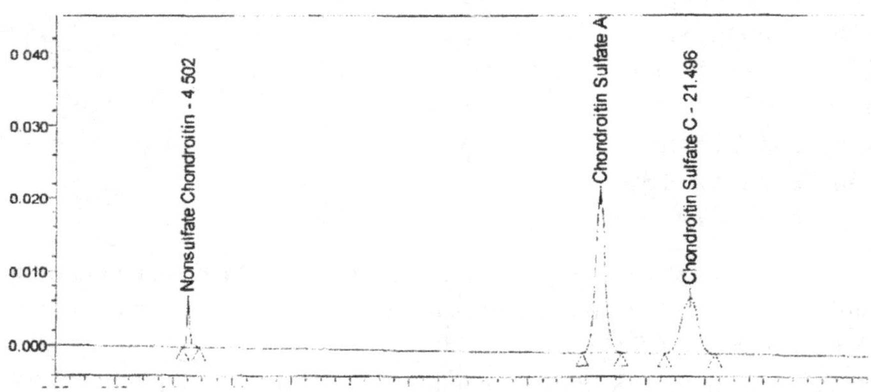

Figure 3.7: HPLC chromatogram of sample solution.

necessary to change the chromatography conditions to the following gradient program, so that the disaccharides from chondroitin sulfate E, D and tri-sulfate chondroitin can also be eluded (see Figure 3.9).

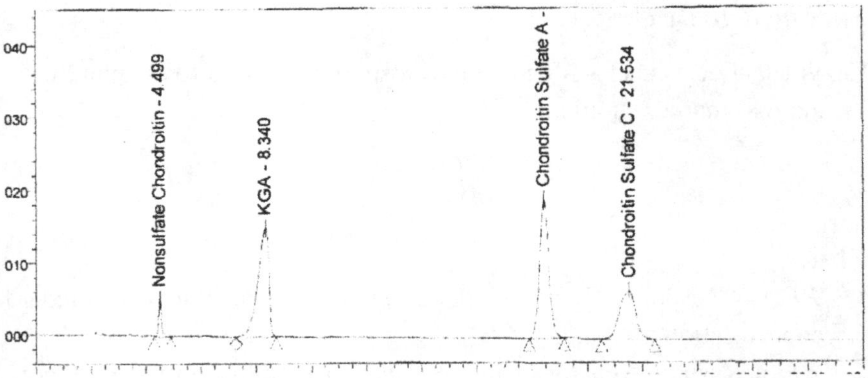

Figure 3.8: HPLC chromatogram of standard solution with internal marker.

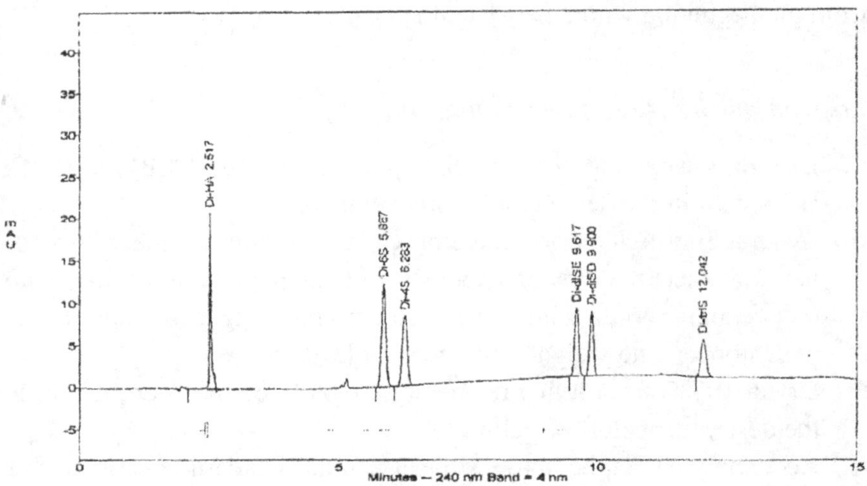

Figure 3.9: UPLC Chromatogram of marine CS.

Gradient:

Time (min)	A%	B%
0	85	15
0–7.0	60	40
7.0–11.0	60	40
11.0–11.5	85	15
11.5–15.0	85	15 End

Enzyme activity check

Enzyme activity check — The ratio of response factor of total chondroitin vs. internal marker should be:

$$\frac{RFcs}{RFi} > 1.5$$

where

$RFcs$ = Response Factor of standard CS (total peak area of standard CS/concentration of standard CS).

RFi = Response Factor of internal marker (peak area of marker/concentration of internal marker).

If enzyme activity check failed, the whole batch test need be retested from the beginning with a new batch enzyme.

Loss on drying (LOD) determination

(a) Dry glass weighing bottle with stopper (Fisher 03–420B) at 105°C. Let it cool in the desiccator before weighing.
(b) Accurately weigh a dried and empty glass weighing bottle with stopper. Then accurately weigh about 1 g of sample and/or standard into the weighing bottle with stopper. Record the weight of empty bottle with stopper, and weight with the sample.
(c) Dry at 105°C for 4 h in a temperature monitored oven. Let it cool in the desiccator before weighing.
(d) Accurately weigh the bottle, stopper and the standard or sample after dry.

Determine the water content in percentage (LOD) by the following formula:

$$LOD = \frac{(Wb - Wa) \times 100\%}{Wsam}$$

where

Wb = Total weight of bottle, stopper and sample or standard before dry.

Wa = Total weight of bottle, stopper and sample or standard after dry.
Wsam = Weight of sample or standard before dry.

Result and calculation

$$CS\ (\%) = \frac{Aa \times Cstd \times Vsam \times 100\%}{As \times Wsam \times (1 - LOD)}$$

or

$$CS(mg/unit) = \frac{Aa \times Cstd \times Vsam \times UW}{As \times Wsam \times (1 - LOD)}$$

Aa = Peak area of sample solution
As = Peak area of standard solution
Cstd = Concentration of standard solution (mg/ml)
Wsam = Weight of sample (mg)
Vsam = Total volume of sample solution (ml)
UW = Unit weight (mg/unit)
LOD = Loss on dry

3.3.2 *Hyaluronic Acid test method*

Hyaluronic Acid (HA) is one of the polysaccharides without a sulfate group.

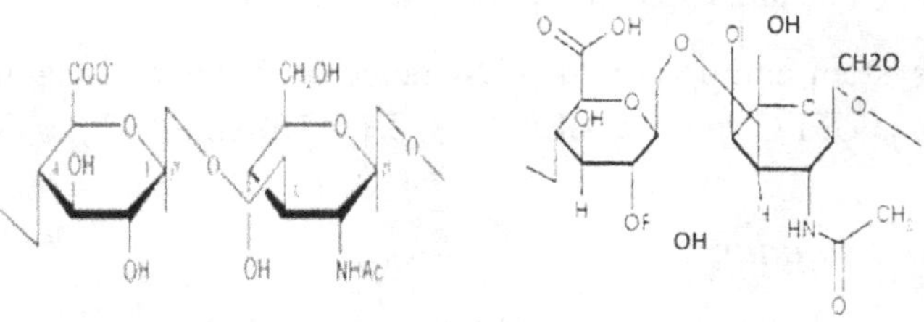

HA CS

(Glucoronic acid-N-Acetyl glucosamine) (Glucoronic acid-N-Acetyl galactose)

The molecular structure of HA is similar to non-sulfate chondroitin, except that the unit skeleton structure of CS is glucoronic acid — N-Acetyl galactose, HA is glucoronic acid — N-Acetyl glucosamine. N-Acetyl glucosamine and N-Acetyl galactose are enantiomers, and they are difficult to be separated by chromatography.

Similar to the CS test method, HA is hydrolyzed using an enzyme first, then the resulting unsaturated disaccharides are identified and quantified by liquid chromatography.

There are two kinds of enzymes that can be considered for hydrolysis of HA: one is hyaluronidase and the other one is chondroitinase ACII. The activity of hyaluronidase provided by SIGMA was not good and it could hydrolyze CS as well. Chondroitinase ACII was chosen to hydrolyze HA. Unlike CS, HA will be hydrolyzed to both unsaturated disaccharide and unsaturated tetrasaccharide. The chromatogram will show two peaks, one is disaccharide, the other one is tetrasaccharide. The sum of the peak areas of both peaks is used to calculate the result.

Apparatus and equipment

5 mL, 25 mL, 50 mL and 100 mL volumetric flasks
Weighing papers
1-spatula
Analytical balance
Disposable pipettes
3cc PTFE syringes with Luer–Lock tip
Gelman Acrodisc 0.45 μm filters
HPLC/UPLC vials and caps with puncturable septa

UPLC system equipped with PDA detector, gradient capability and reversed phase UPLC column, BEH C18, 2.1 × 150 mm, 1.7 μm (Waters).

Reagents and standard

Tris-(hydroxymethyl) aminomethane (Sigma# T-1503)
Sodium acetate, Anhydrous (Sigma# S-8750)
Acetic acid, Glacial (Sigma# A-0808)
Sodium chloride (any source of reagent grade)
Bovine serum albumin (Sigma Cat#A-4378)
HA sodium salt from rooster comb (Sigma)

Chondroitinase AC II Arthro (Seikagaku Bio Business Corporation)
Tetrabutylammonium hydrogen sulfate (aka TBAB)
Nano pure water

Solutions preparation

(1) Enriched tris buffer — Dissolve 3 g of tris (hydroxymethyl) aminomethane, 2.4 g of sodium acetate, 1.46 g of sodium chloride and 50 mg of crystalline bovine serum albumin in 100 mL of 0.13N HCl. The pH should be adjusted to 8.0 by sodium hydroxy and phosphoric acid. Store this solution in refrigerator.
(2) Chondroitinase ACII solution — Dissolve 10 unit of the enzyme in 1.0 mL of nano pure water. Store this solution in <0°C.
(3) Standard solution — Dissolve 50 mg of HA standard in 100 mL of nano pure water. Label this as working standard and store this in refrigerator.
(4) Sample solution — Accurately weigh a certain amount of ground sample or a liquid sample contains about 50 mg of HA in a 100 ml volumetric flask. Add about 60 ml nano pure water and sonicate for 15 min, cool to room temperature, dilute to volume with water, shake and mix well. Take about 5 ml of the solution and centrifuge for 5 min, take about 2 ml of the clear solution, and set aside for later use.
(5) Mobile phase A — Weigh 340 mg of tetrabutylammonium hydrogen sulfate, transfer to a 1,000 ml volumetric flask, add 500 ml nano pure water, sonicate until all dissolved. Use phosphoric acid and potassium phosphate dibasic to adjust pH to 5, add water to 1,000 ml, shake and mix well, filtrate through a 0.2 μm membrane.
Note: Base on the principle described in Chapter 1, Section 1.2.1 "The pH of the mobile phase". HA does not contain a sulfate group, it only contains a carboxylate group on the glucoronic acid side, and the pKa of glucoroic acid is about 3.2. Assuming the pKa of glucoronic acid — N-Acetyl glucosamine unit is similar. In order to make ion pair work efficiently, the mobile phase pH should be higher than 3.2 + 1 = 4.2, here it is recommended that the mobile phase pH adjusted to 5.
(6) Mobile phase B: Acetonitrile

Enzymatic hydrolysis of standard and sample

Pipette 20 μl TRIS buffer solution, 20 μl enzyme solution and 20 μl standard or sample solution, or water (as blank) into a 2 ml HPLC injection vial with a 200 μl insert separately, mix well. Place the vial in a 37°C dry bath for 3 h. Allow to cool to room temperature, carefully transfer the solution into a 2 ml HPLC injection vial. Rinse the 200 μl insert with exactly 100 μl water, twice, and quantitatively transfer the wash solutions into the HPLC vial. Add 740 ml of mobile phase A, shake, and mix well. The solution is ready for injection.

UPLC parameters

Column: Acquity UPLC® BEH C18 1.7 μm, 2.1 × 150 mm
Flow rate: 0.45 ml/min
Injection: 3 μL
Detection: 232 nm
Mobile phase A: 93% Isocratic
Mobile phase B: 7% Isocratic

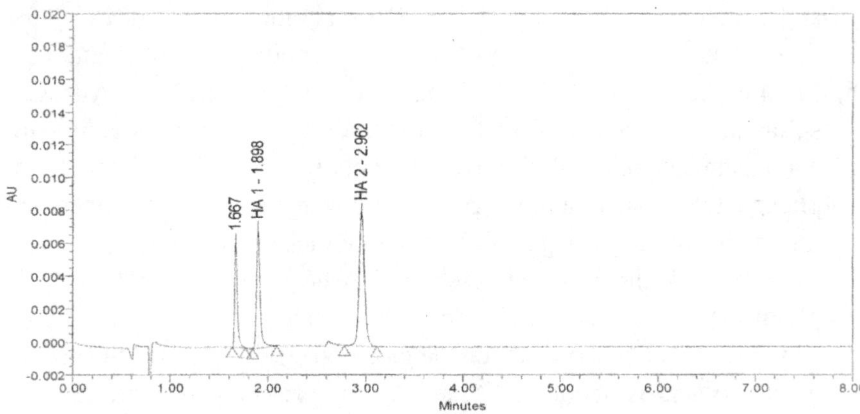

Figure 3.10: Chromatogram of disaccharide (HA1) and tetra saccharide (HA2) after hydrolysis.

Result and calculation

$$Hyaluronic\ acid\ \% = \frac{Aa \times Wstd \times Vsam \times 100\%}{As \times Wsam \times Vstd}$$

or

$$Hyaluronic\ acid\,(mg/unit) = \frac{Aa \times Wstd \times Vsam \times UW}{As \times Wsam \times Vstd}$$

where

Aa = total peak area of sample
As = total peak area of standard
Vsam = total volume of sample solution (ml)
Vstd = total volume of sample solution (ml)
Wsam = sample weight (mg)
Wstd = standard weight (mg)
UW = Unit weight (mg)

As mentioned previously, the unsaturated disaccharides from HA and from non-sulfate chondroitin are enantiomers, and cannot be separated using this chromatography system. Rarely, samples contain both HA and CS. When this is the case, then the peak ratio of HA1/HA2 will be different, the HA1 peak will become much higher. If this happens then the sample should additionally be analyzed using the CS chromatography system (see the previous section), and a CS standard should be compared to the quantify CS A and CS C found in the sample. The non-sulfate chondroitin should be about 5% of the total CS A and CS C. Subtract the estimated amount of non-sulfate chondroitin from the measured HA content to get a true HA content.

3.3.3 *Glucosamine test method*

Glucosamine is often associated with CS and methylsulpremethane (MSM) as a joint health dietary supplement. Glucosamine is a polar compound with poor UV absorbance, does not retain on the reversed phase column, is difficult to be tested using ordinary HPLC-UV methods. Testing glucosamine using IC-ED is a good option.

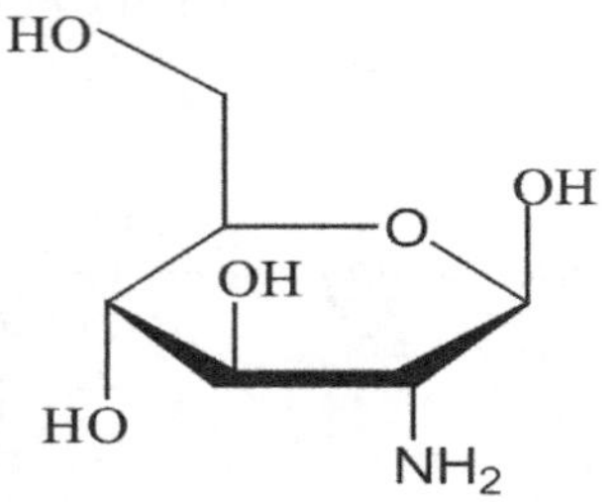

Glucosamine

The method introduced here is a pre-column derivatization method. Glucosamine contains a primary amine group that is easily reacted with isothiocyanate (PITC) to produce a phenylthiourea which can be retained on a reversed phase column and has a UV spectrum. It is an ideal compound to be quantified by HPLC or UPLC.

Apparatus and equipment

HPLC equipped with PDA, gradient capability and reversed phase HPLC column, Betasil C18 250 × 4.6 mm, 5μm (Beckman); or UPLC equipped with PDA detector, gradient capability and reversed phase UPLC column, BEH C18 2.1 × 150 mm, 1.7μm (Waters).

Reagents and solutions

HPLC grade methanol
ACS grade phosphoric acid
ACS grade potassium phosphate dibasic
PITC-No. P-4396 (Sigma, St. Louis, MO)
D-Glucosamine HCl 1294207 SIGMA (Reference Standard)

5% PITC in methanol: Transfer 2.5 mL PITC into a 50 mL volumetric flask. Dilute to volume with methanol and mix well. This solution should be freshly prepared.

pH 8.3 buffer: Weigh 5.22 g potassium phosphate dibasic and transfer into a 100 mL volumetric flask. Add 60 mL DI water and sonicate until completely dissolved. Dilute to volume with DI water. Adjust pH to 8.3 with phosphoric acid.

Mobile phase A: 0.1% phosphoric acid in DI water

Mobile phase B: 0.1% phosphoric acid in methanol for HPLC; in acetonitrile for UPLC

Test procedure

(1) Accurately weigh 50 mg of a glucosamine HCl standard, or an amount of finished product containing an equivalent amount of glucosamine HCL into a 100 mL volumetric flask.
(2) Add 60 mL nano pure water and sonicate 15 min, shake every 5 min. Cool to room temperature, dilute to volume with nano pure water and mix well. Filter this solution through filter paper.
(3) Make 1:10 dilution with nano pure water. The final concentration of glucosamine HCl in the standard or sample solution should be around 0.05 mg/ml.
(4) Pipette 1 ml of standard or sample solution, 1 mL of pH 8.3 buffer and 1 mL of 5% PITC in methanol solution into a 10 mL glass test tube separately. Cap tightly and mix well. Heat at 80°C water bath for 30 min, vortex every 5 min.
(5) Cool in a cold-water bath for 20 min and then centrifuge at 12,000 rpm for 5 min. Take the clear water layer for injection.
(6) For a blank sample, pipette 1 mL water instead of sample or standard solution in step 4.

HPLC parameters

Column: HPLC column, Betasil C18 250 × 4.6 mm, 5 μm
Flow rate: 1.0 mL/min
Injection: 20 μL
Detection: 240 nm
Column temperature: Room temperature

Gradient

Time (min)	A%	B%
0	92	8
14	80	20
16	10	90
23	10	90
23.5	92	8
30	92	8

UPLC parameters

Column: Acquity UPLC® BEH C18, 1.7 μm, 2.1 × 150 mm
Flow rate: 0.4 mL/min
Injection: 2 μL
Detection: 240 nm
Column temperature: 45°C

Gradient

Time (min)	A%	B%
0	95	5
6	85	15
7.8	50	50
8.3	50	50
8.6	95	5
10	95	5

Glucosamine has α and β forms, after derivatization they could be separated by HPLC or UPLC. Chromatograms should show α and β as two peaks, however the α and β structures will eventually reach a dynamic balance, so it does not matter which peak is chosen to use in the calculation. The results are same as long as you select the corresponding peaks from both sample and standard chromatograms. Also, the sum of the two peaks can be used to calculate the result.

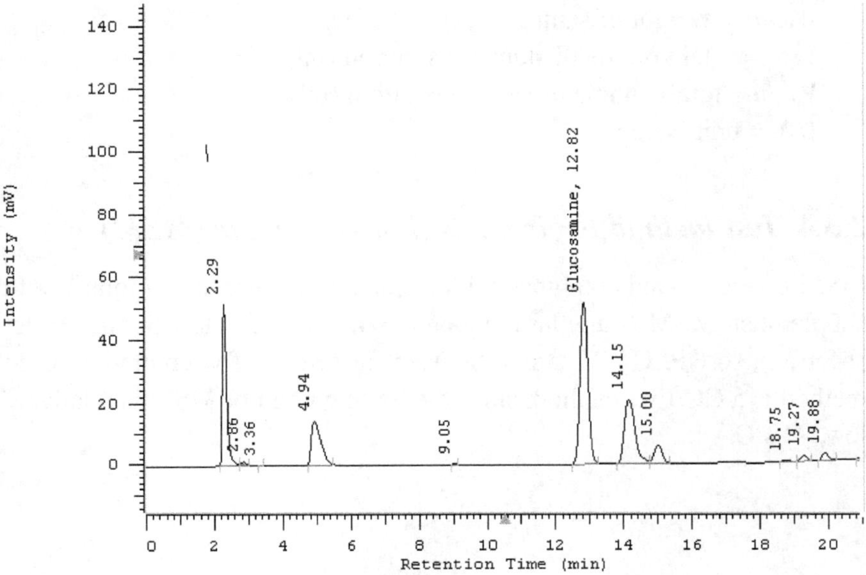

Figure 3.11: HPLC chromatogram of glucosamine after derivatization.

Result and calculation

A blank solution should be injected either after or before the standard solution injection, next compare the chromatograms of standard and blank, find the glucosamine peaks, then calculate the result.

$$Glucosamine\ \% = \frac{Aa \times Wstd \times Vsam \times 100\%}{As \times Wsam \times Vstd}$$

or

$$Glucosamine(mg / unit) = \frac{Aa \times Wstd \times Vsam \times UW}{As \times Wsam \times Vstd}$$

where

Aa = Peak area of sample
As = Peak area of standard
Wstd = Weight of standard (mg)

Wsam = Weight of sample (mg)
Vstd = total volume of standard solution (ml)
Vsam = total volume of sample solution (ml)
UW = unit weight

3.3.4 *Test method for methylsulfonylmethane (MSM)*

MSM is often found combined with CS and glucosamine in a joint health supplement. MSM is a polar compound with no characteristic ultraviolet spectrum, so HPLC-UV cannot be used for testing. The commonly used method is a GC/FID method, since the boiling point of MSM is relatively low, 248°C.

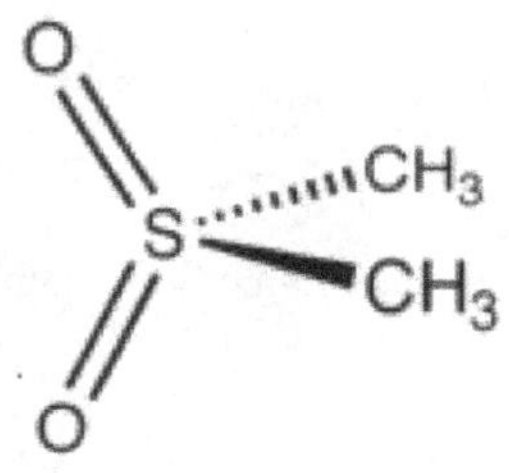

Methylsulfonylmethane

Apparatus and equipment

25 mL and 100 mL volumetric flasks
Weighing papers
Spatula
Analytical balance
Pipettes

GC system with programmable temperature control with Restek Stabil Wax, 30 m × 0.25 mm id, 0.25μm column

Reagent and standard

Methylsulfonylmethane, Acros, Cat# 12778-0050
Nonanoic acid methyl ester, Sigma, Cat# N-5627

Methanol, HPLC Grade
Nano pure water

Test procedure

Internal standard solution — Accurately weigh about 20 mg of nonanoic acid methyl ester into a 100 mL volumetric flask. Add methanol to dissolve and fill to mark, shake and mix well.

Standard preparation — Dissolve about 20 mg MSM standard into 25 mL of the aforementioned internal standard solution quantitatively.

Sample preparation — Accurately weigh a certain amount of ground sample, containing about 20 mg MSM, and transfer to the 50 mL volumetric flasks. Quantitatively pipette 25 mL internal standard solution into the 50 mL volumetric flask, sonicate 15 min with frequent shake. Centrifuge (12,000 rpm) for 5 min, take the top clear solution for injection.

GC condition

Initial temperature: 100°C
Temperature ramp rate = 8°C/min, 20 min to 260°C
Hold time = 5 min
Injector temperature: 250°C
Detector temperature: 250°C
Capillary Column: Restek Stabil Wax, 30 m × 0.25 mm id, 0.25μm
Injection Volume: 2μL
Carry gas: Nitrogen (1 ml/min)

System suitability

Make five injections of the standard solution; the area ratio of MSM/internal standard for the five injections the RSD% should be <3%.

Result and calculation

$$MSM\% = \frac{Cs \times PARu \times Vu \times 100\%}{PARs \times Wu}$$

or

$$MSM(mg/unit) = \frac{Cs \times PARu \times Vu \times UW(mg/unit)}{PARs \times Wu}$$

Cs = Concentration of standard solution (mg/ml)
$PARu$ = The peak rea ratio of MSM/internal standard, in sample solution
$PARs$ = The peak area ratio of MSM/internal standard, in standard solution
Vu = total volume of sample solution (ml)
Wu = sample weigh (mg)
UW = Unit weight (mg/unit)

Chapter 4
Test Methods for Botanicals and Botanical Extracts

In dietary supplements, plant or herbal raw materials can be a dry powder or powdered extracts. Dry powder is the effective part of the original plant after drying, grinding it to a powder and directly using this material as raw materials, or dietary ingredients. Extract powders are the specific plant parts extracted with a specific solvent. The resulting liquid is sprayed on the carrier powder, and dried into a free-flowing powder.

The treatment of these two raw materials is different. The raw plant powder should be extracted by an appropriate solvent into which the active compounds can be dissolved and extracted with refluxing or sonication. With powdered extracts the extraction procedure can be eliminated, and by using a proper solvent, the active compounds can be dissolved efficiently and completely.

Sometimes the carrier material of the extract powder is a ground powder of the original plant. In this case, the raw material should be re-extracted, because the active compounds in the carrier material should not be ignored.

Testing of natural plants or extracts is complex. At present, the most common approach is to quantitatively test the active ingredients or marker compounds in plants. However, the active compounds exist in other plants, or even be synthetic compounds are used in the adulteration of products. Therefore, it is important to verify the original species of the active compounds that are being tested. There are several ways to verify the original species.

(1) Compare chromatographic fingerprints of the sample and standard of the original plant and the UV spectra of major peaks. If the standard chromatogram and UV spectrum of the sample are not confirmed with original plant, then this product may be a problem product. Of course, when dietary supplement samples contain a variety of ingredients, the chromatogram is more complex, so it is better to compare sample chromatograms with a chromatogram that comes from a verified dietary supplement ingredient, in a product matrix.
(2) Compare the proportion of active or marker compounds. The proportion of active compounds may vary with the species of natural products. For example, *ginkgo biloba* contains three groups of flavonol glycosides. After hydrolysis they are mainly converted to quercetin, kaempferol, isorhamnetin three flanonols. The proportion of the three flanonols in natural *ginkgo biloba* should be within a certain range, if the sample is beyond the range, it could be an adulterated product.
(3) Hydrolyze samples and reference standard to convert the many glycosides to fewer aglycones or convert the multiple esters to few carboxylic acids and alcohols, thus making the chromatograms much simpler. Then compare the new peaks created after hydrolysis and their proportions. Also, you can compare the peaks lost or reduced after hydrolysis.
Note: The chromatograms of plant powders and extract powders may be different, so when making comparisons, be sure plant powders from a sample is compared to a standard plant powder. Also, plant extract powders in samples must be compared to standard plant extracts, and same solvent must be used to treat samples and standards.

4.1 Test Method for Isoflavones in Soybean (Kudzu, Red Clover)

Soybean isoflavones are flavonoids, and soybeans contain a significant quantity of soy isoflavones. People who eat soy products regularly have the potential for delaying the occurrence of arteriosclerosis, reducing total blood cholesterol concentration, and reducing the incidence of heart disease. In addition, soy isoflavones also have an estrogenic effect, and may prevent osteoporosis without the side effects of estrogen use.

Soybean isoflavones are mainly, genistein, genistin, acetyl genistin, malonyl genistin, daidzein, daidzin, acetyl daidzin, malonyl daidzin, glyctein, glyctin, acetyl glyctin, malonyl glyctin.

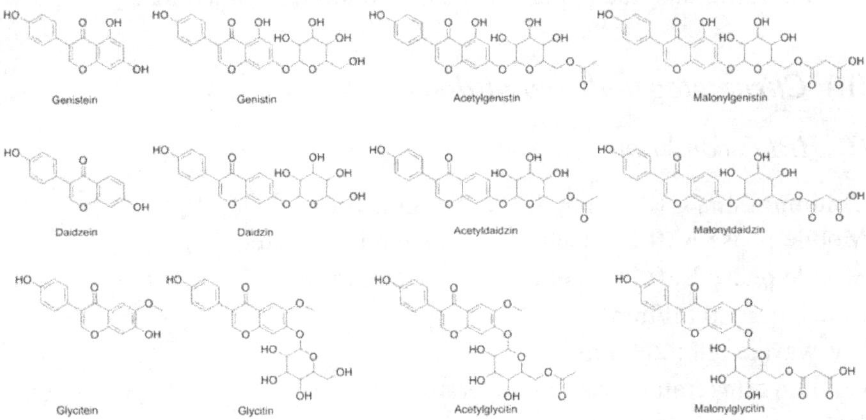

From the aforementioned molecular structure, it can be seen that these molecules are basically weak non-polar compounds, so reversed phase chromatography can be used to perform the testing. With a reverse phase column, the most polar glycosides (daidzin, glyctin and genistin) should be the first peaks of the corresponding groups to elute; the least polar aglycones (daidzein, glycitein and genistein) should be the last peaks of each corresponding group of compounds.

(i) *Test procedure*

Preparation of standard solution — Accurately weight about 10 mg of each six isoflavone standards: daidzein, daidzin, genistein, genistin, gly-citein, glycitin (the acetyl- and malonyl-derivatives will be calculated as daidzin, genistin, glycitin with molecular weight correction). Transfer these to a 100 ml volumetric flask, add 20 ml water, shake 10 min, add 40 ml ethanol, sonicate for 10 min, and cool to room temperature. After cooling, fill with methanol to 100 ml, shake and mix well. This solution is ready to injection.

Preparation of sample solution — Take a certain amount of ground sample containing about 10 mg of any soy isoflavones, transfer to a 100 ml volumetric flask, add 20 ml water, soak for 10 min with shaking, add 40 ml of ethanol, and sonicate for 10 min. Cool to room temperature, fill with methanol to 100 ml, shake and mix well. Centrifuge for 5 min (10,000 rpm), take the upper layer clear solution for injection.

(ii) *Chromatography conditions*

(i) *HPLC condition*

Column: Luna C18, 5 um, 4.6 × 250 mm, 100A
Mobile phase A: 0.1% acetic acid in nano pure water
Mobile phase B: 0.1% acetic acid in acetonitrile
Flow rate: 1.0 ml/min
UV wavelength: 260 nm
Column temperature: room temperature
Injection volume: 20 ul

Gradient:

Time (min)	A%	B%
0	85	15
0–50	65	35
50–60	65	35
60.0–60.5	85	15
70	85	15 End

UPLC conditions

Column: Acquity BEH Phenyl 1.7 um 2.1 × 150 mm
Mobile phase A: 0.1% acetic acid in nano pure water
Mobile phase B: 0.1% acetic acid in acetonitrile
Flow rate: 0.40 ml/min
Column temperature: 45°C
UV wavelength: 260 nm
Injection volume: 2 ul

Gradient:

Time (min)	A%	B%
0	90	10
0–7.0	68	32
7.0–8.5	68	32
8.5–9	50	50
9.0–9.8	50	50
9.8–10.0	90	10
12.0	90	10

Pueraria Lobata also contains soy isoflavones, unlike soybeans, which also contains puerarin, and can be as much as 50% of the total isoflavones. Puerarin can be tested using the same method as soy isoflavones, if the puerarin standard is added to the standard solution. The puerarin peak eluted after glycitin and before genistin.

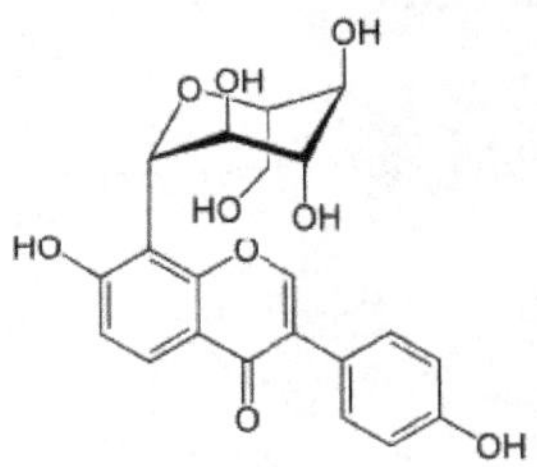

Puerarin

Red clover also contains soy isoflavones, and two other isoflavones, biochanin A and formonetin. By adding these two standards to the soy isoflavones standard solution, the red clover can be tested by the soybean testing procedure. From the molecular structures below, biochanin A and formonetin molecules contain less hydroxy groups than other soy isoflavones, so peak retention times are longer than other soybean isoflavones.

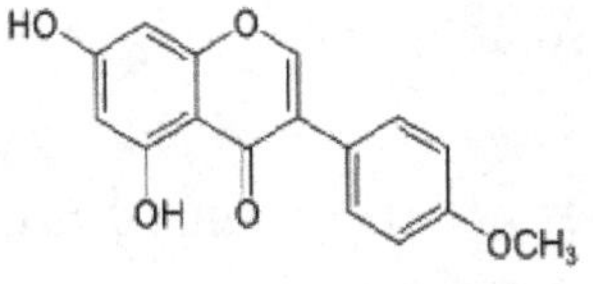

Biochanin A

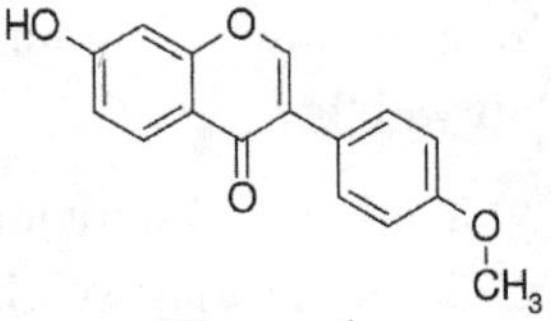

Formonetin

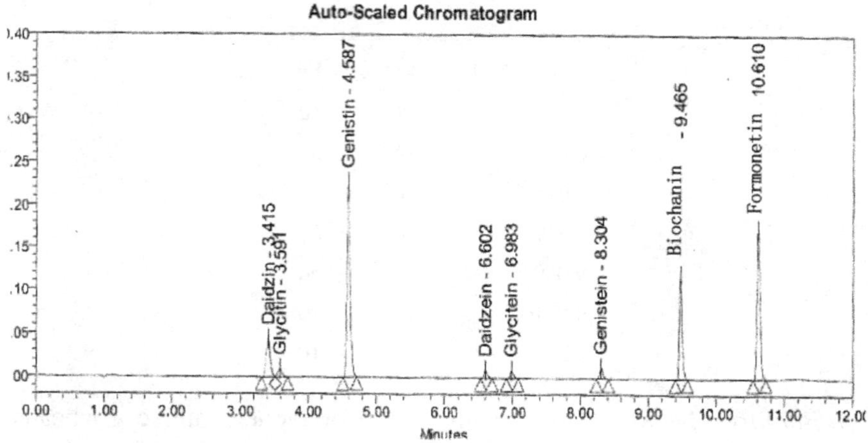

Figure 4.1: UPLC Chromatogram of soy isoflavones.

(iii) *Results and calculation*

$$Individual\ isoflavone\ (\%) = \frac{Aa \times Cs \times Vsam \times 100\%}{As \times Wsam}$$

or

$$Individual\ isoflavone\ (mg/unit) = \frac{Aa \times Cs \times Vsam \times UW}{As \times Wsam}$$

Here
Aa = Peak area of corresponding flavone in sample solution
As = Peak area of corresponding flavone in standard solution
Cs = Concentration of corresponding standard
Wstd = Weight of corresponding standard (mg)
Wsam = Weight of sample (mg)
Vsam = Total volume of sample solution (ml)
UW = Unit weight

The acetyl and malonyl derivatives will be calculated as daidzin, genistin, glycitin with molecular weight correction.

MW:	Daidzein	254.24
	Genistein	270.24
	Glycitein	284.24
	Daidzin	433.4
	Genistin	449.4
	Glycitin	463.4
	Acetyl-Daidzin	476.4
	Acetyl-Genistin	492.4
	Acetyl-Glycitin	506.4
	Malonyl-Daidzin	520.4
	Malonyl-Genistin	536.4
	Malonyl-Glycitin	550.4

Reversed phase column soy isoflavones elute order:

daidzin
glyctein
genistin
malonyl daidzin
malonyl glyctin
acetyl daidzin
malonyl genistin
acetyl glyctin
acetyl genistin
daidzein
glyctein
genistein

4.2 Aflatoxins Determination Using LC/MS/MS

Aflatoxin is a strong carcinogen found in grains and legumes. US FDA guideline has set 20 ppb maximum level for total aflatoxins B1, B2, G1 and G2. It is a major challenge for analytical chemists. But the modern LC/MS/MS instrument can help to meet the guideline.

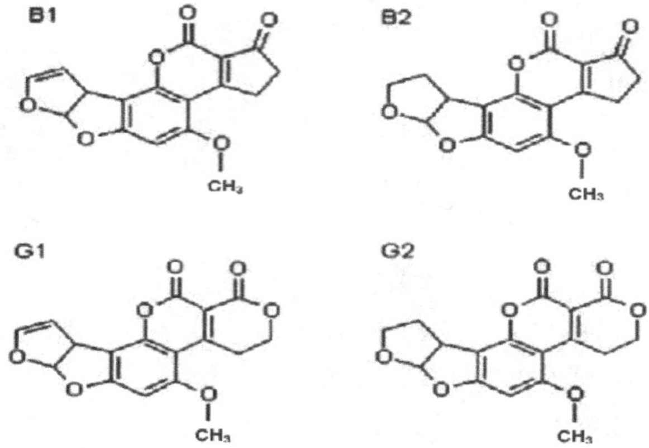

From the aforementioned molecular structure, it can be seen that B1 has one additional double bond than B2, as does G1and G2. G1 and G2 have one more oxygen atom than the corresponding B1 and B2. So, these four molecules can be separated by reversed phase C18 column with the elution order of B1, B2, G1 and G2.

(i) ***Test procedure***

Standard solution preparation — Accurately transfer 500 mg of an aflatoxin standard solution (Sigma-P9441) to 100 ml volumetric flask, add about 60 ml of methanol, shake well and then add methanol to 100 ml. Label as "Aflatoxin stock standard solution".

Transfer 50 μL stock standard solution to 50 ml volumetric flask, add methanol to the mark, shake well, label as "High concentration standard solution" (used for instrument calibration and quantify high concentration samples). Dilute the high concentration standard solution 10 times with methanol, obtain a low concentration standard solution, label as "Low concentration standard solution" (used for quantifying the lower concentration samples).

Concentration of the standard solutions:

	High conc.	Low conc.
Aflatoxin B1	50 ppb	5 ppb
Aflatoxin B2	15 ppb	1.5 ppb
Aflatoxin G1	50 ppb	5 ppb
Aflatoxin G2	15 ppb	1.5 ppb

Sample solution preparation — Weigh 2 g of ground samples into a 50 ml of volumetric flask, add 30 ml methanol, vortex for 2 min, and sonicate for 20 min. Cool to room temperature, add methanol to the mark, shake well, centrifuge for 10 min (10,000 r/min). Transfer 1 ml of clear solution to an injection vail as sample solution; transfer 900 μl to another vail and spike 100 μl of high contraction standard solution as spiked sample solution, shake well.

(ii) *UPLC conditions*

Column: Acquity UPLC® HSS C18, 1.8μm, 2.1 × 150 mm
Flow rate: 0.40 ml/min
Mobile phase A: 0.01% acetic acid in nano pure water
Mobile phase B: 0.01% acetic acid in acetonitrile
Injection volume: 1.0 μl
Column temperature: 45°C

Gradient:

Time (min)	A%	B%
0	70	30
0–4.0	40	60
4.0–4.5	40	60
4.5–4.8	70	30
7.0	70	30

MS/MS parameters (from Waters TQS)

Model	MRM
Polarity	ES+
Inter Channel Delay(sec)	–1.000
InterScan Time (sec)	–1.000
Span (Da)	0.0
Start Time (min)	1.0
End Time (min)	6.0

Aflatoxin B1:

C	Prnt (Da)	Dau (Da)	Dwell (s)	Cone (V)	Coll (eV)	Delay (s)
1	312.65	213.18	0.020	46.00	58.00	−1.000
2	312.65	241.02	0.020	46.00	52.00	−1.000
3	312.65	284.71	0.020	46.00	32.00	−1.000

Aflatoxin B2:

C	Prnt (Da)	Dau (Da)	Dwell (s)	Cone (V)	Coll (eV)	Delay (s)
1	314.46	242.90	0.020	48.00	56.00	−1.000
2	314.46	258.96	0.020	48.00	44.00	−1.000
3	314.46	286.91	0.020	48.00	38.00	−1.000

Aflatoxin G1:

Ch	Prnt (Da)	Dau (Da)	Dwell (s)	Cone (V)	Coll (eV)	Delay (s)
1	328.58	199.75	0.020	42.00	56.00	−1.000
2	328.58	214.57	0.020	42.00	42.00	−1.000
3	328.58	242.91	0.020	42.00	38.00	−1.000

Aflatoxin G2:

Ch	Prnt (Da)	Dau (Da)	Dwell (s)	Cone (V)	Coll (eV)	Delay (s)
1	330.52	216.84	0.020	46.00	50.00	−1.000
2	330.52	244.92	0.020	46.00	34.00	−1.000

Aflatoxin G2 only can find two ion pair.

(iii) *Results and calculation*

Refer to Chapter 1, Section 1.1.5 “Qualitative and quantitative testing of LC-MS/MS”.

4.3 Ginsenosides Test Method

4.3.1 *Ginsenosides Test Method by HPLC*

Current research indicates that polysaccharides may be the active components in ginseng. But traditionally ginsenosides are used to identify and quantify ginseng and ginseng products. At least 150 different ginsenosides have been found, but at present, the industry mainly tests the following seven ginsenosides:

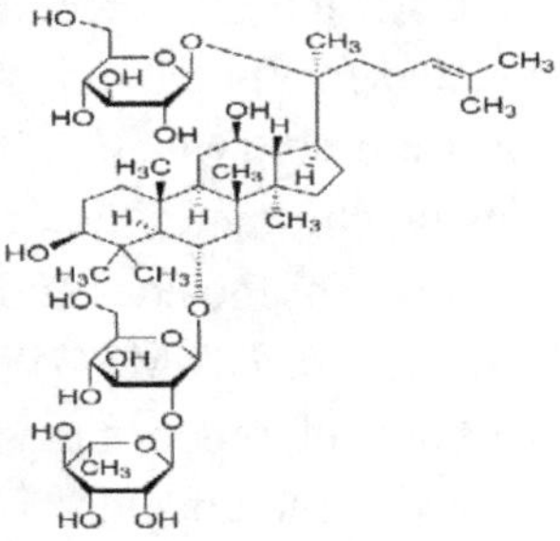

Genosenoside Re

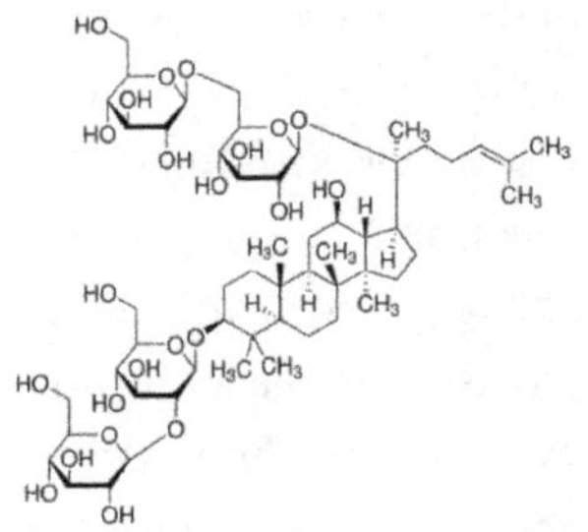

Ginsenoside Rb1

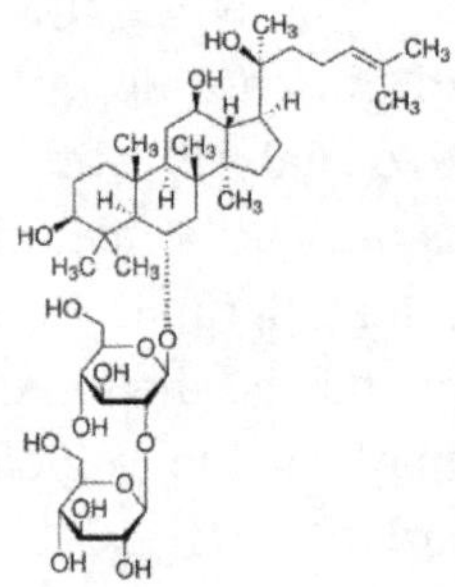

Gensenoside Rf

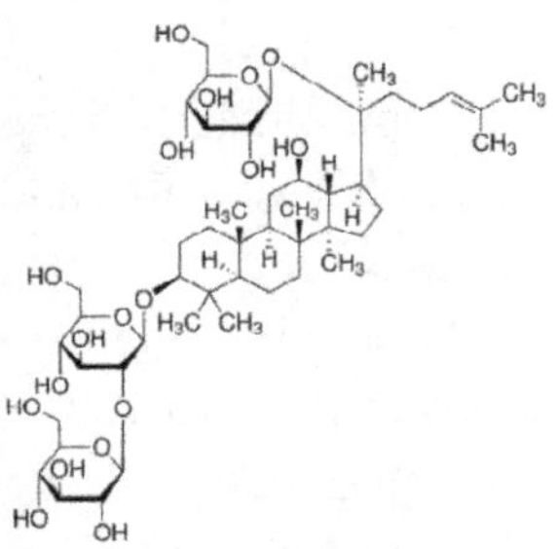

Ginsenoside Rd

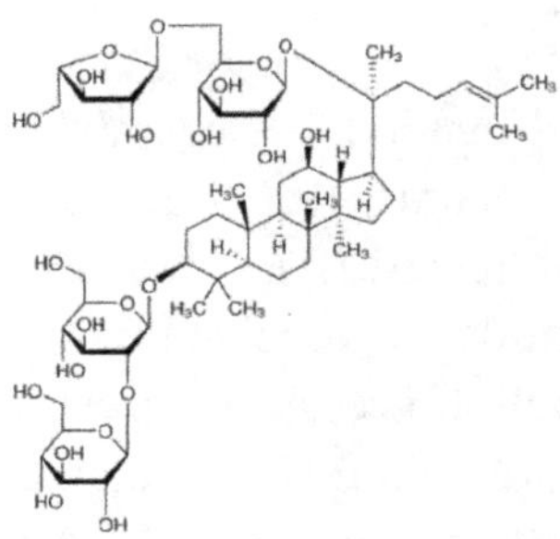

Ginsenoside Rc

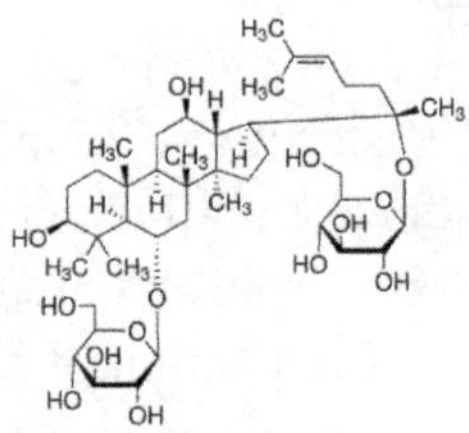

Gensenoside Rg1

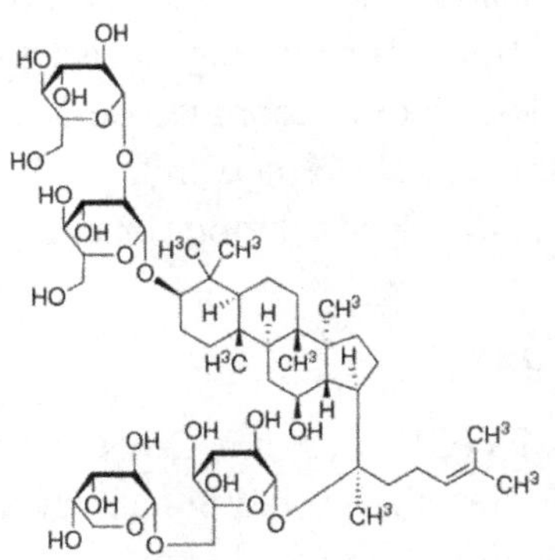

Ginsenoside Rb2

The main test methods are HPLC and GC. The HPLC method is a direct injection method. The GC method using a trimethyl silane reaction with hydroxy groups of ginsenosides to reduce the boiling point, and then uses GC to separate and quantify the ginsenosides.

Neither GC nor HPLC methods can test all of the ginsenosides, because not all reference standards are available. Current quality control tests generally measure only test 6–7 ginsenosides.

The HPLC-UV method is the most widely used. All the UV spectra of ginsenosides are similar. Usually, 205 nm is selected for the quantitative analysis. Since most of the ginsenoside standards are not available, it is difficult to identify each individual ginsenoside using chromatographic retention times. Some peaks may have several co-eluting ginsenosides and cannot be distinguished due to the common UV spectrum. LC-MS/MS may be able to identify some ginsenosides even without reference standards. The UPLC-UV method introduced here may need some updates.

(i) *Test procedure*

Preparation of standard solution — Accurately weigh approximately 5 mg of each ginsenoside standards, Rg1, Re, Rf, Rb1, Rb2, Rd, and Rc, and transfer it to a 25 ml volumetric flask. Add 15 ml methanol/water (70/30), sonicate until all standards are dissolved. Dilute to volume with same solvent, shake and mix well. If necessary, further dilutions can be made.

Preparation of sample solution — Weigh a certain amount of ginseng or ginseng extract samples which contain about 20 mg of ginsenosides, transfer it to 50 ml of volumetric flask, and add 30 ml of methanol/water (70/30). Sonicate for 10 min for ginseng extract samples, or 40 min for ginseng powder samples. Cool to room temperature, fill to volume with the aforementioned solvent, shake and mix well. Centrifuge for 5 min (10,000 r/min) and take the clear solution for injection.

(ii) *UPLC conditions*

Column: Acquity Hss T3 (C18), 1.8 um, 2.1 × 150 mm
Mobile phase A: 0.1% phosphoric acid in nano pure water
Mobile phase B: 0.1% phosphoric acid in acetonitrile
Flow rate: 0.4 ml/min
Injection volume: 2 ul
UV wavelength: 205 nm
Run time: 12 min
Column temperature: 45°C

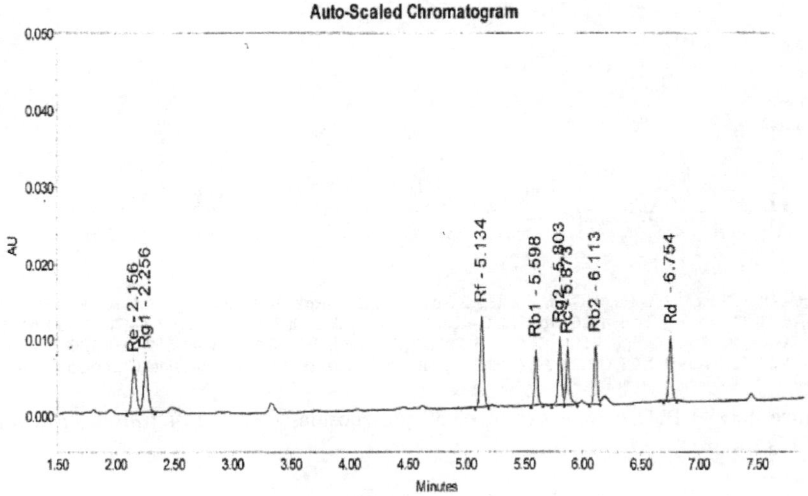

Figure 4.2: UPLC chromatogram of ginsenosides.

Gradient

Time (min)	A%	B%
0–2.0	72	28
2.0–7.0	50	50
7.0–7.5	50	50
7.5–8.0	30	70
8.0–8.5	30	70
8.5–9.0	72	28
12.0	72	28

The following UPLC method is from Hee-Won Park and others published in *Journal of Ginseng Research*, 2013, 37(4), 457–467.

Column: Waters ACQUITY BEH C8, 2.1 mm × 100 mm, 1.7 um
Column temperature: 40°C
Flow rate: 0.6 ml/min
Mobile phase A: 0.001% phosphoric acid in water
Mobile phase B: 0.001% phosphoric acid in acetonitrile

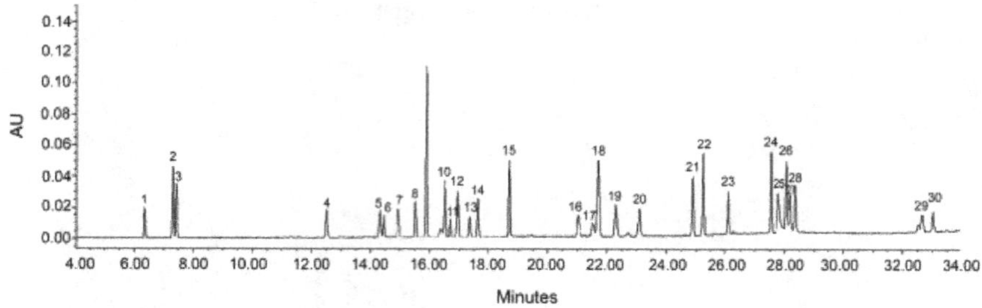

NG-R1, 1; G-Rg1, 2; G-Re, 3; G-Rf, 4; 20(S)-G-Rh1, 5; 20(S)-G-Rg2, 6; 20(R)-G-Rg2, 7; G-Ro, 8; G-Rb1, 9; G-Rc, 10; G-Ra1, 11; G-F1, 12; G-Rb2, 13; G-Rb3, 14; G-Rd, 15; G-Rg6, 16; G-Rk3, 17; G-F4, 18; G-Rh4, 19; G-F2, 20; 20(S)-G-Rg3, 21; 20(R)-G-Rg3, 22; C-Y, 23; C-K, 24; G-Rk1, 25; G-Rg5, 26; 20(S)-G-Rh2, 27; 20(R)-G-Rh2, 28; G-Rk2, 29; G-Rh3, 30. NG, notoginsenoside; G, ginsenoside; C, compound.

Figure 4.3: UPLC chromatogram of 30 ginsenosides (*Journal of Ginseng Research*, 2013, 37(4), 457–467).

Gradient:

Time (min)	A%	B%
0–0.5	85	15
14.5	70	30
15.5	68	32
18.5	62	38
24.0	57	43
27.0	45	55
31.0	45	55
35.0	30	70
38.0	10	90
38.1	85	15
43.0	85	15

(iii) *Results and calculation*

$$Ginsenoside\,(\%) = \frac{Aa \times Cs \times Vsam \times 100\%}{As \times Wsam}$$

or

$$Ginsenoside\ (mg/unit) = \frac{Aa \times Cs \times Vsam \times UW}{As \times Wsam}$$

Here
Aa = Peak area of corresponding ginsenoside in sample solution
As = Peak area of corresponding ginsenoside in standard solution
Cs = Concentration of corresponding standard
Wsam = Weight of sample (mg)
Vsam = Total volume of sample solution (ml)
UW = *Unit weight*

Total ginsenosides = Sum of each measured individual ginsenoside.

Ginsenosides UV sensitivity is low, and can easily be interfered at 205 nm. It is difficult to test samples containing low levels ginsenosides and with a complex sample matrix. At this point, using LC-MS/MS method can be considered.

4.3.2 *LC-MS/MS method*

Standard and sample solution preparation is the same as LC-UV method. Adjust the final concentration of each ginsenoside to approximately 20 ppb.

UPLC condition

Column: Acquity Hss T3 (C18), 1.8 um, 2.1 × 150 mm
Mobile phase A: 0.1% formic acid in nano pure water
Mobile phase B: 0.1% formic acid in acetonitrile
Flow rate: 0.4 ml/min
Injection volume: 2 ul
Column temperature: 45°C

Gradient:

Time (min)	A%	B%
0	72	28
0–2.0	71	29
2.0–9.0	54	46
9.0–9.2	30	70
9.2–9.8	30	70
9.8–10.0	72	28
12.0	72	28

MS/MS parameters (from Waters TQS)

Function 1: MRM of 3 mass pairs, time 6.2–7.2 ES-(Ginsenoside Rg2)

Model	MRM
Polarity	ES-
Inter Channel Delay (sec)	–1.000
InterScan Time (sec)	–1.000
Span (Da)	0.0
Start Time (min)	6.2
End Time (min)	7.2

Ginsenoside Rg2

Ch	Prnt (Da)	Dau (Da)	Dwell (s)	Cone (V)	Coll (eV)	Delay (s)
1	783.34	100.92	0.025	100.00	34.00	–1.000
2	783.34	475.23	0.025	100.00	36.00	–1.000
3	783.34	637.30	0.025	100.00	26.00	–1.000

Function 2: MRM of 3 mass pairs, time 1.5–2.5 ES-(Ginsenoside Rg1)

Model	MRM
Polarity	ES-
Inter Channel Delay (sec)	–1.000
InterScan Time (sec)	–1.000
Span (Da)	0.0
Start Time (min)	1.5
End Time (min)	2.5

Ginsenoside Rg1

Ch	Prnt (Da)	Dau (Da)	Dwell (s)	Cone (V)	Coll (eV)	Delay (s)
1	799.34	100.92	0.05	98.00	32.00	–1.000
2	799.34	475.24	0.05	98.00	32.00	–1.000
3	799.34	637.31	0.05	98.00	20.00	–1.000

Function 3: MRM of 3 mass pairs, time 4.5–6.1 ES-(Ginsenoside Rf)

Model	MRM
Polarity	ES-
Inter Channel Delay (sec)	–1.000
InterScan Time (sec)	–1.000
Span (Da)	0.0
Start Time (min)	4.5
End Time (min)	6.1

Ginsenoside Rf

Ch	Prnt (Da)	Dau (Da)	Dwell (s)	Cone (V)	Coll (eV)	Delay (s)
1	799.34	100.92	0.05	88.00	36.00	–1.000
2	799.34	475.24	0.05	88.00	38.00	–1.000
3	799.34	637.31	0.05	88.00	26.00	–1.000

Function 4: MRM of 3 mass pairs, time 8.0–9.5 ES-(Ginsenoside Rd)

Model	MRM
Polarity	ES-
Inter Channel Delay (sec)	–1.000
InterScan Time (sec)	–1.000
Span (Da)	0.0
Start Time (min)	8.0
End Time (min)	9.5

Ginsenoside Rd

Ch	Prnt (Da)	Dau (Da)	Dwell (s)	Cone (V)	Coll (eV)	Delay (s)
1	945.38	88.94	0.05	100.00	44.00	–1.000
2	945.38	100.98	0.05	100.00	46.00	–1.000
3	945.38	783.28	0.05	100.00	36.00	–1.000

Function 5: MRM of 3 mass pairs, time 1.5–3.0 ES-(Ginsenoside Re)

Model	**MRM**
Polarity	ES-
Inter Channel Delay (sec)	–1.000
InterScan Time (sec)	–1.000
Span (Da)	0.0
Start Time (min)	1.5
End Time (min)	3.0

Ginsenoside Re

Ch	**Prnt (Da)**	**Dau (Da)**	**Dwell (s)**	**Cone (V)**	**Coll (eV)**	**Delay (s)**
1	945.38	100.38	0.05	100.00	42.00	–1.000
2	945.38	475.23	0.05	100.00	40.00	–1.000
3	945.38	637.29	0.05	100.00	32.00	–1.000

Function 6: MRM of 3 mass pairs, time 6.3–7.8 ES-(Ginsenoside Rc)

Model	**MRM**
Polarity	ES-
Inter Channel Delay (sec)	–1.000
InterScan Time (sec)	–1.000
Span (Da)	0.0
Start Time (min)	6.3
End Time (min)	7.8

Ginsenoside Rc

Ch	**Prnt (Da)**	**Dau (Da)**	**Dwell (s)**	**Cone (V)**	**Coll (eV)**	**Delay (s)**
1	1077.38	100.92	0.025	100.00	56.00	–1.000
2	1077.38	783.31	0.025	100.00	38.00	–1.000
3	1077.38	945.34	0.025	100.00	38.00	–1.000

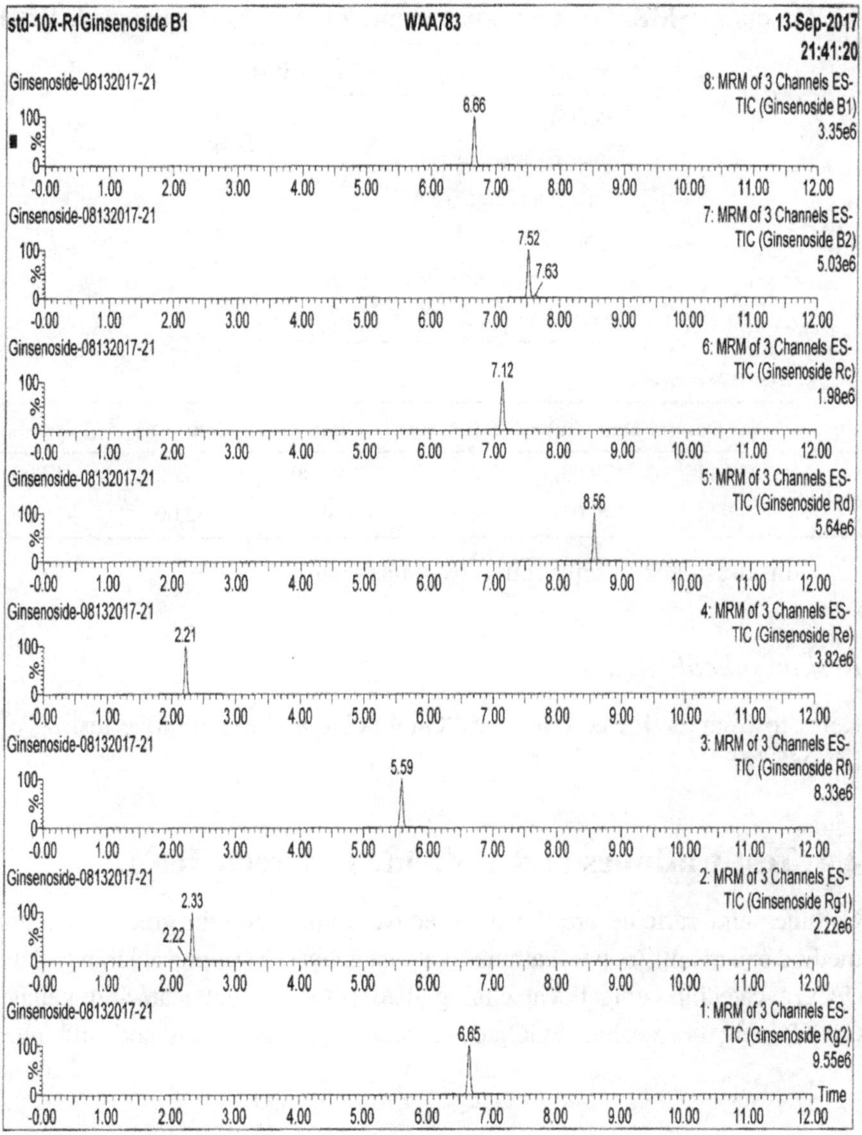

Figure 4.4: TIC chromatogram of ginsenosides.

Function 7: MRM of 2 mass pairs, time 7.0–8.5 ES-(Ginsenoside Rb2)

Model	MRM
Polarity	ES-
Inter Channel Delay (sec)	–1.000
InterScan Time (sec)	–1.000
Span (Da)	0.0
Start Time (min)	7.0
End Time (min)	8.5

Ginsenoside Rb2

Ch	Prnt (Da)	Dau (Da)	Dwell (s)	Cone (V)	Coll (eV)	Delay (s)
1	1077.44	89.03	0.025	94.00	56.00	–1.000
2	1077.44	149.06	0.025	94.00	42.00	–1.000

Ginsenoside Rb2 only found two mass pairs.

Result and calculation

Refer to Chapter 1, Section 1.1.5 "Qualitative and quantitative testing of LC-MS/MS".

4.4 Test Cathines and Caffeine in Green Tea

Cathines and caffeine are the main active components in green tea. This method can quantify seven cathines, gallocatechin (GC), epigcatechin gallate (ECG), catechin, epigallocatechin gallate (EGCG), gallocatechin gallate (GCG), epigallocatechin (EGC), epicatechin (EC), gallic acid and caffeine.

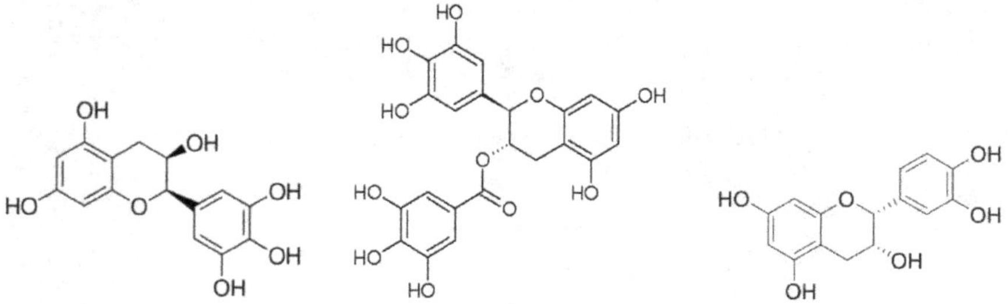

EGC GCG EC

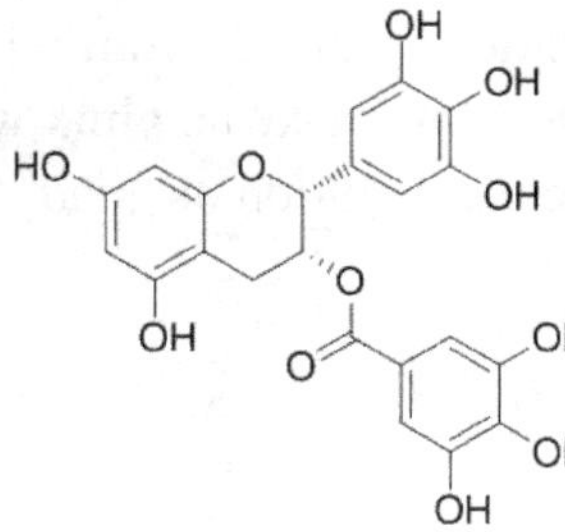

EGCG

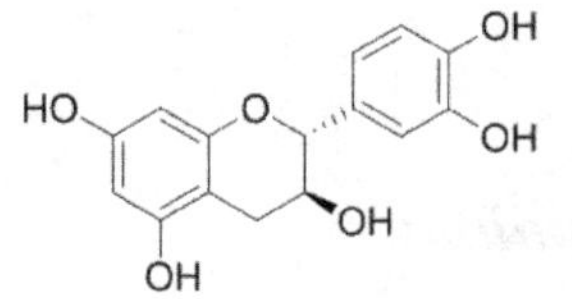

Catechin

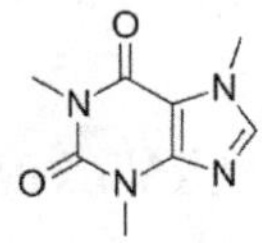

Caffeine

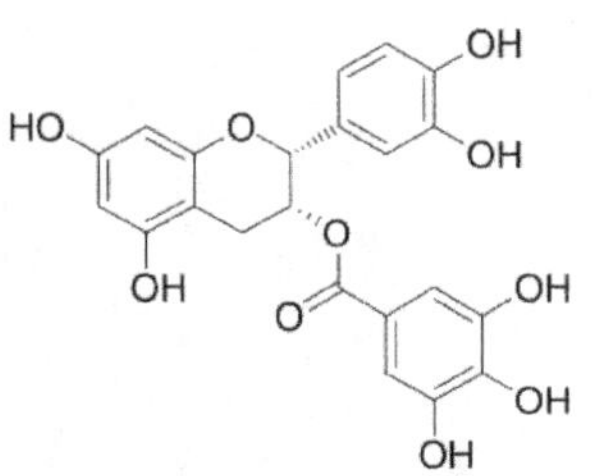

ECG

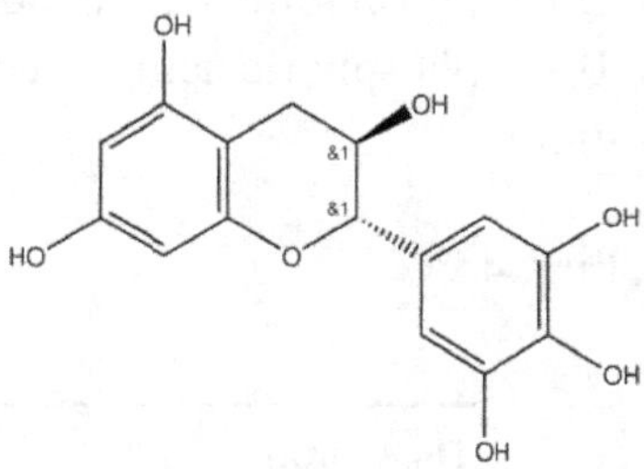

GC

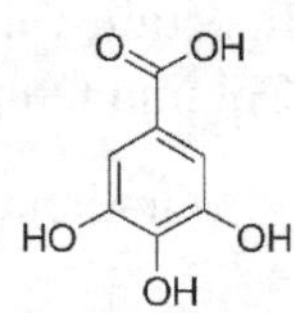

Gallic acid

From the aforementioned molecular structures it can be seen that all tea polyphenols are weak non-polar compounds. All of them contain aromatic low energy π electrons, so a phenyl column was selected to separate and quantify the polyphenols in green tea (see Chapter 1, Section 1.1.1, "Types of stationary phases").

(i) *Test procedure*

Preparation of standard solution — Accurately weigh about 10 mg of each of the catechin standards, GC, EGC, EC, GCG, ECG, EGCG, catechin, gallic acid and caffeine. Transfer it to a 100 ml volumetric flask, add 60 ml of 0.1% phosphoric acid, 5% acetonitrile in water solution, shake with a wrist action shaker until all standards are dissolved. Fill the aforementioned solution to 100 ml, shake and mix well. If necessary, further dilutions can be made.

Preparation of sample solutions — Accurately weigh a certain amount of ground sample containing about 10 mg of any aforesaid catechins or caffeine, and transfer it to 100 ml of volumetric flask. Add about 15–20 ml of warm water (70°C), sonicate for 2 min, and add 50 ml of 0.1%

phosphoric acid, 5% acetonitrile in water solution, shake 15 min with a wrist action shaker. Fill to 100 ml with same solvent, shake and mix well. Centrifuge for 5 min (10,000 r/min). The clear solution is ready for injection.

(ii) *UPLC condition*

Column: Acquity BEH Phenyl, 1.7 um, 2.1 × 150 mm
Mobile phase A: 0.1% phosphoric acid in nano pure water
Mobile phase B: 0.1% phosphoric acid in acetonitrile
Flow rate: 0.4 ml/min
Injection volume: 1 ul
Column temperature: 45°C

Gradient:

Time (min)	A%	B%
0	97	3
0–7.0	65	35
7.0–8.0	55	45
8.0–8.5	55	45
8.5–8.8	97	3
11.0	97	3 End

Note: Some green tea samples only require testing of caffeine. In this case the chromatographic method used should be verified to be able to separate caffeine and catechins, because some caffeine test methods may have problems separating caffeine and catechins.

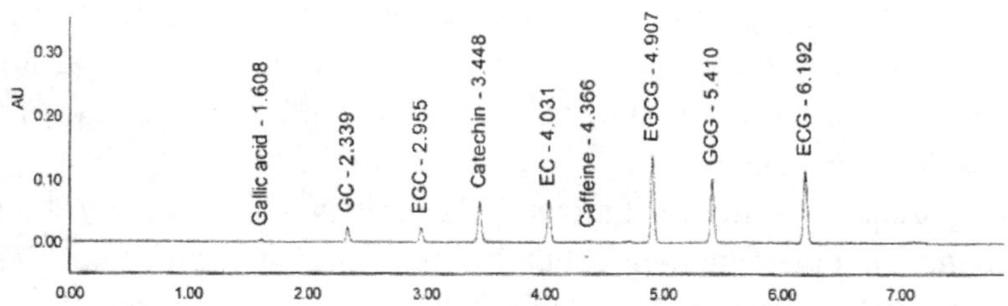

Figure 4.5: UPLC chromatogram of catechins and caffeine in green tea.

(iii) *Results and calculation*

$$Individual\ catechin(\%) = \frac{Aa \times Wstand \times Vsam \times 100\%}{As \times Vstd \times Wsam}$$

or

$$Individual\ catechin\ (mg/unit) = \frac{Aa \times Wsand \times Vsam \times UW}{As \times Vstd \times Wsam}$$

Here
Aa = Peak area of corresponding ginsenoside in sample solution
As = Peak area of corresponding ginsenoside in standard solution
Wsand = Weight of standard (mg)
Wsam = Weight of sample (mg)
Vstd = Total volume of standard solution (ml)
Vsam = Total volume of sample solution (ml)
UW = Unit weight (mg)

Total catechins = Sum of each measured individual catechin.

Relatively, catechin is more stable than other polyphenols in green tea, so you can consider using a single catechin as reference standard. All other catechins can be quantified by using conversion factors. The conversion factor can be calculated by the following formula.

$$Conversion\ factor\ Rn,\ (n = 1-6) = \frac{Aa \times Cs}{As \times Ca}$$

Here
Aa = Peak area of corresponding green tea polyphenol
As = Peak area of standard catechin
Cs = Concentration of standard catechin
Ca = Concentration of corresponding green tea polyphenol

The content of each catechin can be calculated as follows:

$$Individual\ catechin(\%) = \frac{Aa \times Wstand \times Vsam \times 100\%}{As \times Vstd \times Wsam \times Rn}$$

or

$$Individual\ catechin\ (mg/unit) = \frac{Aa \times Wsand \times Vsam \times UW}{As \times Vstd \times Wsam \times Rn}$$

Here
Aa = Peak area of corresponding polyphenol in sample solution
As = Peak area of standard (catechin) in standard solution
Vsam = Total volume of sample solution (ml)
Vstd = Total volume of standard solution (ml)
Wsand = Standard weight (mg)
Wsam = Sample weight (mg)
Rn = Conversion factor of corresponding polyphenol

The catechin standard solution should be stable for some time. In order to ensure the stability of catechin standard solution, you can add stable caffeine in the standard solution as a reference compound, calculate the peak area ratio of the two compounds, and record it. The standard solution can be used for each test until the ratio is out of the control range. This means the catechin is being degraded, so prepare a new standard solution.

4.5 Testing Theaflavin in Black Tea

Fermentation and processing of green tea produces black tea. Catechins in green tea are oxidized into theaflavin and other phenolic compounds, such as thearubigin, tea brown pigments, etc. The content of theaflavin is often measured as an indicator of the quality of black tea.

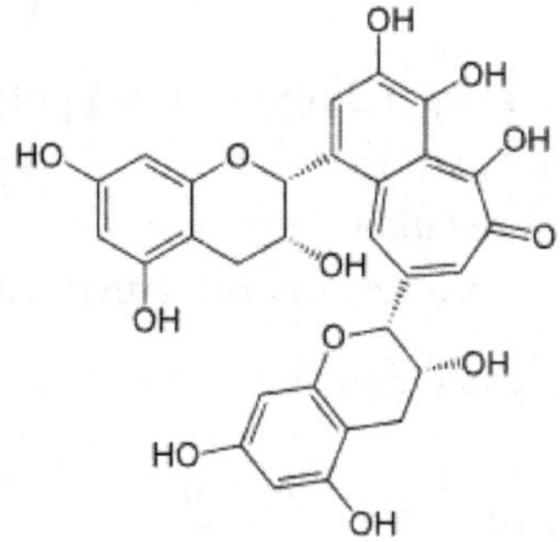

Theaflavin

C18 or phenyl columns can be used to separate and quantify theaflavin.

(i) *Testing procedure*

Solvent A preparation — 900 ml of water plus 99 ml of methanol, 1 ml of phosphoric acid, shake well.

Preparation of standard solution — Accurately weigh about 5 mg of theaflavin standard, transfer it to a 50 ml volumetric flask, add 30 ml of solvent A, shake with wrist action shaker for 10 min, then sonicate for 5 min. Cool to room temperature, fill solvent A to mark, and shake well. Label as "Theaflavin stock solution". Transfer 1 ml of stock standard solution into a 50 ml volumetric flask, add solvent A to 50 ml, shake and mix well. The standard solution is ready for injection.

Preparation of sample solution — Weigh a certain amount of ground sample containing about 2 mg theaflavin, transfer it to a 100 ml volumetric flask, add 60 ml of solvent A, shake with a wrist action shaker for 10 min. Put the flask in a water bath at 70°C, sonicate for 5 min if the sample is an extract material; sonicate for 20 min for black tea powder. Cool to room temperature, add solvent A to 100 ml, shake well, centrifuge (12,000 rpm) 5 min, transfer 1 ml of the clear sample solution into a 10 ml volumetric flask, then dilute to 10 ml with solvent A.

(ii) *UPLC conditions*

Mobile phase A: 0.1% phosphoric acid in nano pure water
Mobile phase B: 0.1% phosphoric acid in acetonitrile
Flow rate: 0.4 ml/min
Injection volume: 2 ul
UV wavelength: 380 nm
Run time:12 min
Column temperature: 45°C
Column: Acquity Hss T3 (C18), 1.8 um, 2.1 × 150 mm

Gradient:

Time (min)	A%	B%
0	95	5
0–1.0	95	5
1.0–7.0	65	35
7.0–8.0	58	42
8.0–8.8	58	42
8.8–9.0	95	5
12.0	95	5 Finish

(iii) *Results and calculation*

$$Theaflavin(\%) = \frac{Aa \times Wstand \times Vsam \times 100\%}{As \times Vstd \times Wsam}$$

or

$$Theaflavin\ (mg/unit) = \frac{Aa \times Wsand \times Vsam \times UW}{As \times Vstd \times Wsam}$$

Here
Aa = Peak area of sample
As = Peak area of standard
Wsand = Weight of standard (mg)
Wsam = Weight of sample (mg)
Vstd = Total volume of standard solution (ml)
Vsam = Total volume of sample solution (ml)
UW = Unit weight (mg)

4.6 Determination of Total Rosavins in Rhodiola Rosea by UPLC

A reversed phase chromatography method with photodiode array detector is used to determine the total rosavins content in Rhodiola rosea. Quantitation is carried out using an external standard calibration.

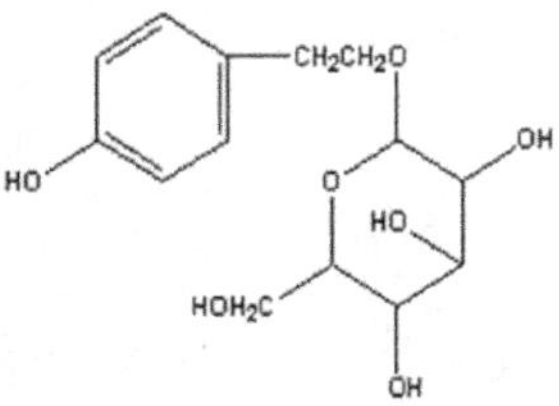

Salidroside

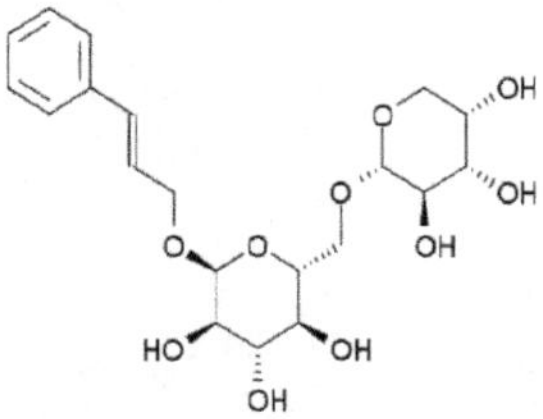

Rosavin

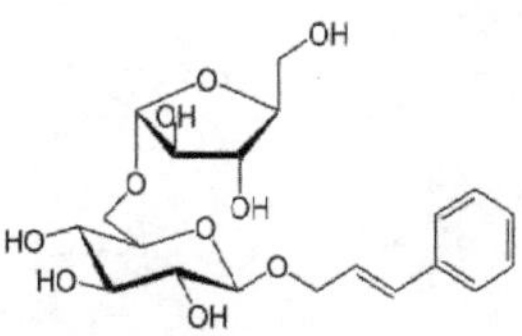

Rosarin

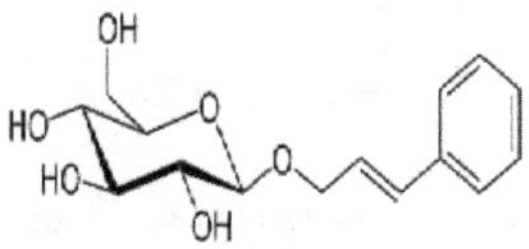

Rosin

From the previous molecular structure it can been seen that the molecules of rosavin, rosarin and rosin are similar with a styrene monomer group. A phenyl column can be used to separate them.

(i) *Test procedure*

Preparation of standard solution — Accurately weigh about 10 mg salidroside, rosavin, rosaring and rosin standards. Transfer it to a 100 ml volumetric flask, add about 60 ml of methanol, sonicate until all standards dissolved. Fill with methanol to the mark, shake and mix well. Transfer 5 ml of the solution into a 50 ml volumetric flask, dilute to 50 ml with methanol, and mix well. This solution is ready for injection.

Preparation of sample solution — Weight a certain amount of ground sample containing about 1 mg of any aforementioned compound, transfer it to a 100 ml volumetric flask, add 15 ml warm water (70°C), sonicate for 5 min. Add 50 ml of ethanol, shake, and sonicate for 10 min if the sample is an extract material; sonicate for 40 min for Rhodiola Rosea powder. Cool to room temperature, add methanol to mark, shake and mix well. Centrifuge (10,000 r/min) for 5 min. Take the clear solution for injection.

(ii) *UPLC conditions*

Column: Acquity BEH Phenyl 1.7 um, 2.1 × 150 mm

Mobile phase A: 0.1% phosphoric acid in nano pure water

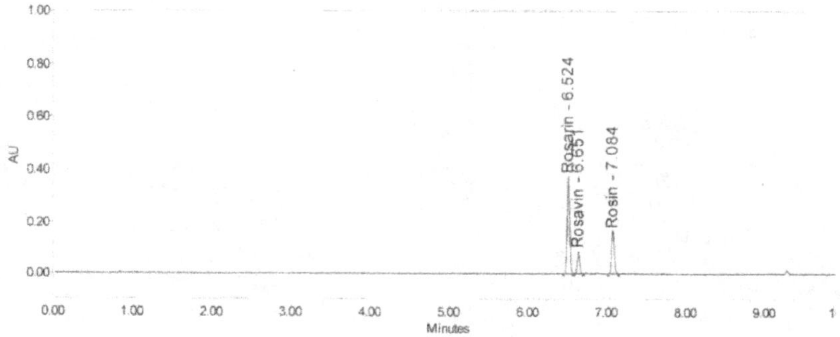

Figure 4.6: UPLC chromatogram of rosavin, rosarin and rosin. Salidroside standard was not added, so there is no salidroside peak in the chromatogram. The salidroside peak should be eluted much earlier.

Mobile phase B: 0.1% phosphoric acid in acetonitrile
Flow rate: 0.40 ml/min
Column temperature: 45°C
UV wavelength: 250 nm
Injection volume: 2 ul

Gradient:

Time (min)	A%	B%
0	95	5
0–7.0	70	30
7.0–7.8	95	5
10.0	95	5 End

(iii) *Results and calculation*

$$Individual\ rosavins\ (\%) = \frac{Aa \times Wstand \times Vsam \times 100\%}{As \times Vstd \times Wsam}$$

or

$$Individual\ rosavins\ (mg/unit) = \frac{Aa \times Wsand \times Vsam \times UW}{As \times Vstd \times Wsam}$$

Here
Aa = Peak area of corresponding *rosavin* in sample solution
As = Peak area of corresponding *rosavin* in standard solution
Wsand = Weight of standard (mg)
Wsam = Weight of sample (mg)
Vstd = Total volume of standard solution (ml)
Vsam = Total volume of sample solution (ml)
UW = Unit weight (mg)

The total rosavins content is the sum of each measured individual rosavin.

4.7 Valerian Test Method

Valerican (*Valeriana officinalis, Caprifoliaceae*) contains four active compounds, Valerenal, Hydroxyvalerenic acid, Valerenic acid and Acetoxyvalerenic acid. HPLC-PDA method can be used quantify each of the compounds.

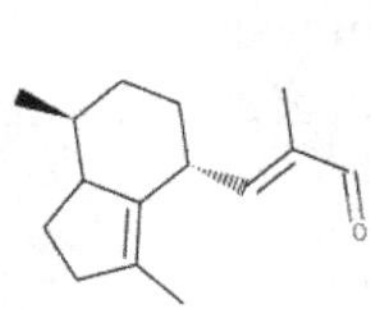

Valerenal

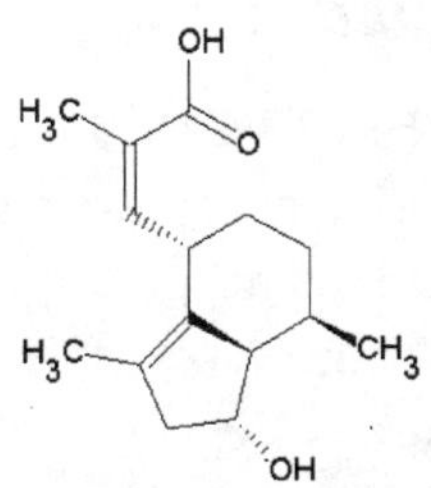

Hydroxyvalerenic acid

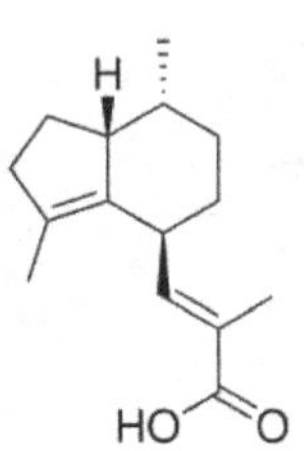

Valerenic acid

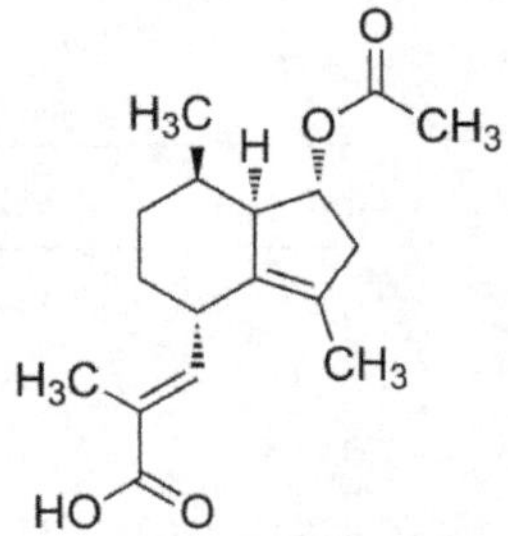

Acetoxyvalerenic acid

(i) *Test procedure*

Preparation of standards solution — Accurately weigh about 5 mg of valerenal, hydroxyvalerenic acid, valerenic acid and acetoxyvalerenic acid standards. Transfer it to a 50 ml volumetric flask, add about 5 ml warm water (70°). Soak and vortex for 5 min, add 30 ml ethanol, shake and sonicate until all standards dissolved. Cool to room temperature, add methanol to the mark, and mix well. If necessary, further dilutions can be made with methanol.

Preparation of sample solution — Weigh a certain amount of ground sample, containing about 5 mg any of the aforesaid analytes. Transfer it to a 50 ml volumetric flask, add 5 ml warm water (70°), soak and sonicate for 5 min. Add 30 ml ethanol, shake and sonicate for 10 min (for valerian extract); 40 min (for valerian powder). Cool to room temperature, add methanol to mark, and shake well. Centrifuge for 5 min (10,000 r/min), and take the clear solution for injection. If necessary, further dilutions can be made with methanol.

(ii) *UPLC conditions*

Column: Acquity Hss T3 C18, 1.8 um, 2.1 × 150 mm
Mobile phase A: 0.1% phosphoric acid in water
Mobile phase B: 0.1% phosphoric acid in acetonitrile
Flow rate: 0.40 ml/min
Column temperature: 45°C
UV wavelength: 218 nm
Injection volume: 2 ul

Gradient:

Time (min)	A%	B%
0	60	40
0–7.0	10	90
7.0–7.8	10	90
7.8–8.0	60	40
10.0	60	40 Finish

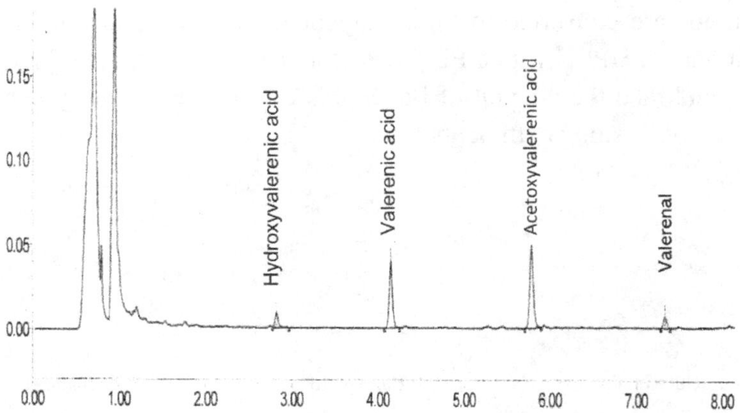

Figure 4.7: UPLC chromatogram of valerian.

(iii) *Results and calculation*

$$Individual\ active\ compound\ (\%) = \frac{Aa \times Wstand \times Vsam \times 100\%}{As \times Vstd \times Wsam}$$

or

$$Individual\ active\ comp.\ (mg/unit) = \frac{Aa \times Wsand \times Vsam \times UW}{As \times Vstd \times Wsam}$$

Here
Aa = Peak area of corresponding active compound in sample solution
As = Peak area of corresponding active compound in standard solution
Wsand = Weight of corresponding active compound standard (mg)
Wsam = Weight of sample (mg)
Vstd = Total volume of standard solution (ml)
Vsam = Total volume of sample solution (ml)
UW = Unit weight (mg/unit)

4.8 Testing of Ginkgo Flavonol Glycosides in Ginkgo Extract and Ginkgo Leave Powder

Ginkgo biloba contains a large number of flanvonol glycosides, and it is difficult to quantify each individual flavonoid. After acidic hydrolysis, all flavonoids are converted to three aglycones: quercetin, kaempferol and isorhamnetin. HPLC with a PDA detector can quantify all the three aglycones, and then the amount of flavonoids can be calculated by using the average conversion coefficients.

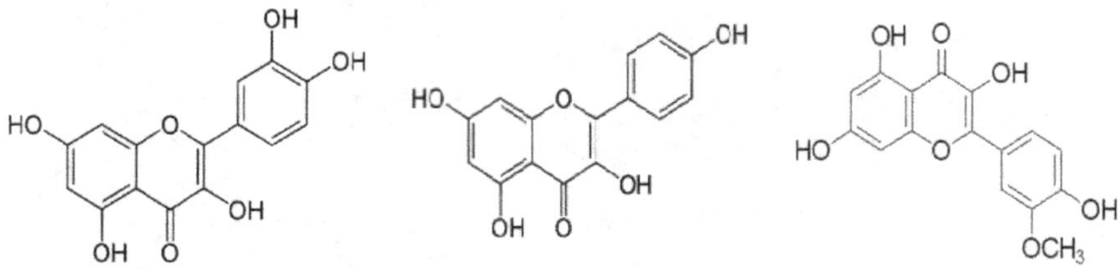

Quercetin Kaempferol Isorhamnetin

According to the aforementioned molecule structures, the three molecules contain different numbers of hydroxy and methoxy groups, and can be separated using C18 columns.

(i) *Test procedure*

Preparation of standard solution — Accurately weigh 15 mg of quercetin and kaempferol, and 5 mg of isorhamnetin. Transfer it to a 100 ml volumetric flask, add 60 ml of methanol, sonicate until all standards are dissolved. Cool to room temperature, then add methanol to the mark, shake well, and dilute the solution with methanol as need.

Preparation of sample solution — Accurately weigh a certain amount of ground sample (5 g of ginkgo leaf powder, or 300 mg extract materials) containing about 10–70 mg of ginkgo flavonoids, transfer it to a 250 ml of reflux flask, add 20 ml water, 50 ml of ethanol, and sonicate for 10 min. Add 8 ml concentration of HCl and a small magnetic stirring rod, start to reflux under 100°C water bath with magnetic rod stirring for 2 h. Cool to room temperature, transfer the extract to a 100 ml volumetric flask, rinse the reflux flask and slag with methanol, combine rinse solution and extract solution to reach 100 ml volume. Shake and mix well. Filter the solution through a 0.45 μm filter paper, the filtrate is ready for injection.

(ii) *HPLC conditions*

Column: Waters Symmetry C18, 3.5 μm, 4.6 × 150 mm
Flow rate: 1 ml/min

Injection volume: 10 μl
UV wavelength: 270 nm
Column temperature: 35°C
Mobile phase: Methanol/0.5%phosphoric acid in water (47:53)

(iii) *Results and calculation*

$$Individual\ aglycone\ (\%) = \frac{Aa \times Wstand \times Vsam \times 100\% \times R}{As \times Vstd \times Wsam}$$

or

$$Individual\ aglycone\ (mg/unit) = \frac{Aa \times Wsand \times Vsam \times UW \times R}{As \times Vstd \times Wsam}$$

Here
Aa = Peak area of corresponding aglycone in sample solution
As = Peak area of corresponding aglycone in standard solution
Wsand = Weight of corresponding aglycone standard (mg)
Wsam = Weight of sample (mg)
Vstd = Total volume of standard solution (ml)
Vsam = Total volume of sample solution (ml)
UW = Unit weight (mg/unit)
R = Average Conversion factor (aglycone glycosides/aglycone)
quercetin glycosides/Quercetin = 2.054
kaempferol glycosides/ kaempferol = 2.588
isorhamnetin glycosides/isorhamnetin = 2.437
Total ginkgo flavonoids = Sum of each individual flavonoids

4.9 Determination of Ginkgoterpenoids in Dietary Supplements by GC/FID

Ginkgo biloba contains two groups of active compounds: ginkgo flavonoids and ginkgoterpenoids.

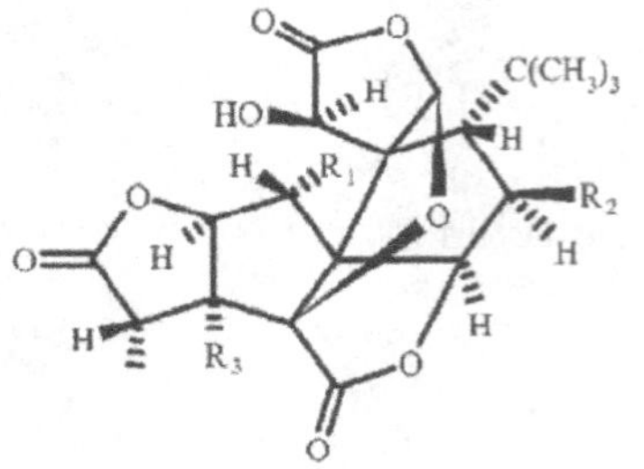

Ginkgolide A	$R_1 = H$,	$R_2 = H$,	$R_3 = OH$
Ginkgolide B	$R_1 = OH$,	$R_2 = H$,	$R_3 = OH$
Ginkgolide C	$R_1 = OH$,	$R_2 = OH$,	$R_3 = OH$
Ginkgolide J	$R_1 = H$,	$R_2 = OH$,	$R_3 = OH$
Ginkgolide M	$R_1 = OH$,	$R_2 = OH$,	$R_3 = H$

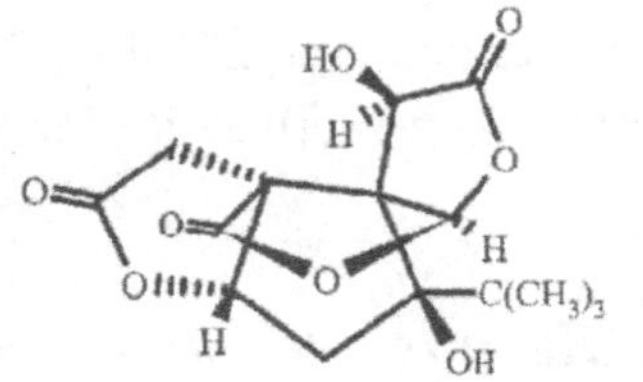

Bilobalide

As shown earlier, the ginkgoterpenoid molecules have a few unconjugated double bonds, with poor UV absorption. There are no specific spectrum features, plus the content of ginkgoterpenoids in *ginkgo biloba* are relatively low, so an HPLC-UV method is not a good choice. Some laboratories conduct HPLC-ELSD to test ginkgoterpenoids. This approach is acceptable if the ELSD linearity is good. Here we will introduce a GC-FID method for testing ginkgoterpenoids.

After extraction, trimethyl silane is used to derivativatize the ginkgoterpenoid molecules to reduce the boiling points. Then GC-FID is utilized to separate and quantify each of the ginkgoterpenoids.

(i) *Apparatus and equipment*

Hewlett-Packard 5890 with FID detection
GC column, J&W 19091J-02, HP-5, 25 m × 0.318 mm × 0.17 μm
Ultrasonic water bath
Analytical balance
2 mL glass vial with screw cap (PTFE/SIL)
Weighing paper

(ii) *Reagents and standards*

DHEA (dehydroisoandrosterone, internal standard), *Sigma,* D-4000
Bilobalide, 95%, Sigma, S-9031

Ginkgolide A, 90%, Sigma, G-4028
Ginkgolide B, 90%, Sigma, G-6910
Ginkgolide C, 98.5%, MP, 199661
Ginkgolide J, 86.9%, ChromaDex, ASB-00007186
Acetonitrile (ACN), HPLC Grade
N, N-Dimethylformamide (DMF), HPLC Grade
N, O-bis (trimethylsilil) trifluoroacatamide (BSTFA) with 1% of trimethyl chlorosilane (TMCS), reagent grade

(iii) *Procedure*

Internal Standard Solution (ISTD) — Accurately weigh 15 mg of DHEA, dissolve with 10 mL of DMF in a 25 mL volumetric flask. Fill to the mark with DMF and mix well.

Standard preparation — Accurately weigh 10 mg of bilobalide and Ginkgolide A, 5 mg each of Ginkgolide B, C and J. Accurately transfer all of them to a 10 mL volumetric flask, add 1 mL of DMF and sonicate for 5 min to dissolve all the standards. Then fill to the mark with acetonitrile and mix well. Label as "Standard stock solution". The standard stock solution will be stable for 6 months under frozen conditions.

Take 500 μL of standard stock solution into a 2 mL injection vial, add 200 μL of ISTD and 200 μL of BSTFA with 1% of TMCS, then cap tightly, mix well, and incubate it in 100°C water bath for 20 min. Cool to room temperature. This standard solution is ready for injection.

Sample preparation for ginkgo leaf powder — Weigh about 8.0 g pulverized leaf, put into a 150 mL reflux flask, and extract under reflux for 15 min with 30 mL 30% methanol in water. Then filter the supernatant into a 200 mL of round-bottom flask, repeat the extraction twice. Combine all extract in the 200 ml round-bottom flask, dry the combination extract with a vacuum evaporator. During the evaporation procedure, an additional amount of methanol can be added to make the drying go faster. Take 1 mL of DMF to the round-bottom flask, and sonicate for 15 min to dissolve the residual. Add 9 mL ACN and shake vigorously for 2 min. Transfer it to a test tube, centrifuge at 2,500 rpm for 5 min. Transfer 500 μL of clear solution into a 2 mL injection vial, add 200 μL of ISTD and 200 μL of BSTFA with 1% of TMCS, then cap tightly, mix well, and incubate it in 100°C water bath for 20 min. Cool to room temperature, and it is ready for injection.

Sample preparation for *ginkgo biloba* extract and finished products containing *ginkgo biloba* extract — Accurately weigh around 500 mg of ginkgo extract powder (or equivalent amount of ground finished products) into a 25 mL volumetric flask. Add 2.0 mL of DMF and sonicate for 10 min. Add 8 mL of ACN sonicate for 15 min and vigorously shake every 5 min. Transfer it to a 10 mL centrifuge tube, and centrifuge at 2,500 rpm for 5 min. Pipette 500 μL of clear solution into a 2 mL injection vial, add 200 μL of ISTD and 200 μL of BSTFA with 1% of TMCS, then cap tightly, mix well, and incubate it in 100°C water bath for 20 min. Cool to room temperature. This sample solution is ready for injection.

(iv) *GC conditions*

Instrument: Hewlett-Packard GC 5890 with FID
Column: J&W 19091 J-012, HP-5, 25 m × 0.318 mm × 0.17μm
Column oven temperature: Initial Oven Temperature: 200°C hold for 1 min, at rate of 2°C/min to 260°C, then to 290°C at 15°C/min, hold for 2 min
Detector: 300°C
Injector: 250°C
Injection Volume: 1μL

(v) *Calculation*

$$Individual\ ginkgoterpenoid\ (\%) = \frac{Cs \times PARu \times Vsam \times 100\%}{PARs \times Wsam}$$

or

$$Individual\ ginkgoterpenoid\ (mg/unit) = \frac{Cs \times PARu \times Vsam \times UW}{PARs \times Wsam}$$

Here

Cs = Concentration of corresponding ginkgoterpenoid standard (mg/m)

Wsam = Weight of sample (mg)

PARs = Peak area of corresponding ginkgoterpenoid vs. peak area of internal standard in sample solution

PARu = Peak area of corresponding ginkgoterpenoid vs. peak area of internal standard in standard solution

Vsam = Total volume of sample solution (ml)

UW = Unit weight (mg/unit)

Total of ginkgoterpenoids = Summarize the content of each terpenoid

4.10 Ginger Test Method

The main active compounds found in ginger are capsaicin, gingerols, shogaols, gingerdione and gingerdiol.

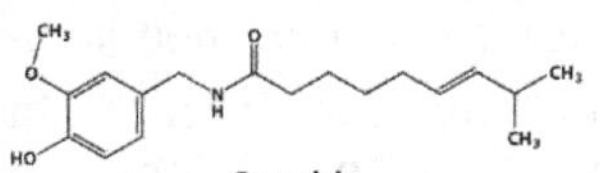

Capsaicin

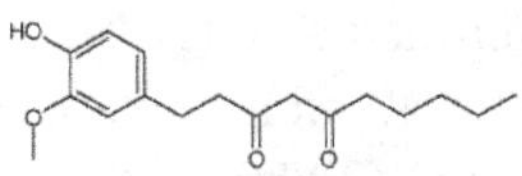

6-gingerdiol

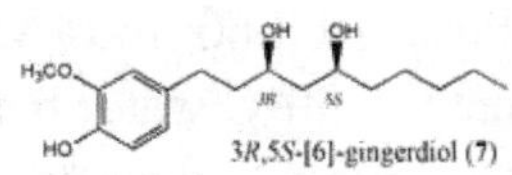

3R,5S-[6]-gingerdiol (7)

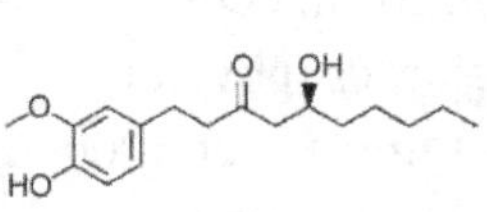

6-Gingerol

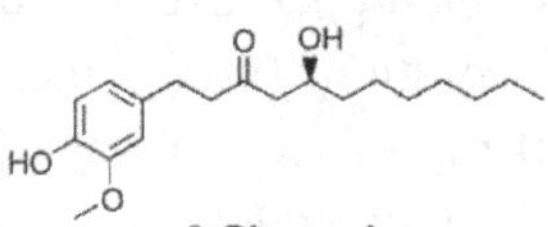

8-Gingerol

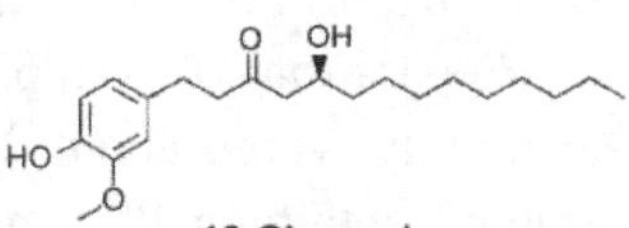

10-Gingerol

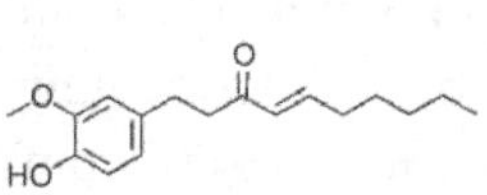

6-Shogaol

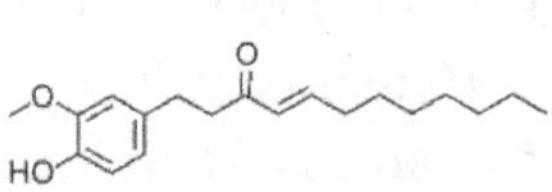

8-Shogaol

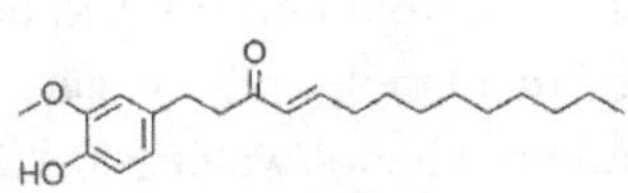

10-Shogaol

From the aforementioned molecular structure it can be seen that this group of compounds contain a phenolic group, so the UV sensitivity is relatively high. Using PDA detector, general test needs should be able to be met. Either C18 or phenyl column can be used to test the ginger samples. The standards of the aforementioned compounds are available on the standards market. The most accurate method will use the individual standards to quantify each active compound. However, some laboratories test ginger using only a single capsaicin standard. Obviously, there will be some differences in the results measured by the two methods.

(i) *Test procedure*

Preparation of stock standard solutions — Accurately weigh about 5 mg of capsaicin, 6-, 8-, 10-gingerol, 6-,8-,10-shogaol, 6-gingerdione and 6-gingerdiol standard separately. Transfer it to 25 ml volumetric flasks for each standard. Add 15 ml of water/methanol (20/80) to each flask, sonicate until the standards are completely dissolved, fill the same water/methanol solvent to 25 ml marker, shake and mix well. These are the standard stock solutions.

Preparation of standard solutions — Transfer 3 ml of the capsaicin stock solution, and 1 ml of 6-, 8-, 10-gingerol,6-,8-,10-shogaol,6-gingerdione and 6-gingerdiol stock solutions to a 50 ml of volumetric flask, add water/methanol (20/80) to 50 ml mark, shake and mix well. This standard solution is ready for injection.

Preparation of sample solution (for ginger powder) — Accurately weigh about 1 g of ginger dry powder. Transfer it to a 100 ml volumetric flask. Add 60 ml of water/methanol (20/80), vortex for 1 min, then sonicate in 50°C water bath for 40 min, shaking every 5 min for 10 sec. After cooling, add water/methanol (20/80) to the mark, mix well, centrifuge at 10,000 r/min) for 5 min. Take the upper level of liquid for injection.

Preparation of sample solution (for ginger extract powder) — Accurately weigh about 200 mg of extract powder samples, or ground sample containing 200 mg extract powder equivalent. Transfer it to a 100 ml volumetric flask, add 10 ml of water, vortex for 3 min, add 40 ml of methanol, and sonicate for 10 min in 50°C water bath. After cooling, add methanol/water (80:20) to mark, shake well, centrifuge (10,000 rpm) for 5 min, and take the clear liquid for injection.

(ii) *HPLC conditions*

Column: Phenomenex LUNA C18 (2) 5 μm 4.6 × 250 mm 100A
Mobile phase A: 0.1% phosphoric acid in water
Mobile phase B: 0.1% phosphoric acid in acetonitrile
Column temperature: Room temperature
UV wavelength: 282 nm
Flow rate: 1.0 ml/min
Injection volume: 20 ul

Gradient:

Time (min)	A%	B%
0	65	35
0–15	0	100
15–20	0	100
20–21	65	35
30	65	35 Finish

Order of peak elution

6-gingerdiol
6-gingerol
Capsaicin
8-gingerol
6-shogaol
6-gingerdione
10-gingerol
8-shogaol
10-shogaol

(iii) *Results and calculation*

$$Individual\,compond(\%) = \frac{Aa \times Wstand \times Vsam \times 100\%}{As \times Vstd \times Wsam}$$

or

$$Individual\,compond(mg/unit) = \frac{Aa \times Wsand \times Vsam \times UW}{As \times Vstd \times Wsam}$$

Here

Aa = Peak area of corresponding compound in sample solution
As = Peak area of corresponding compound in standard solution
Wsand = Weight of corresponding standard (mg)
Wsam = Weight of sample (mg)
Vstd = Total volume of standard solution (ml)
Vsam = Total volume of sample solution (ml)
UW = Unit weight (mg/unit)

Total content = The sum of each individual compound

4.11 Echinacea Test Method

Echinacea and echinacea extracts are common ingredients in dietary supplements. The main functions of these ingredients are to enhance immunity and to take advantage of their anti-inflammatory effects. Modern testing methods quantitatively test four main effective compounds (or marker compounds), caftaric acid, chlorogenic acid, echinocoside and cichoric acid.

Historically, species of echinacea have been used for medicinal purposes like *echinacea purpurea* and *echinacea angusfolia*. Both species contain the above four ingredients, but the proportions are different, so the differences can be distinguished in the chromatography (see Figures 4.8 and 4.9).

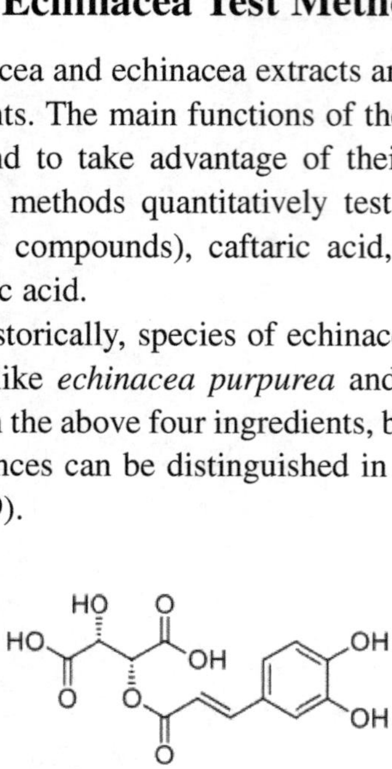

Caftaric acid

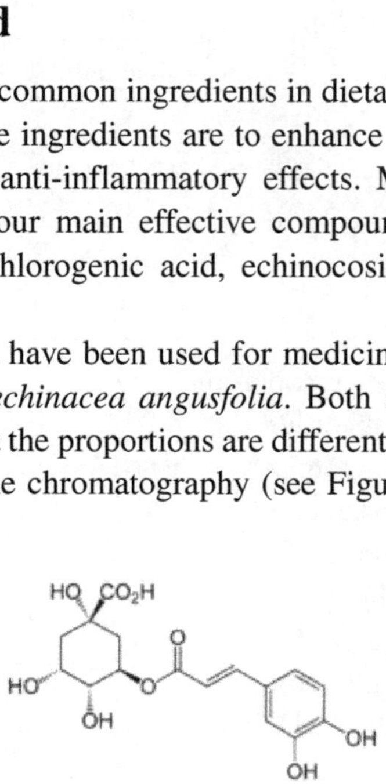

Chlorogenic acid

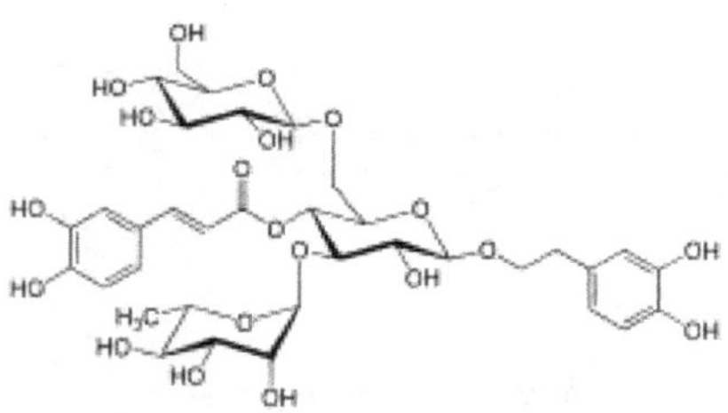

Echinocoside

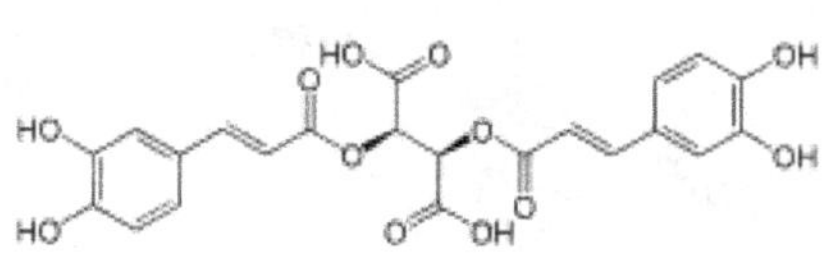

Cichoric acid

All the aforementioned compounds contain an aromatic group. As each molecule is quite different, it is easy to separate and quantify them by either using C18 or phenyl columns with a PDA detector.

(i) *Test procedure*

Prepare solvent A — To 700 ml of ethanol add 300 ml of nano pure water, shake, and mix well.

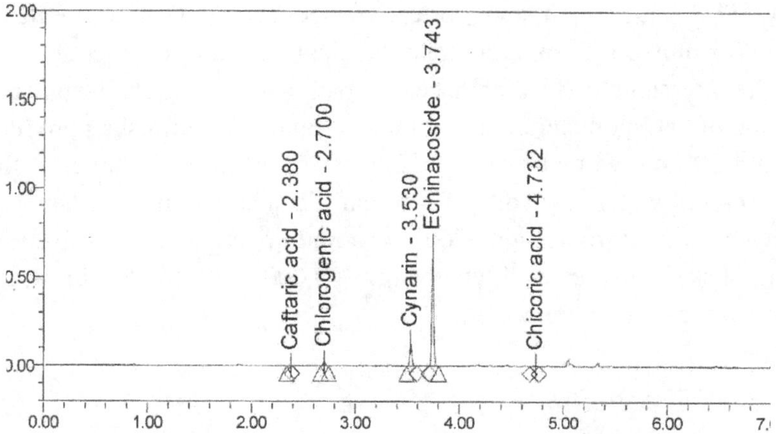

Figure 4.8: UPLC chromatogram of *echinacea purpurea.*

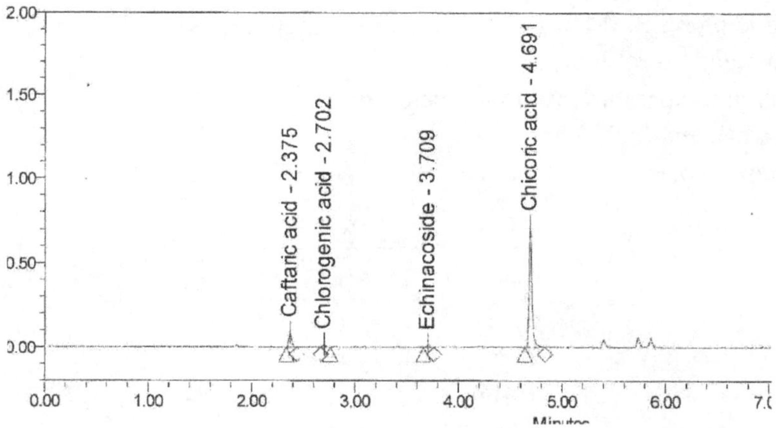

Figure 4.9: UPLC chromatogram of *echinacea angusfolia.*

Prepare standard solution — Accurately weigh about 5 mg of caftaric acid, chlorogenic acid, chinocoside and cichoric acid standards, and transfer to a 50 ml volumetric flask. Add 30 ml solvent A, sonicate until all standards are dissolved, fill solvent A to mark, shake, and label as "Stock standard solution". Transfer 1 ml of stock standard solution into a 25 ml volumetric flask, dilute to volume with solvent A.

Prepare sample solution (for echinacea powder) — Weigh about 1 g of echinacea powder, transfer it to a 100 ml volumetric flask. Accurately transfer 50 ml of solvent A to the flask, vortex for 2 min, sonicate 40 min in a 50°C water bath and vortex 10 sec every 10 min. Centrifuge (10,000 r/min) for 5 min, and take the clear solution for injection.

Prepare sample (for echinacea extract) — Accurately weigh about 200 mg of extract material or a sufficient amount of a finished product to contain 200 mg extract material. Transfer to 50 ml of volumetric flask, add 10 ml of water, and vortex for 5 min. Then add 30 ml of ethanol, and sonicate for 5–10 more min. Cool to room temperature, add solvent 1 to mark, shake and mix well, centrifuge (10,000 rpm) for 5 min, and the clear solution can be injected.

(ii) *HPLC conditions*

Column: Prodigy ODS (3) C18 5 μm 4.6 × 250 mm 100A
Mobile phase A: 0.1% phosphoric acid in water
Mobile phase B: 0.1% phosphoric acid in acetonitrile
Flow rate: 1.0 ml/min
Column temperature: room temperature
UV wavelength: 330 nm
Injection volume: 20 ul

Gradient:

Time (min)	A%	B%
0	90	10
0–15	70	30
15–16	50	50
16–16.5	90	10
25.0	90	10

(iii) *Results and calculation*

$$Individual\ active\ compond(\%) = \frac{Aa \times Wstand \times Vsam \times 100\%}{As \times Vstd \times Wsam}$$

or

$$Individual\ active\ compond\ (mg/unit) = \frac{Aa \times Wsand \times Vsam \times UW}{As \times Vstd \times Wsam}$$

Here
Aa = Peak area of corresponding compound in sample solution
As = Peak area of corresponding compound in standard solution
Wsand = Weight of corresponding standard (mg)
Wsam = Weight of sample (mg)
Vstd = Total volume of standard solution (ml)
Vsam = Total volume of sample solution (ml)
UW = Unit weight (mg/unit)
Total content = The sum of each individual content

4.12 Test Method for Hydroxy Citric Acid in *Garcinia Combogia*

Hydroxy citric acid originally came from the Indian plant *garcinia combogia*. It is claimed to inhibit the conversion of carbohydras to energy, so it is used as a weight control dietary supplement.

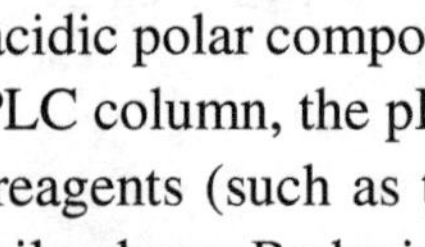

Hydroxy citric acid

Hydroxy citric acid contains three carboxylic acid groups and two hydroxy groups, so it is an acidic polar compound. To extend the retention time in a reversed phase HPLC column, the pH in the mobile phase needs to be reduced, or ion pair reagents (such as tetrabutyl ammonium salts) need to be added to the mobile phase. Reducing pH of mobile phase is an easier way, so it can be tried first. If interferes from the sample matrix cannot be separated, then the ion pairing method may be required. These two methods are optional, as long as the interferences can be separated.

(i) *Test procedure*

Prepare standard solution — Accurately weigh about 20 mg of hydroxy citric acid standard, transfer it to a 100 ml volumetric flask and add water to dissolve the standard. Then dilute to volume with water and shake and mix well. The standard solution is ready to inject.

Prepare sample solution — Weigh a certain amount of ground sample containing about 20 mg of hydroxy citric acid, transfer it to a 100 ml volumetric flask, add 60 ml of water, vortex 1 min. Then sonicate for 10 min for extract materials; sonicate for 40 min for garcinia combogia powder. Cool to room temperature, add water to volume, shake and mix well. Centrifuge (12,000 r/min) for 5 min, then take the clear solution for injection.

(ii) *UPLC conditions*

Column: Acquity UPLC® HSS T3, 1.8 μm, 2.1 × 150 mm
Mobile phase A: 0.5% phosphoric acid in nano pure water
Mobile phase B: 0.5% phosphoric acid in acetonitrile
Mobile phase A/mobile phase B = 97/3 isocratic
Flow rate: 0.4 ml/min
Column temperature: 45°
UV wavelength: 210 nm
Injection volume: 2.0 ul

(iii) *Results and calculation*

$$Hydroxy\,citric\,acid(\%) = \frac{Aa \times Wstand \times Vsam \times 100\%}{As \times Vstd \times Wsam}$$

or

$$Hydroxy\,citric\,acid\ (mg/unit) = \frac{Aa \times Wsand \times Vsam \times UW}{As \times Vstd \times Wsam}$$

Here
Aa = Peak area of sample
As = Peak area of standard
Wsand = Weight of standard (mg)
Wsam = Weight of sample (mg)
Vstd = Total volume of standard solution (ml)
Vsam = Total volume of sample solution (ml)
UW = Unit weight (mg/unit)

4.13 Test Method for Coumarin

Coumarin is found in many natural plants and has a sweet fragrance. It is often used in cosmetics, tobacco and the alcohol industry as an additive. A large dose may cause cancer.

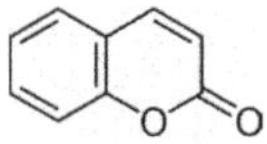

Coumarin

Coumarin is a non-polar compound that can be analyzed by HPLC using reversed phase C18 or phenyl columns.

(i) *Test procedure*

Preparation of standard solution — Accurately weigh about 10 mg of coumarin standard, transfer it to a 100 ml volumetric flask, add 60 ml of methanol, sonicate until the standard completely dissolved. Then add methanol to volume, and shake well. Further dilutions can be made with methanol if needed. Coumarin exhibits a strong UV absorption, so the concentration of standard solution could be as low as 0.1 ppm.

Preparation of sample solution — Weigh a certain amount of powdered sample containing about 10 mg of coumarin. Transfer it to a 100 ml volumetric flask, and add 10 ml of water, vortex 5 min. Next, sonicate for 5 min, add about 60 ml of ethanol, and sonicate for 10 min. Cool to room temperature, fill methanol to volume, shake and mix well, then centrifuge (12,000 r/min) for 5 min. Take the clear solution for injection.

(ii) *UPLC conditions*

Column: Acquity UPLC® BEH C18 1.7 μm, 2.1 × 150 mm
Mobile phase A: 0.1% phosphoric acid in water
Mobile phase B: 0.1% phosphoric acid in acetonitrile
Flo rate: 0.4 ml/min
Column temperature: 45°C
UV wavelength: 276 nm
Injection volume: 1 μl

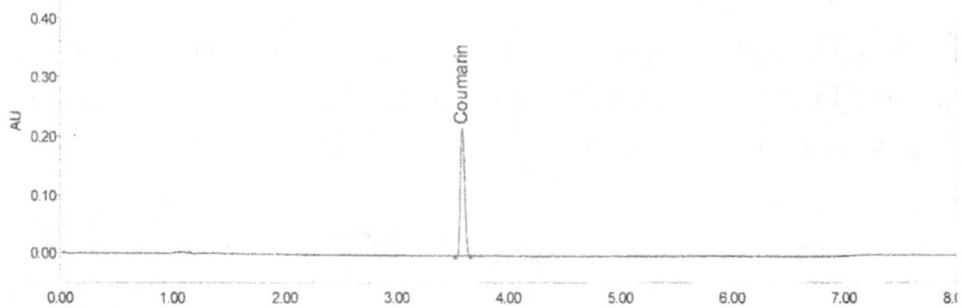

Figure 4.10: UPLC chromatogram of coumarin.

Gradient:

Time (min)	A%	B%
0	90	10
0–6	40	60
6–7	40	0
7.0–7.5	90	10
7.5–10	90	10

(iii) *Results and calculation*

$$Coumarin\ \% = \frac{Aa \times Wstand \times Vsam \times 100\%}{As \times Vstd \times Wsam}$$

or

$$Coumarin\ (mg/unit) = \frac{Aa \times Wsand \times Vsam \times UW}{As \times Vstd \times Wsam}$$

Here
Aa = Peak area of sample
As = Peak area of standard
Wsand = Weight of standard (mg)
Wsam = Weight of sample (mg)
Vstd = Total volume of standard solution (ml)
Vsam = Total volume of sample solution (ml)
UW = Unit weight (mg/unit)

4.14 Test Anthocyanidins and Anthocyanins in Bilberry

The European bilberry contains anthocyanidins and anthocyanins, which are high-quality antioxidants, and can potentially help improve vision, especially night blindness. European bilberry mainly contains five types of anthocyanidins (see molecular structure below) and their glycosides with different kinds of sugars at different position. All these compounds are pH sensitive; the colors will change when the pH is changed.

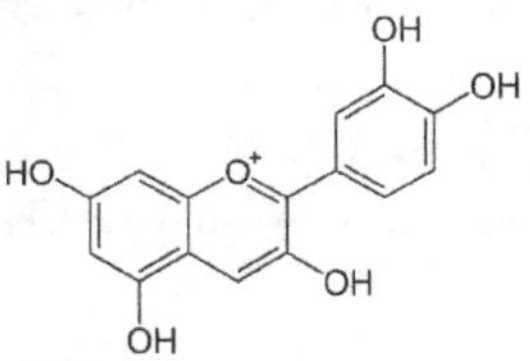

Cyanidin

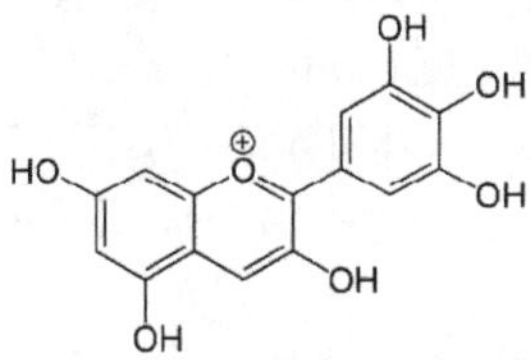

Delphin

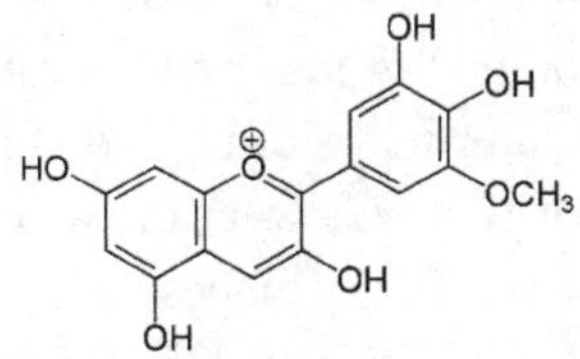

Petunidin

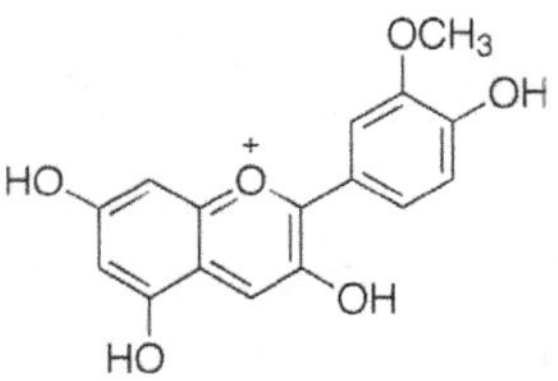

Peonidin

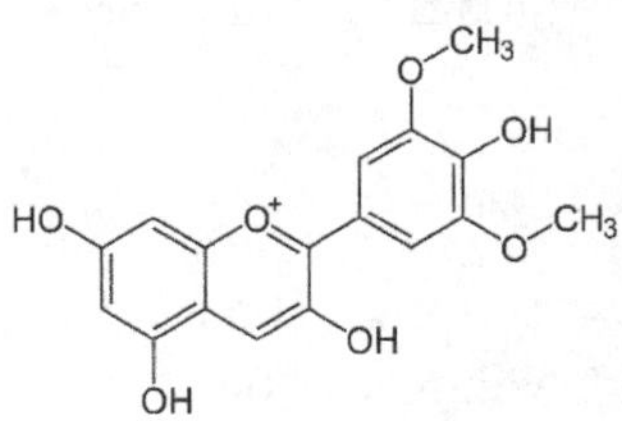

Malvidin

Reversed phase chromatography can separate more than 20 anthocyanidins and anthocyanins from bilberry. See Figure 4.11 (chromatogram from Indena — Anthocynines and Anthocyindins test method).

There are two test methods:

(1) UV spectroscopy to quantitatively test anthocyanidins and their glycosides.
(2) Qualitative and quantitative testing of anthocyanins and their glycosides with liquid chromatography.

(i) *Method (1)*

Quantitative testing by spectroscopy (this method is derived from the Institute for Nutraceutical Advancement (INA) method).

(i) *Apparatus and equipment*

Calibrated analytical balance accurate to ±0.1mg
Pipette
Spectrophotometer
Volumetric flasks, assorted sizes

(ii) *Reagents and solution*

pH 1.0 buffer — Dissolve 1.49 g KCl into 100 mL DI water. Carefully pour 1.7 mL concentrated HCl into 100 mL volumetric flask, add DI water to volume, and shake well. This is 0.2 N HCl solution. Mix 25 mL of the KCl solution with 67 mL of the 0.2 N HCl solution. Adjust to pH 1.0 ± 0.1, if necessary.

pH 4.5 Buffer — Dissolve 1.64 g sodium acetate in 100 mL DI water. Adjust to pH 4.5 ± 0.1 with HCl.

(iii) *Procedure*

(1) Accurately weigh about 75 mg of powdered bilberry extract into a 100 mL volumetric flask. Add about 80 mL of DI water to the flask and sonicate for 15 min or until dissolved. Allow the solution to cool to room temperature and fill water to volume, mix well. If the solution appears to have turbidity, centrifuge a portion of it to help remove particulates.
(2) Remove a 1.0 mL aliquot of the bilberry solution and place it into a 25 mL volumetric flask. Dilute to volume with pH 1.0 buffer and mix.
(3) Remove another 1.0 mL aliquot of the bilberry solution and place it into a 25 mL volumetric flask. Dilute to volume with pH 4.5 buffer and mix.
Centrifuging sample preparations may improve method precision. (*Note*: Solutions are stable at room temperature for 4 h.)
(4) Zero spectrophotometer with distilled water.
(5) Measure UV absorbance at 510 nm and 700 nm for both pH 1.0 and pH 4.5 sample solutions.

(6) Calculate result — Calculate the difference in absorbance between the two pH solutions using the following equation.

$$Absorbance\ difference = (A_{510nm},\ pH\ 1.0 - A_{700nm},\ pH\ 1.0) - (A_{510nm},\ pH\ 4.5 - A_{700nm},\ pH\ 4.5)$$

Calculate the %(w/w) of total anthocyanins in the sample:

$$\%(w/w) = (A/\varepsilon L) \times MW \times DF \times (V/Wt) \times 100\%$$

Here
A = Absorbance difference
ε = Cyd-3-glu molar absorbance difference (26,900)
L = cell path length (usually 1 cm)
MW = Cyd-3-glu molecular weight (449.2)
DF = dilution factor
V = final volume (mL)
Wt = Sample weight (mg)

(ii) *Method (2)*

Qualitative and quantitative testing of anthocyanins and their glycosides with liquid chromatography method.

The UV method can quantitatively test the content of total anthocyanins and anthocyanins, but it is not capable of determining which plant species the anthocyanins come from, or what the specific anthocyanin components are. Since the price of bilberry is higher than other berries, there are many adulterated products in the market, with other raw materials instead of European bilberry. So, it is necessary to use a chromatographic method to obtain a complete chromatogram in order to determine the source of anthocyanins. Figure 4.11 is a standard European bilberry chromatogram, which is different from other berries. The quantitative results can be obtained by comparing peak area with a known quantity of standards.

(i) *Test procedure*

Preparation of standard solution — Accurately weigh about 100 mg of Indena 30% European bilberry extract, transfer it to a 50 ml volumetric flask, add about 30 ml of 1% hydrochloric acid in methanol solution, sonicate until all standard dissolved. Add methanol to 50 ml, shake well for injection. If necessary, the solution may be diluted with methanol until the appropriate concentration is achieved.

Preparation of sample solution — Accurately weigh a sample equivalent of 30 mg anthocyanins and transfer to a 50 ml volumetric flask. If the sample is an extract, follow the preparation procedure of the standard solution described earlier.

If the sample is a raw fruit or a dried powder, proceed with the following steps: Transfer the sample to a 50 ml volumetric flask, add 40 ml of methanol containing 1% hydrochloric acid, sonicate for 1 h. After cooling add methanol to the mark, shake and mix well. Centrifuge (10,000 r/min) for 5 min and take the clear solution for injection. If necessary, further dilutions can be made with methanol until the appropriate concentration is reached.

(ii) *HPLC conditions*

Column: Prodigy ODS (2), 5 μm 4.6 × 150 mm
Mobile phase A: 10% formic acid in nano pure water
Mobile phase B: Methanol
Flow rate: 1 ml/min
Column temperature: room temperature
UV wavelength: 460 nm
Injection volume: 10 μl

Gradient:

Time (min)	**A%**	**B%**
0–5	90	10
5–40	35	65
40–42	0	100
42–45	0	100
45–46	90	10
46–55	90	10

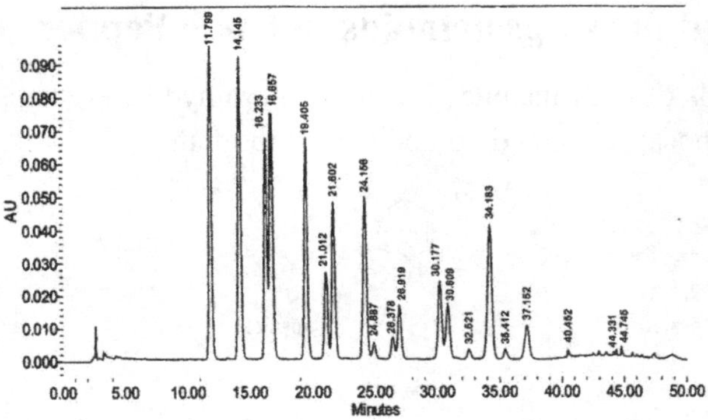

COMPOUND	RETENTION TIME
Delphinidin-3-O-galactosid	11.80
Delphinidin-3-O-glucoside	14.15
Cyanidin-3-O-galactoside	16.23
Delphinidin-3-O-arabinoside	16.66
Cyanidin-3-O-glucoside .	19.41
Petunidin-3-O-galactoside	21.01
Cyanidin-3-O-arabinoside	21.60
Petunidin-3-O-glucoside	24.16
Delphinidin	24.89
Peonidin-3-O-galactoside	26.38
Petunidin-3-O-arabinoside	26.92
Peonidin-3-O-glucoside	30.18
Malvidin-3-O-glucoside	30.81
Peonidin-3-O-arabinoside	32.52
Malvidin-3-O-galactoside	34.18
Cyanidin	35.41
Malvidin-3-O-arabinoside	37.15
Petunidin	40.45
Peonidin	44.33
Malvidin	44.75

Figure 4.11: HPLC chromatogram of bilberry, from Indena — Anthocyanidins and anthocyanins test method.

Following the chromatography conditions as described may not obtain exactly same chromatogram as shown earlier, but it must be consistent with the standard chromatogram run by the same system.

(iii) *Result and calculation*

$$Total\ anthocyanins\ \% = \frac{Aa \times Cs \times Vsam \times 100\%}{As \times Wsam}$$

or

$$Total\ anthocyanins\ (mg/unit) = \frac{Aa \times Cs \times Vsam \times UW}{As \times Wsam}$$

Here
As = Total peak area of standard
Aa = Total peak area of sample
Cs = Concentration of standard solution (mg/ml)
Vsam = Total volume of sample solution (ml)
Wsam = Sample weight (mg)
UW = Average unit weight

4.15 Test Method for Capsaicinoids in Chile Pepper

The total capsaicinoids of chili includes capsaicin, nordihydrocapsaicin, dihydrocapsaicin, homocapsaicin and homodihydrocapsaicin.

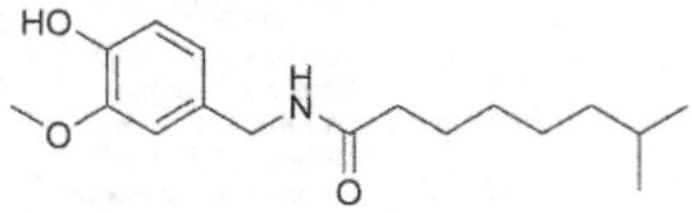
Nordihydrocapsaicin

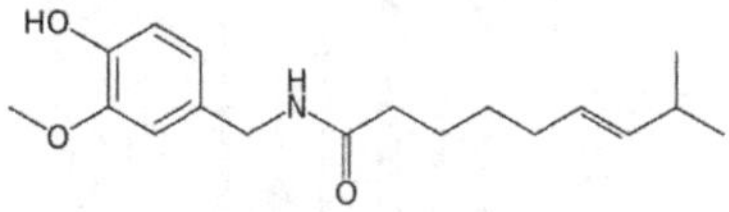
Capsaicin

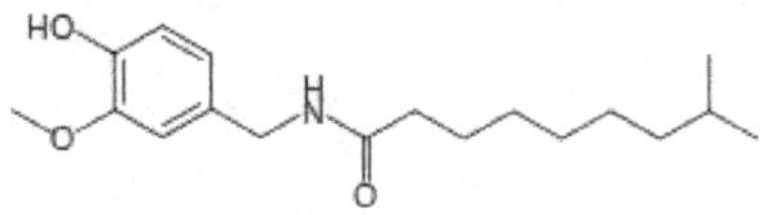
Dihydrocapsaicin

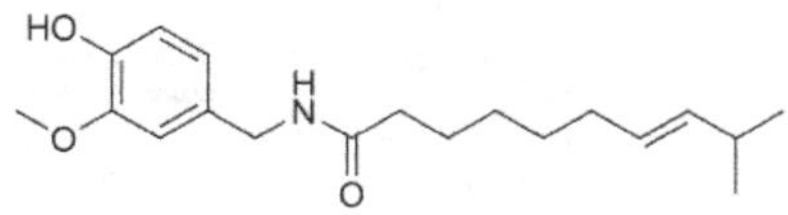
Homocapsaicin

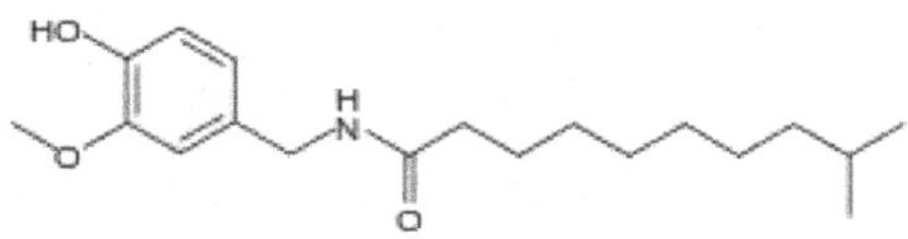
Homodihydrocapsaicin

The five compounds can be separated by using reversed phase C18 HPLC column. According to the polarity of the shortest carbon chain, nordihydrocapsaicin should be eluted first, followed by capsaicin, dihydrocapsaicin, homocapsaicin and homodihydrocapsaicin. By knowing the peak elution order, then based on the UV spectrum of the peaks, you can identify each of the capsaicinoids peaks. According to the molecular structure above, the UV spectrums and the sensitivities of all capsaicinoids should be very close. In the actual test, a single capsaicin standard is used to identify and quantify other capsainoids. The content of each capsaicinoids is corrected using the molecular weight. Adding all capsaicinoids measured together will determine the total capsainoids.

(i) *Test procedure*

Preparation of standard solution — Accurately weigh about 5 mg of standard capsaicin, transfer it to a 100 ml volumetric flask, add about 60 ml of methanol to dissolve the standard, then fill methanol to 100 ml volume, mix well. Further dilutions with methanol can be made if needed.

Preparation of sample solution — If the sample is an extract or product containing an extract, weigh a certain amount of sample containing about 15 mg capsainoides, transfer it to a 100 ml volumetric flask, and add 10 ml of water. Sonicate for 5 min, add 60 ml of ethanol, and then sonicate for another 5 min. After cooling add methanol to the volume. After shaking, centrifuge (10,000 r/min) for 5 min, the top clear solution can be directly injected. If necessary, further dilutions can be made with methanol and then injected.

If the sample is chili or chili powder, weigh a certain amount of sample containing about 15 mg capsainoids, transfer it to a 200 ml volumetric flask, accurately add 90 ml of sodium acetate saturated 95% ethanol solution, and put in a 60°C water bath. Stir with a magnetic rod for 5 h. After cooling, accurately add 10 ml of methanol, shake well and centrifuge (10,000 r/min) for 5 min. Upper-level solution can be injected directly. If needed the solution can also be diluted with methanol before injection.

(ii) *HPLC conditions*

Column: Phenomenex Luna C18 (2) 5 μm 4.6 × 250 mm 100A
Flow rate: 1.0 mL/min
Injection volume: 10 μL
UV wavelength: 282 nm
Mobile phase A: Nano pure water
Mobile phase B: Acetonitrile
Mobile phase C: Methanol

A%	B%	C%
60	20	20 Isocratic

Run time: 25 min

(iii) *Results and calculation*

$$Individual\ capsaicinoid(\%) = \frac{Aa \times Wstand \times Vsam \times R \times 100\%}{As \times Vstd \times Wsam}$$

or

$$Individual\ capsaicinoid\ (mg/unit) = \frac{Aa \times Wsand \times Vsam \times R \times UW}{As \times Vstd \times Wsam}$$

Here

Aa = Peak area of corresponding capsaicinoid in sample solution
As = Peak area of capsaicin standard
Wsand = Weight of capsaicin standard (mg)
Wsam = Weight of sample (mg)
Vstd = Total volume of standard solution (ml)
Vsam = Total volume of sample solution (ml)
UW = Unit weight (mg/unit)
R = Molecular weight correction factors

Capsaicin MW: 305.4
Non-dihydrocapsaicin MW: 293.4, (R) = 293.4/305.4 = 0.961
Dihydrocapsaicic MW: 307.4, (R) = 307.4/305.4 = 1.01
Homocapsaicin MW: 319.4, (R) = 319.4/305.4 = 1.05
Homodihydrocasaticin MW: 321.5, (R) = 321.5/305.4 = 1.06

Total capsaincinoids = Sum of individual capsaicinoid

4.16 Test Method for Icariins and Epimedins in Epimedium

The active ingredients of epimedium are epimedosids and epimedins. Icariin and epimedin C are the main components.

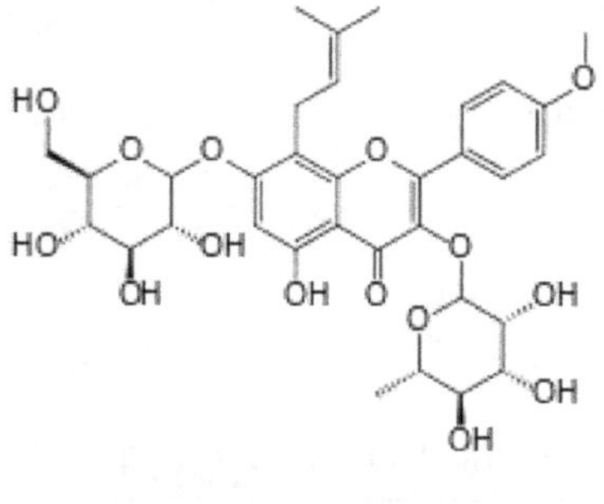

Icariin

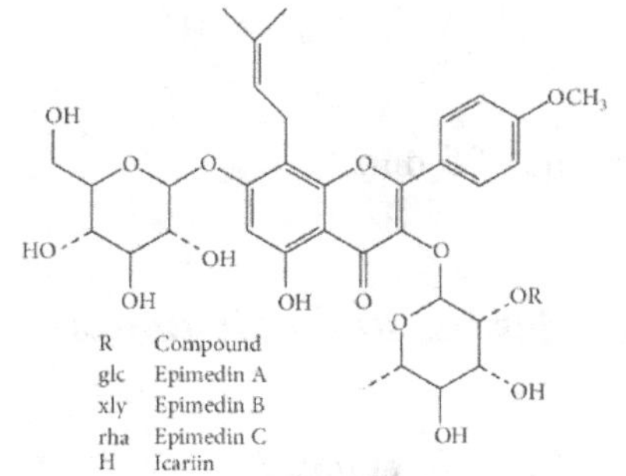

Epimedins

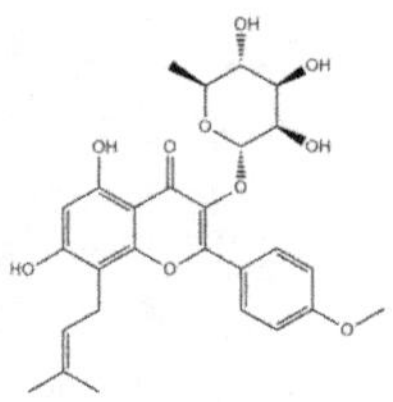

Epimedoside A

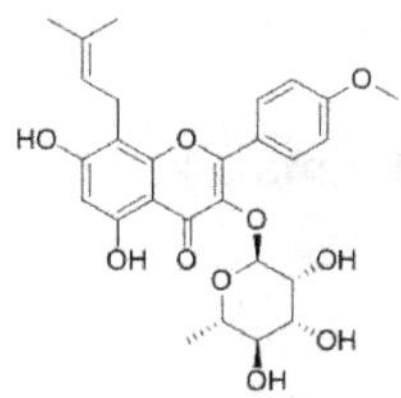

BaohuosideII

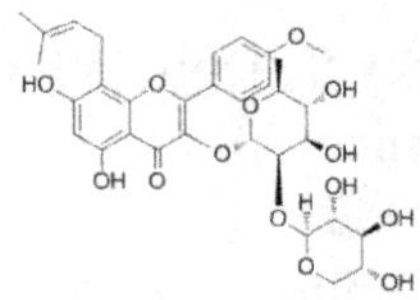

Sagittatoside B

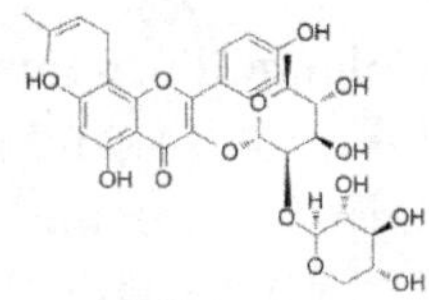

Icarisoside C

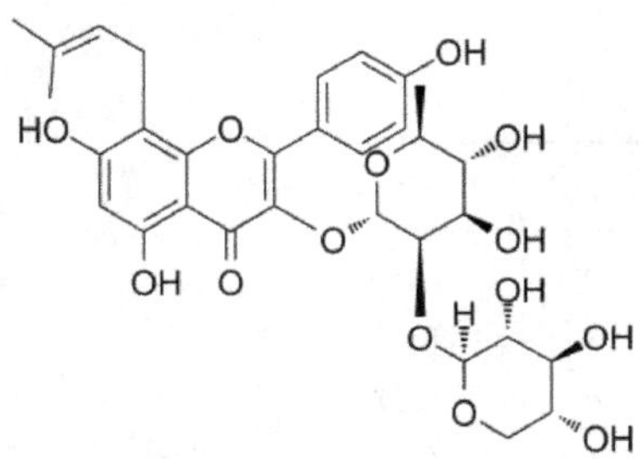

Icarisoside F

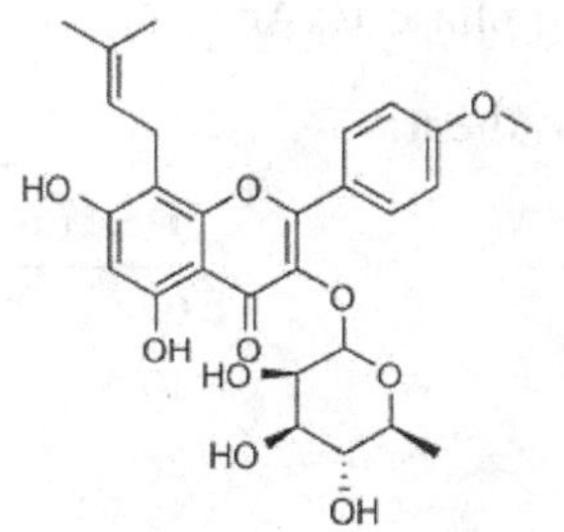

Baohuoside I

From the aforementioned molecular structures it can be seen that the active ingredients of epimedium are relatively non-polar compounds, and can be separated and quantified by reversed phase chromatography.

(i) *Test procedure*

Preparation of standard solution — Accurately weigh about 5 mg of icariin standard, transfer it to a 25 ml of volumetric flask, add methanol, sonicate until all standard dissolved. Then add methanol to volume, and shake well. If needed, further dilutions can be made with methanol.

Preparation of sample solution — Weigh a certain amount of sample containing about 10 mg of icariin, transfer it to 50 ml volumetric flask, add 5 ml of water, and sonicate for 5 min. Add 30 ml of ethanol, sonicate 10 min for extract materials; or 40 min for epimedium powder. Cool to room temperature, add methanol to volume, shake and mix well, then centrifuge (10,000 r/min) for 5 min. Take the top clear solution for injection. If necessary, methanol can be used to make further dilutions.

(ii) *HPLC conditions*

Column: Phenomenex Synergi 250 × 4.6 mm, 4 μm,
Flow rate: 1.0 mL/min
Injection volume: 10 μL
UV wavelength: 272 nm
Mobile phase A: 0.1% phosphoric acid in water
Mobile phase B: Acetonitrile

Gradient:

Time (min)	A%	B%
0	80	20
10	75	25
26	62	38
38	55	45
39.5	55	45
40.0	80	20
46.0	80	20 Finish

(iii) *Results and calculation*

According to molecular structures, all icariin and epimedins are flavonoid glycosides, so the UV spectrums and the sensitivity should be similar. Therefore, you can use a single icariin standard to identify and quantify all the compounds combine shown in Figures 4.12 and 4.13. The calculated results can be corrected by molecular weight.

$$\textit{Individual}\ \text{epimedosids/epimedins}\ (\%) = \frac{Aa \times Wstand \times Vsam \times R \times 100\%}{As \times Vstd \times Wsam}$$

or

$$\textit{Individual}\ \text{epimedosids/epimedins}\ (mg/unit) = \frac{Aa \times Wsand \times Vsam \times R \times UW}{As \times Vstd \times Wsam}$$

Here

Aa = Peak area of corresponding in epimedosids/epimedins in sample solution

As = Peak area of icariin standard
Wsand = Weight of icariin standard (mg)
Wsam = Weight of sample (mg)
Vstd = Total volume of standard solution (ml)
Vsam = Total volume of sample solution (ml)
UW = Unit weight (mg/unit)
R = Molecular correction factors

Total epimedosids/epimedins = Sum of individual epimedosids and epimedins.

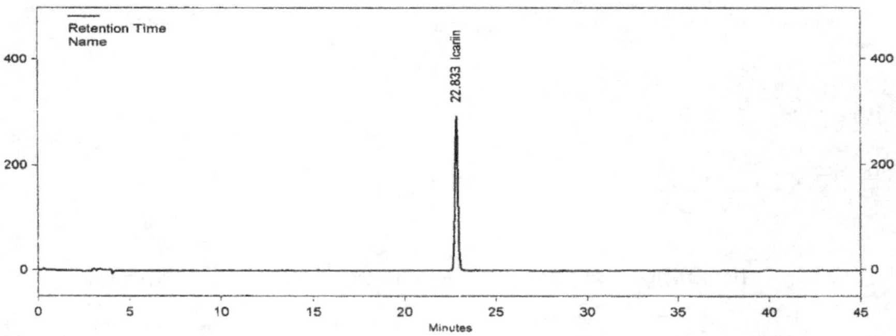

Figure 4.12: Icariin chromatogram.

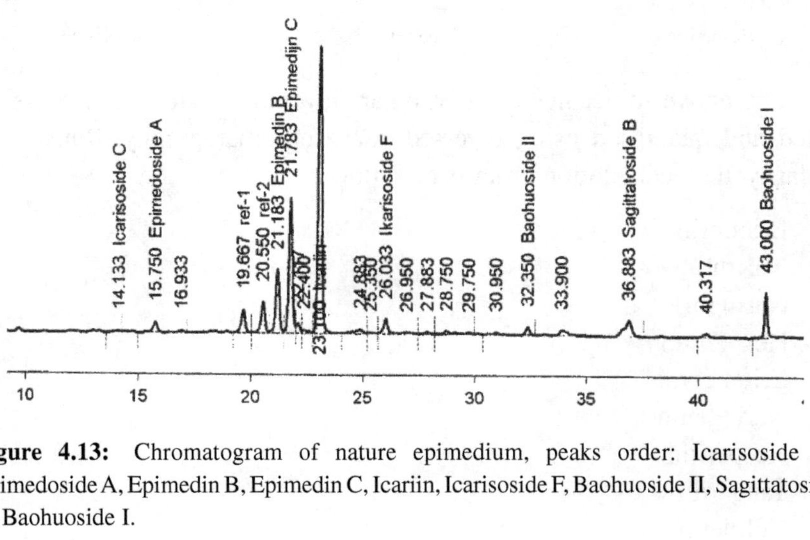

Figure 4.13: Chromatogram of nature epimedium, peaks order: Icarisoside C, Epimedoside A, Epimedin B, Epimedin C, Icariin, Icarisoside F, Baohuoside II, Sagittatoside B, Baohuoside I.

4.17 Citribioflavonoids Test Method

There are more than 10 known citrus bioflavonoids. This test method is able to identify and quantify nine of the citrus bioflavonoids including eriocitrin, narirutin, naringin, hesperidin, hesperitin, eriodictyol, naringenin, nobiletin and tangeritin.

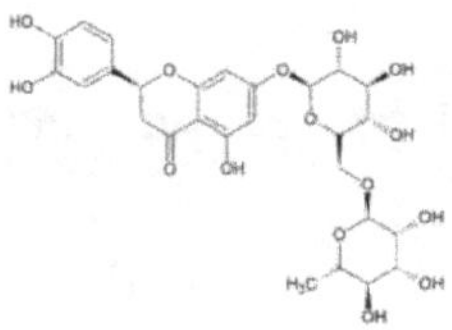

Eriocitrin

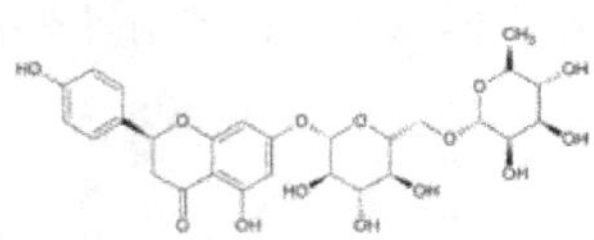

Narirutin

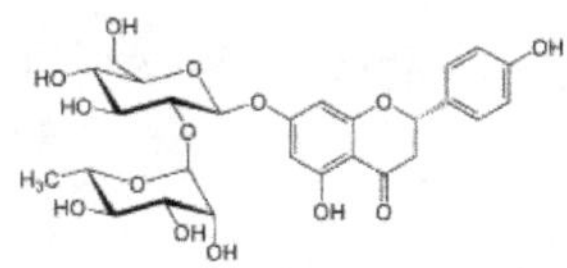

Naringin

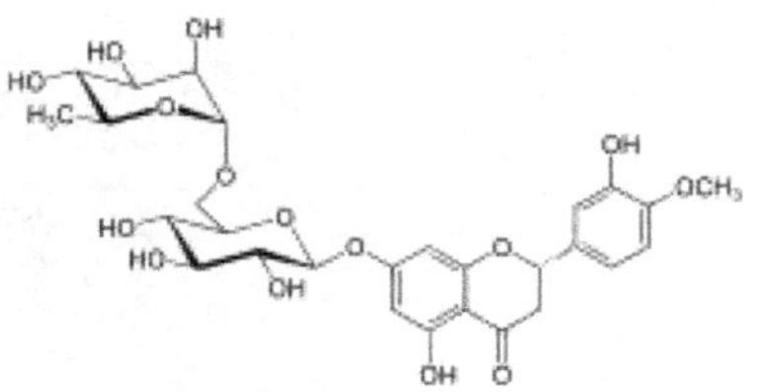

Hesperidin

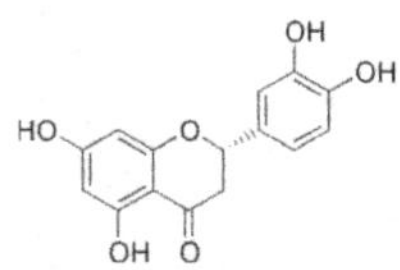

Eriodictyol

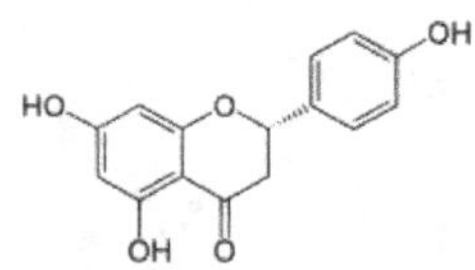

Naringenin

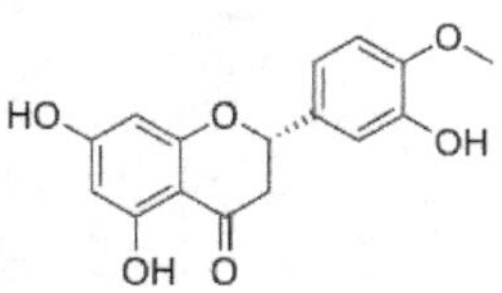

Hesperitin

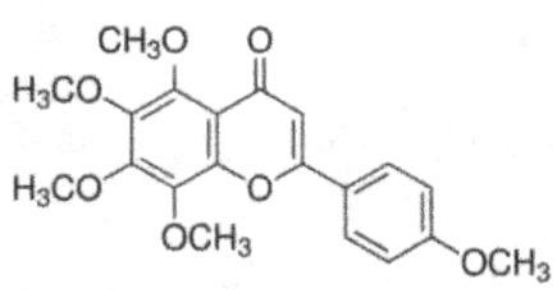

Tangeritin

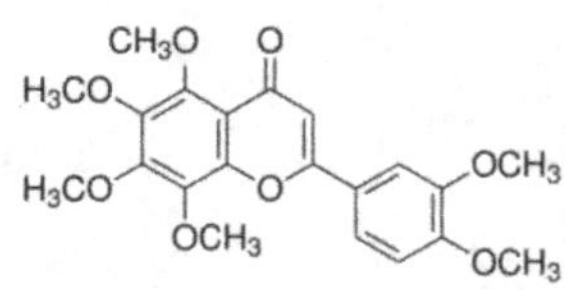

Nobiletin

The above molecules are non-polar flavonoids, which can be separated and quantified using reversed phase chromatography. Ranked by polarity, the peak elution order is as follows:

Eriocitrin
Narirutin
Naringin
Hesperidin
Eriodictyol
Naringenin
Hesperitin
Tangeritin
Nobiletin

(i) *Test procedure*

Preparation of standard solution — Accurately weigh about 2.5 mg of each naringin, eriodictyol, hesperitin, tangeritin, and nobiletin, respectively, transfer to individual 10 ml volumetric flasks, and add 3 ml of dimethyl sulfoxide/methanol (50/50) in each flask. Sonicate until all standards are dissolved, add methanol to volume, and shake well. In addition, accurately weigh 25 mg of hesperidin, transfer to a 50 ml volumetric flask, add 15 ml of dimethyl sulfoxide/methanol (50/50)/methanol, and sonicate to dissolve. Add methanol to the volume, and shake well.

Transfer 1 ml of naringin, eriodictyol, hesperitin, tangeritin and nobiletin stock solutions to a 50 ml volumetric flask, then add 5 ml of hesperidin stock solution, fill with methanol to volume, shake and mix well. The standard solution is ready for injection.

Preparation of sample solution — Accurately weigh a certain amount of ground sample containing about 10 mg of the total citrus bioflavonoids, transfer it to 100 ml of volumetric flask, add 30 ml of dimethyl sulfoxide/methanol (50/50), and sonicate for 20 min. Cool to room temperature, add methanol to volume, shake and mix well, then centrifuge (10,000 r/min) for 5 min. The clear solution can be injected.

(ii) *UPLC conditions*

Column: Acquity HSS T3 C18 100 × 2.1 mm
Floe rate: 0.5 ml/min
Injection volume: 2 μL
UV wave length: 280 nm
Mobile phase A: 0.1% phosphoric acid in nano pure water
Mobile phase B: Acetonitrile

Gradient:

Time (min)	A%	B%
0	82	18
4	58	30
9.0	30	70
9.0–9.8	30	70
9.8–10.0	82	18
12.0	82	18 Finish

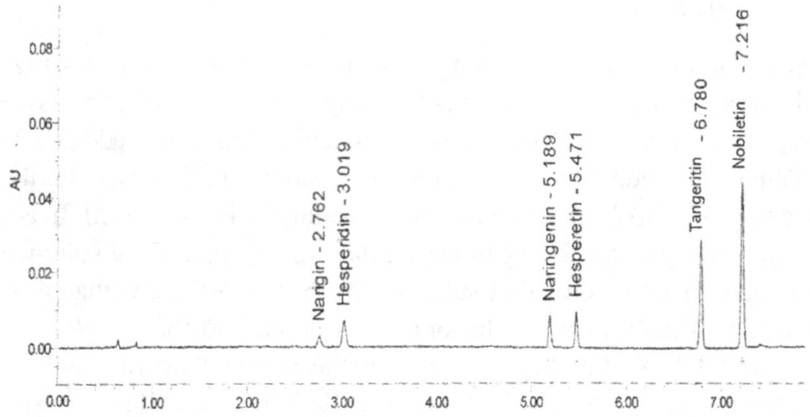

Figure 4.14: UPLC chromatogram of citrus bioflavonoids.

(iii) *Results and calculation*

$$Individual\,citrus\,bioflavonoid\ (\%) = \frac{Aa \times Wstand \times Vsam \times 100\%}{As \times Vstd \times Wsam}$$

or

$$Individual\,citrus\,bioflavonoid\ (mg/unit) = \frac{Aa \times Wsand \times Vsam \times UW}{As \times Vstd \times Wsam}$$

Here
Aa = Peak area of corresponding citrus bioflavonoid in sample solution
As = Peak area of corresponding citrus bioflavonoid in standard solution
Wsand = Weight of corresponding citrus bioflavonoid standard (mg)
Wsam = Weight of sample (mg)
Vstd = Total volume of standard solution (ml)
Vsam = Total volume of sample solution (ml)
UW = Unit weight (mg/unit)

Calculation for citrus bioflavonoids without standards:
Eriocitrin, narirutin and eriodictyol can be calculated as hesperitin followed by molecule correction.

$$Individual\,citrus\,bioflavonoid\ (\%) = \frac{Aa \times Wstand \times Vsam \times 100\% \times R}{As \times Vstd \times Wsam}$$

or

$$Individual\ citrus\ bioflavonoid\ (mg/unit) = \frac{Aa \times Wsand \times Vsam \times UW \times R}{As \times Vstd \times Wsam}$$

Here
Aa = Peak area of Eriocitrin/narirutin/eriodictyol in sample solution
As = Peak area of hesperitin in standard solution
Wsand = Weight of hesperitin standard (mg)
Wsam = Weight of sample (mg)
Vstd = Total volume of standard solution (ml)
Vsam = Total volume of sample solution (ml)
UW = Unit weight (mg/unit)
R = molecule correction factor
eriocitrin/hesperitin: 596.5/302.28 = 1.97
narirutin/hesperitin: 580.5/302.28 = 1.92
eriodictyol/hesperitin: 288.25/302.28 = 0.954

Total citrus bioflavonoids = Sum of individual citrus bioflavonoid

4.18 Test Method for Aucubin

Aucubin is an iridoid golyside extracted from eucommia ulmoides bark. Its main function is as an anti-inflammatory and a pain reliever.

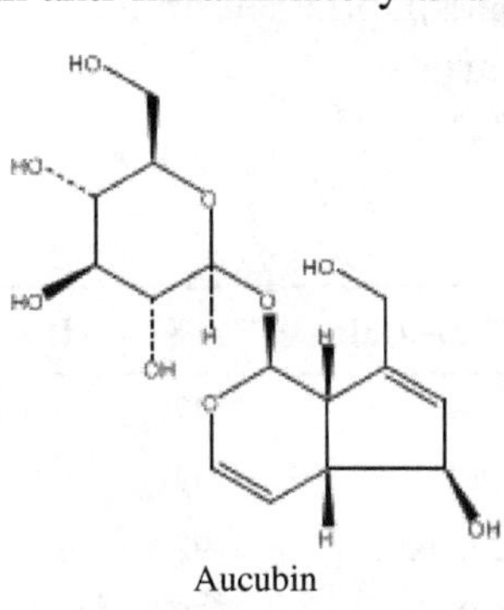

Aucubin

Aucubin is a relatively non-polar compound with two unconjugated double bonds, and it has a limited UV response. HPLC or UPLC with PDA detector can be used to analyze aucubin in a relative high concentration solution.

(i) *Test procedure*

Solvent A prepare — To 250 ml of methanol add 750 ml nano pure water, sonicate for 10 min.

Preparation of standard solution — Accurately weigh about 10 mg of aucubin standard, transfer to a 50 ml volumetric flask, add 30 ml of solvent A, sonicate until completely dissolved. Fill to volume with solvent A, shake and mix well. The solution is ready for injection.

Preparation of sample solution — Weigh a certain amount of sample containing about 20 mg of aucubin, transfer to 100 ml volumetric flask, add 60 ml of solvent A, and sonicate 10 min or extract materials materials or for eucommia ulmoides bark, sonicate for 50 min. Cool to room temperature, add solvent A to volume, shake and mix well. Then centrifuge (10,000 r/min) for 5 min, and take the clear solution for injection.

(ii) *UPLC conditions*

Column: Acquity HSS T3 C18, 1.8 μm, 2.1 × 150 mm
Flow rate: 0.4 ml/min
Injection volume: 2μL
UV wavelength: 210 nm
Mobile phase A: 0.1% phosphoric acid in nano pure water
Mobile phase B: Acetonitrile
Column temperature: 45°C

Gradient:

Time (min)	A%	B%
0	97	3
2.0	97	3
2.0–6.0	92	8
6.0–6.8	50	50
6.8–7.8	50	50
7.8–8.0	97	3
8.0–10.0	97	3

(iii) *Result and calculation*

$$Aucubin\ (\%) = \frac{Aa \times Wstand \times Vsam \times 100\%}{As \times Vstd \times Wsam}$$

or

$$Aucubin\ (mg/unit) = \frac{Aa \times Wsand \times Vsam \times UW}{As \times Vstd \times Wsam}$$

Here
Aa = Peak area of aucubin in sample solution
As = Peak area of aucubin in standard solution
Wsand = Weight of aucubin standard (mg)
Wsam = Weight of sample (mg)
Vstd = Total volume of standard solution (ml)
Vsam = Total volume of sample solution (ml)
UW = Unit weight (mg/unit)

4.19 Test Method for Hawthorn

This method can separately and quantitatively measure the three active ingredients found in hawthorn, vitexin, Isovitexin and Vitexin-2-O-rhamniside.

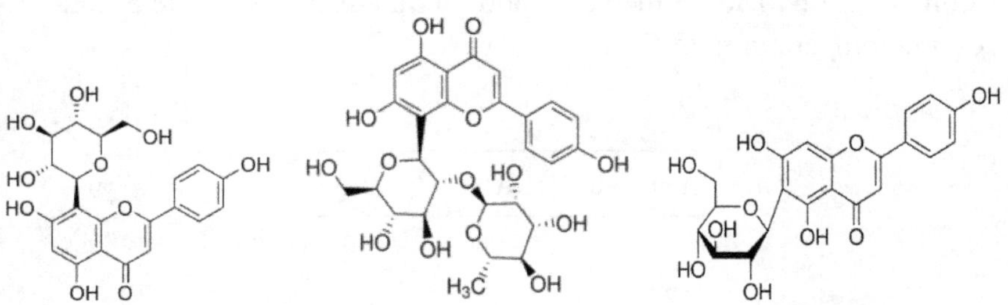

Vitein   Vitexin-2-O-rhamniside   Isovitexin

(i) *Test procedure*

Preparation of standard solution — Accurately weigh about 5 mg of vitexin, isovitexin and vitexin-2-O-rhamniside and transfer it to 50 ml volumetric flask. Add 30 ml of methanol, sonicate for 5 min, cool, and add methanol to the volume. The solution can be injected.

Preparation of sample solution (for extract) — Accurately weigh a certain amount ground sample containing 5 mg of any above compound. Transfer it to 50 ml of volumetric flask, add 10 ml of water then sonicate for 5 min. Add 30 ml of ethanol and sonicate for another 10 min. After cooling add methanol to the volume, shake well, and centrifuge (10,000 rpm) for 5 min. Take the clear solution for injection.

Preparation of sample solution (for hawthorn powder) — Accurately weigh a certain amount ground sample containing 5 mg of any above compound, and transfer it to a 100 ml volumetric flask. Add exactly 50 ml of methanol, cap the flask, and sonicate for 40 min. Cool to room temperature, centrifuge (10,000 rpm) for 5 min, and take the clear solution for injection.

(ii) *UPLC conditions*

Column: Acquity UPLC® BEH C18, 1.7 μm, 2.1 × 100 mm
Flow rate: 0.4 mL/min
Injection volume: 1 μL
UV wavelength: 340 nm
Mobile phase A: 0.1% phosphoric acid in water
Mobile phase B: 130 ml methanol add 70 ml ethanol, sonicate 5 min
Column temperature: 45°C

Gradient:

Time (min)	A%	B%
0	90	10
0–7.0	75	25
7.0–7.2	75	25
7.2–7.8	40	60
7.8–8.0	90	10
10.0	90	10 Finish

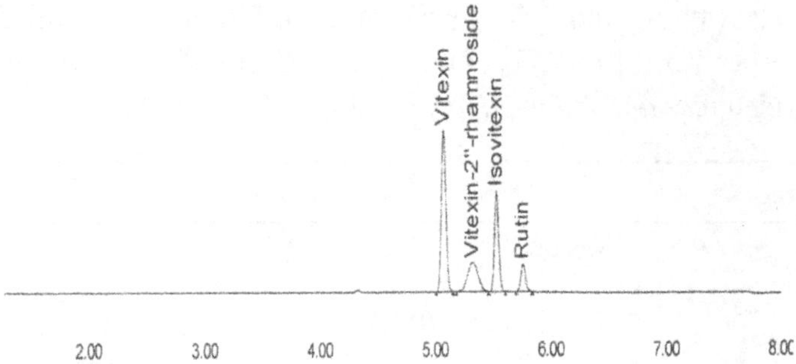

Figure 4.15: UPLC chromatogram of hawthorn.

(iii) *Results and calculation*

$$Individual\ active\ compound\ (\%) = \frac{Aa \times Wstand \times Vsam \times 100\%}{As \times Vstd \times Wsam}$$

or

$$Individual\ active\ compound\ (mg/unit) = \frac{Aa \times Wsand \times Vsam \times UW}{As \times Vstd \times Wsam}$$

Here
Aa = Peak area of corresponding active compound in sample solution
As = Peak area of corresponding active compound in standard solution
Wsand = Weight of corresponding standard (mg)
Wsam = Weight of sample (mg)
Vstd = Total volume of standard solution (ml)
Vsam = Total volume of sample solution (ml)
UW = Unit weight (mg/unit)

4.20 Test Method for Monacolins in Red Yeast Rice

Red yeast rice contains a variety of monacolins, which may help lower cholesterol and serum lipids. Monacolin K is a prescription drug, lovastatin, for lowering cholesterol. Monacolins have K, J, M, ×, etc., all have similar efficacies. The following table lists the molecular structure, molecular weight and UV spectrum of different monacolins. This is an excerpt from Li, Y.G., Zhang, F., Wang, Z.T. *et al. Journal of Pharmaceutical and Biomedical*, 35(2004), 1101–1112.

Structure	Name	R	MW	UV(λ_{xxx})
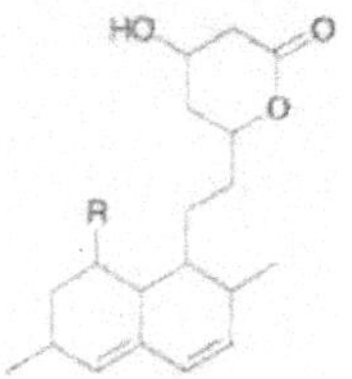	1. Monacolin K (MK)	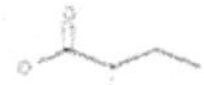	404	230, 237, 246
	2. Monacolin J (MJ)	OH	320	230, 237, 247
	3. Monacolin L (ML)	H	304	230, 237, 247
	4. Monacolin X (MX)	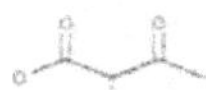	418	230, 237, 247
	5. Monacolin M (MM)	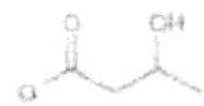	406	
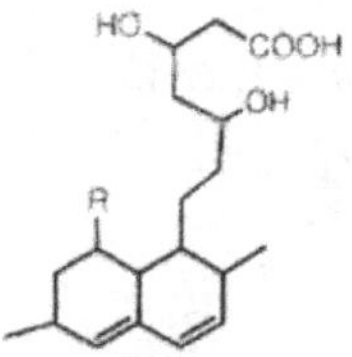	1a. MK acid form (MKA)	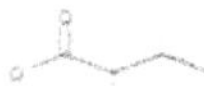	422	
	2a. MJ acid form (MJA)	OH	338	
	3a. ML acid form (MLA)	H	322	
	4a. MX acid form (MXA)	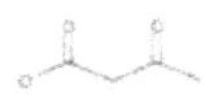	436	
	5a. MM acid form (MMA)	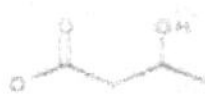	424	

(i) *Test procedure*

Solvent A preparation — To 250 ml of water add 750 ml of ethanol, shake well.

Preparation of standard solution — Accurately weight about 5 mg of monacolin K (Lovastatin), transfer it to a 50 ml volumetric flask, add about 30 ml of solvent A, vortex until it is all dissolved. Then fill the flask with solvent A to volume, and shake well. This solution can be injected. If necessary, further dilutions can be made with solvent A.

Preparation of sample solution — Weigh a certain amount of ground sample containing about 5 mg of monacolin K. Transfer to a 100 ml of volumetric flask, and quantitatively transfer 50 ml solvent A to the flask. Cap the flask and sonicated it for 90 min, then cool to room temperature. Next, centrifuge (10,000 rpm) for 5 min, and take the clear solution for injection. If necessary, further dilutions can be made using solvent A.

(ii) *UPLC conditions*

Column: Acuity UPLC®, BEH C18, 1.7 μm, 2.1 × 150 mm
Flow rate: 0.4 mL/min
Injection volume: 2 μL
UV wavelength: 237 nm
Mobile phase A: 0.1% phosphoric acid in nano pure water
Mobile phase B: Acetonitrile
Column temperature: 45°C

Gradient:

Time (min)	A%	B%
0	75	25
0–13.0	20	80
13.0–15.5	10	90
15.0–15.8	10	90
15.8–16.0	75	25
16.0–18.0	75	25 End

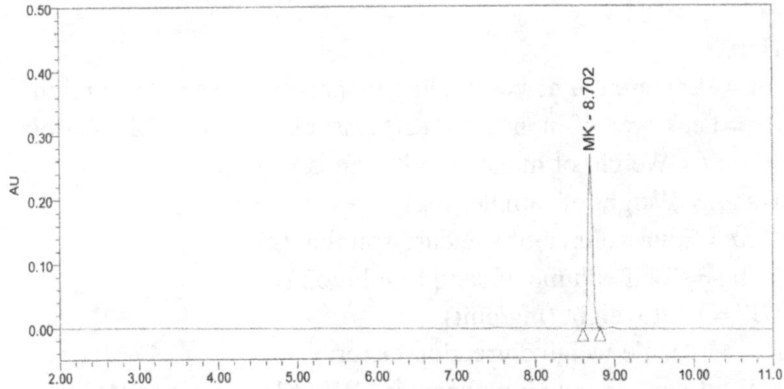

Figure 4.16: Chromatogram of lovastatin.

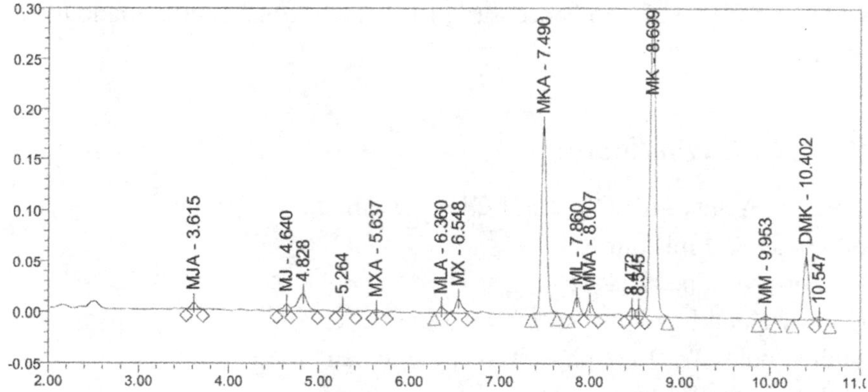

Figure 4.17: Chromatogram of red yeast rice.

(iii) *Results and calculation*

Each monacolin is calculated as monacolin K, followed by a molecular weight correction.

$$Individual\ monacolin\ (\%) = \frac{Aa \times Wstand \times Vsam \times 100\% \times R}{As \times Vstd \times Wsam}$$

or

$$Individual\ monacolin\ (mg/unit) = \frac{Aa \times Wsand \times Vsam \times UW \times R}{As \times Vstd \times Wsam}$$

Here
Aa = Peak area of corresponding monacolin in sample solution
As = Peak area of monacolin K (lovastatin) in standard solution
Wsand = Weight of monacolin K standard (mg)
Wsam = Weight of sample (mg)
Vstd = Total volume of standard solution (ml)
Vsam = Total volume of sample solution (ml)
UW = Unit weight (mg/unit)
R = Molecule weigh correction factor:
MW of corresponding monacolin/MW of lovastatin (404)

Total monacolins = Sum of each individual monacolin measured

4.21 Test Method for Milk Thistle

Silymrin is the main components of milk thistle, contains, silychristin, silydianin, silbinin A, silbinin B, isosilbinin A and isosilybinin B.

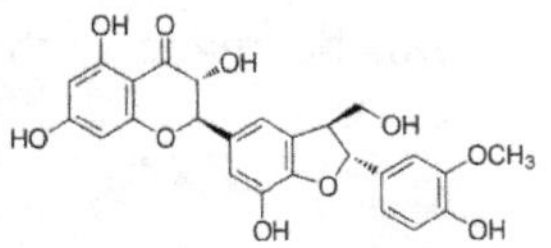
Silychristin

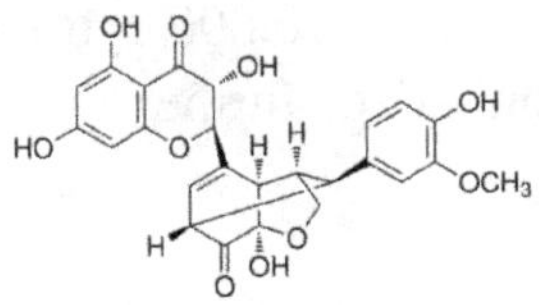
Silydianin

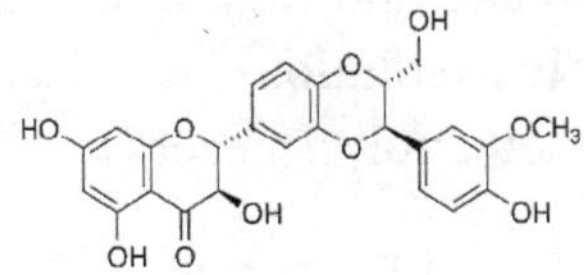
Silbinin A

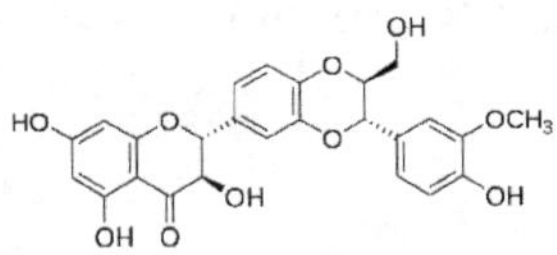
Silbinin B

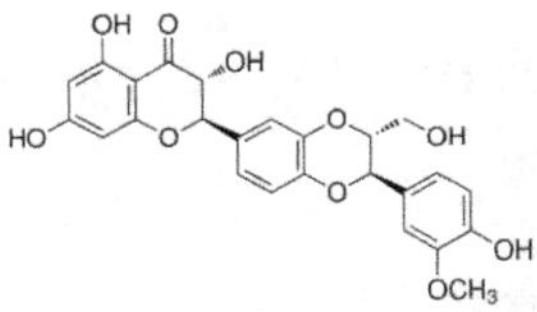
Isosilbinin A

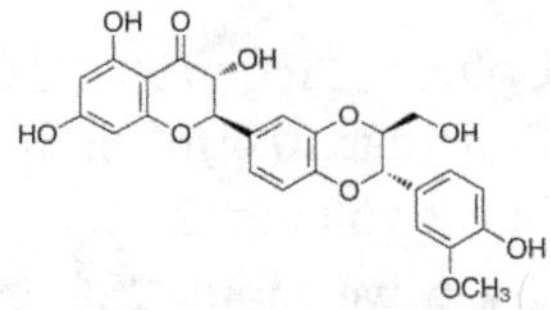
Isosilybinin B

The above compounds are relatively non-polar compounds and can be separated and measured by using HPLC C18 chromatography. Silbinin A and silbinin B are a pair of stereoisomers that can also be separated by C18 column.

(i) *Test procedure*

Preparation of standard solution (I) — Accurately weigh about 10 mg of silbinin standard, transfer it to a 50 ml of volumetric flask, and add about 30 ml of methanol. Vortex until it is all dissolved, then add methanol to the volume, and shake well. Label this solution as "Silbinins standard solution". If necessary, further dilutions can be made with methanol.

Preparation of standard solution (II) — Accurately weigh about 20 mg of silymrin standard, transfer it to another 50 ml volumetric flask, and add about 30 ml of methanol. Vortex and sonicate until all of the standard is dissolved. Fill with methanol to volume, shake well and label as "Silymrin standard solution". If necessary, further dilutions can be made with methanol.

Preparation of sample solution — Accurately weigh a certain amount of ground sample containing about 10 mg of silbinin or 20 mg of silmyrin. Transfer it to a 50 ml of volumetric flask, add 10 ml of water, and sonicate for 5 min. Then add 30 ml of ethanol and sonicate for another 10 min for extract materials, or milk thistle powder, sonicate for 40 min. Cool to room temperature and add methanol to the mark. Shake and mix well, centrifuge (10,000 rpm) for 5 min, and take the clear solution for injection. Also, further dilutions can be made with methanol, if necessary.

(ii) *UPLC conditions*

Column: Acquity UPLC®, HSS T3 C18, 1.8 μm, 2.1 × 150 mm
Flow rate: 0.4 mL/min
Inject volume: 2 μL
UV wavelength: 286 nm
Mobile phase A: 0.1% phosphoric acid in water
Mobile phase B: Acetonitrile
Column temperature: 45C°

Gradient:

Time (min)	A%	B%
0	85	15
0–5.0	75	25
5.0–11	45	55
11–12.5	45	55
12.5–13.0	85	15
13.0–16.0	85	15 Finish

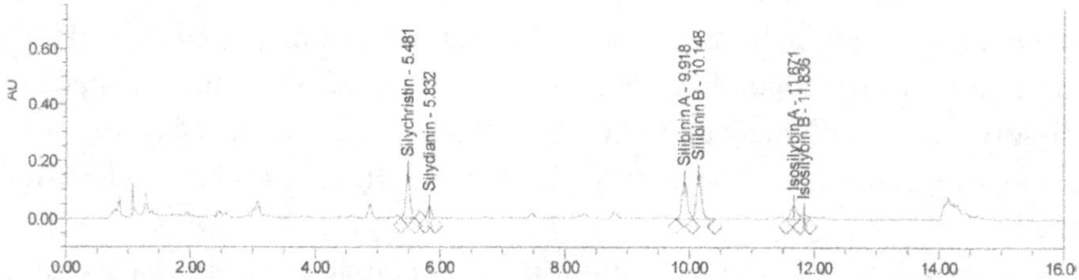

Figure 4.18: UPLC chromatogram of milk thistle.

(ii) *Results and calculation*

Calculation (1):

Use standard solution (I) as reference standard, compare peak area of each individual silymarin with peak area of silybinin standard, and calculate the content of each silmyrin component, adjusted by molecular weight. Add all individual silymarin content together get total silymarins.

$$Individual\,silmyrin\ (\%) = \frac{Aa \times Wstand \times Vsam \times 100\% \times R}{As \times Vstd \times Wsam}$$

or

$$Individual\,silmyrin\ (mg/unit) = \frac{Aa \times Wsand \times Vsam \times UW \times R}{As \times Vstd \times Wsam}$$

Here

Aa = Peak area of corresponding silymarin in sample solution

As = Peak area of silbinin in standard solution

Wsand = Weight of silbinin standard (mg)

Wsam = Weight of sample (mg)

Vstd = Total volume of standard solution (ml)

Vsam = Total volume of sample solution (ml)

UW = Unit weight (mg/unit)

R = Molecule weigh correction factor

Total silmyrin content = Sum of each individual silmyrin concentration.

Calculation (2):

Use total peak areas of silymrin in sample solution to compare with the total peak area of silymrin in standard solution (II), calculate the total silmyrin content.

$$Total\,silmyrin\ (\%) = \frac{Aa \times Wstand \times Vsam \times 100\%}{As \times Vstd \times Wsam}$$

or

$$Total\,silmyrin\ (mg/unit) = \frac{Aa \times Wsand \times Vsam \times UW}{As \times Vstd \times Wsam}$$

Here
Aa = Total peak area of silymarin in sample solution
As = Total peak area of silymarin in standard solution
Wsand = Weight of silymarin standard (mg)
Wsam = Weight of sample (mg)
Vstd = Total volume of standard solution (ml)
Vsam = Total volume of sample solution (ml)
UW = Unit weight (mg/unit)

Note: All the peaks should be intergraded at 286 nm, and each peak must be confirmed by UV spectrum.

4.22 Determination of Eleutheroside B and E in Siberian Ginseng

The active components of Siberian ginseng are eleutheroside A, B, C, D, E, F and G, eleutheroside B and E are the main components.

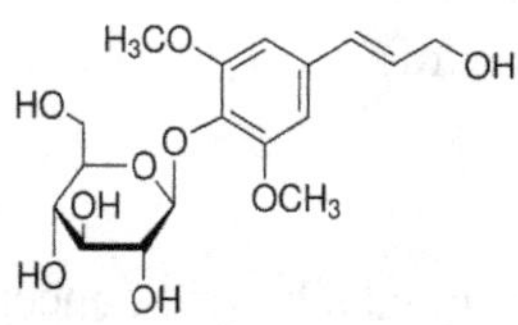

Eleutherosid B

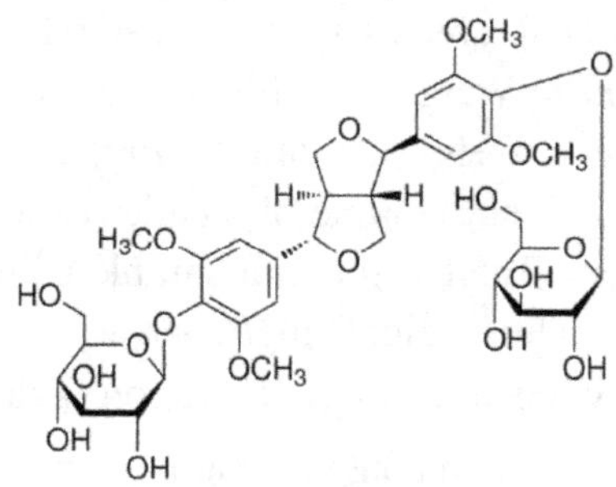

Eleutheroside E

The molecule structure of eleutheroside B and E are quite different, C18 HPLC column can be used to separate and quantify them.

(i) *Test procedure*

Preparation of standard solution — Accurately weigh approximately 5 mg of eleutheroside B and 5 mg of E, and transfer it to a 100 ml volumetric flask. Add 60 ml of methanol, sonicate until the standards are completely dissolved, then add methanol to the mark, shake and mix well. This solution is ready for injection. If necessary, can make further dilutions with methanol.

Preparation of sample solution — Accurately weigh a certain amount of ground sample containing about 5 mg of eleutheroside B or E. Transfer it to a 100 ml volumetric flask, and add 10 ml of water. Sonicate this for 5 min, then add 50 ml methanol, sonicate for another 10 min for extract sample, or 40 min for Siberian ginseng powder. Cool to room temperature, fill with methanol to mark, shake and mix well. Then centrifuge (10,000 rpm) for 5 min. The clear solution is ready for injection. If necessary, further dilutions can be made with methanol.

(ii) *UPLC conditions*

Column: Acquity UPLC® HSS Ts C18 1.8 μm, 2.1 × 150 mm
Column temperature: 45°C
Flow rate: 0.4 ml/min
Injection volume: 2 μL
UV wavelength: 220 nm
Mobile phase A: 0.1% phosphoric acid in water
Mobile phase B: 0.1% phosphoric acid in acetonitrile

Gradient:

Time (min)	**A%**	**B%**
0	95	5
0–5.0	75	25
5.0–6.0	65	35
6.0–6.7	65	35
6.7–7.0	95	5
7.0–9.0	95	5 Finish

(iii) *Results and calculation*

$$Eleutheroside\ B/E\ (\%) = \frac{Aa \times Wstand \times Vsam \times 100\%}{As \times Vstd \times Wsam}$$

or

$$Eleutheroside\ B/E\ (mg/unit) = \frac{Aa \times Wsand \times Vsam \times UW}{As \times Vstd \times Wsam}$$

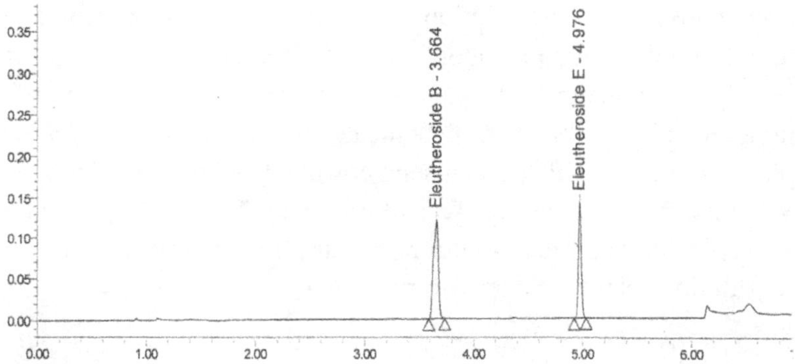

Figure 4.19: UPLC chromatogram of eleutheroside B and E.

Here

Aa = Peak area of eleutheroside B/E in sample solution

As = Peak area of eleutheroside B/E in standard solution

Wsand = Weight of eleutheroside B/E standard (mg)

Wsam = Weight of sample (mg)

Vstd = Total volume of standard solution (ml)

Vsam = Total volume of sample solution (ml)

UW = Unit weight (mg/unit)

Total eleutherosides% = Eleutherosids B% + Eleutherosids E%

4.23 Test Method for Organic Acids in Cranberry

Cranberry, strawberry, blueberry, raspberry, and other fruits contain organic acids. Cranberry mainly contains quinic acid, shikimic acid, malic acid and citric acid.

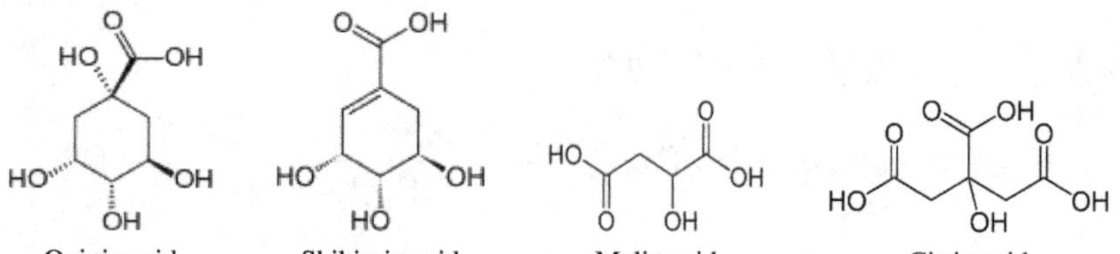

Quinic acid   Shikimic acid   Malic acid   Citric acid

In Chapter 1, Section 1.1.2 "Mobile phase application", the reduction of polarity of organic acids resulting in an increase in the retention time on reversed phase column, which facilitates the separation of compounds, was discussed. In general, the lower the pH of the mobile phase, the longer the retention time for organic acid analytes. Therefore, consider using a strong acid to prepare mobile phases, such as diluted trifluoroacetic acid or hydrochloric acid. However, the pH should not be less than 1 to protect the column from being hydrolyzed. If lowering the pH does not solve the interference problems, consider using ion pairs to extend the retention time. Adding strong alkalines like tetrabutyl ammonium salts into the mobile phase can be helpful.

(i) *Test procedure*

Preparation of shikimic acid stock solution — Accurately weigh about 10 mg of shikimic acid standard, transfer to 25 ml volumetric flask, add water to dissolve and fill to 25 ml. Shake, and mix the solution well, and label it as "Shikimic acid stock solution".

Preparation of standard solution — Accurately weigh about 10 mg of quinine acid, malic acid and citric acid standard, and transfer them to 100 ml volumetric flask. Then accurately transfer 1 ml of the shikimic acid stock solution into the 100 ml volumetric flask, add water to dissolve and fill to 100 ml with water. Shake and mix this well. The solution is ready for injection.

Preparation of sample solution — Weigh a certain amount of evenly mixed sample that contains about the same amount of organic acids as the standard solution. Transfer this to a 100 ml volumetric flask, add 60 ml of water and sonicate for 10 min for extract materials, or 40 min for berry samples. Cool to room temperature, fill water to the volume. Shakes and mix well. Then centrifuge (10,000 rpm) this for 5 min, and take the clear solution for injection.

(ii) *UPLC conditions*

Column: Acquity UPLC®, HSS T3, 1.8 μm, 2.1 × 150 mm
Flow rate: 0.4 mL/min
Injection volume: 2 μL

UV wavelength: 210 nm
Column temperature: 45°C
Mobile phase A: 0.1% hydrochloric in water, use potassium phosphate solution and diluted hydrochloric acid to adjust pH to 1.
Mobile phase B: Acetonitrile
Mobile phase A: Mobile phase B = 97:3

(iii) *Results and calculation*

$$Individual\ organic\ acid\ (\%) = \frac{Aa \times Wstand \times Vsam \times 100\%}{As \times Vstd \times Wsam}$$

or

$$Individual\ organic\ acid\ (mg/unit) = \frac{Aa \times Wsand \times Vsam \times UW}{As \times Vstd \times Wsam}$$

Here
Aa = Peak area of corresponding organic acid in sample solution
As = Peak area of corresponding organic acid in standard solution
Wsand = Weight of corresponding organic acid standard (mg)
Wsam = Weight of sample (mg)
Vstd = Total volume of standard solution (ml)
Vsam = Total volume of sample solution (ml)
UW = Unit weight (mg/unit)
Total organic acid content = The sum of each individual organic acid.

4.24 Determination of Baicalin and Baicalein in Huangqin by HPLC

Huangqi contains a variety of flavones and flavonoids, the main components are baicalin and baicalein. Baicalin is a glycoside of baicalein, so the UV spectrum of two compounds is similar. The baicalin molecule contains sugar, and is more polar than baicalein, so it will elute before baicalein with reversed phase HPLC column. This method uses a C18 column to separate baicalin, baicalein and other flavones.

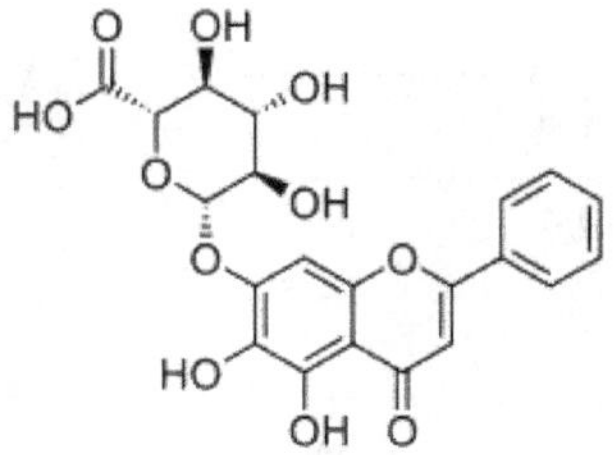

Baicalin

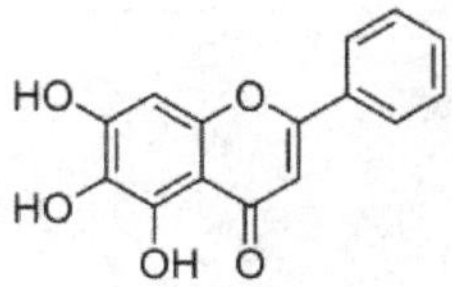

Baicalein

(i) *Test procedure*

Preparation of standard solution — Accurately weigh about 10 mg of baicalin and 2 mg of baicalein and transfer to a 100 ml volumetric flask. Add 60 ml of methanol, sonicate until the standards are completely dissolved, then add methanol to volume. Shake and mix well. Transfer 10 ml of the above solution to a 50 ml volumetric flask, dilute to volume with methanol, and mix well. This solution is ready for injection.

Preparation of sample solution — Weigh a certain amount of ground sample containing about 2 mg of baicalin, transfer it to a 100 ml volumetric flask, add 10 ml of water, and sonicate for 5 min. Add 50 ml ethanol, sonicate another 10 min for extract materials or 40 min for huangqin powder samples. After cooling, fill with methanol to the mark, shake well, and centrifuge (10,000 rpm) for 5 min. Take the clear solution for injection.

(ii) *UPLC conditions*

Column: Acquity UPLC®, BEH C18, 1.7 μm, 2.1 × 150 mm
Flow rate: 0.4 mL/min
Injection volume: 1 μL
UV wavelength: 275 nm
Mobile phase A: 0.1% phosphoric acid in water
Mobile phase B: Acetonitrile
Column temperature: 45°C

Gradient:

Time (min)	A%	B%
0	80	20
0–8.0	35	65
8.0–9.0	35	65
9.0–9.5	80	20
12.0	80	20 Finish

(iii) *Results and calculation*

$$Baicalin/baicalein(\%) = \frac{Aa \times Wstand \times Vsam \times 100\%}{As \times Vstd \times Wsam}$$

or

$$Baicalin/baicalein\ (mg/unit) = \frac{Aa \times Wsand \times Vsam \times UW}{As \times Vstd \times Wsam}$$

Here
Aa = Peak area of baicalin/baicalein in sample solution
As = Peak area of baicalin/baicalein in standard solution
Wsand = Weight of baicalin/baicalein standard (mg)
Wsam = Weight of sample (mg)

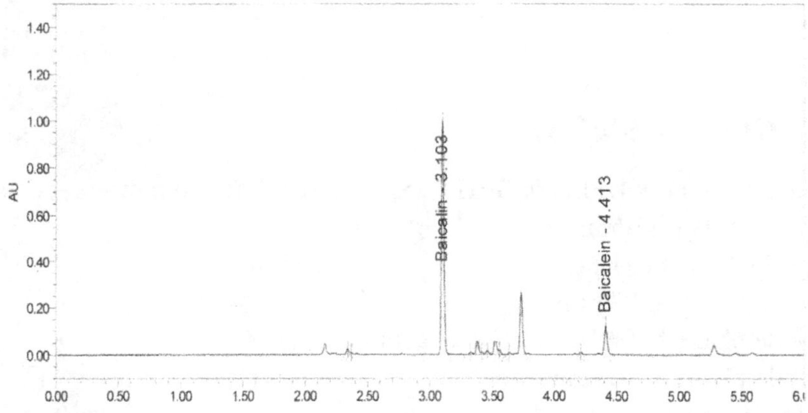

Figure 4.20: UPLC chromatogram of huangqin.

Vstd = Total volume of standard solution (ml)
Vsam = Total volume of sample solution (ml)
UW = Unit weight (mg/unit)

4.25 Test Method for Apigenin

Apigenin is found in many plans, and is a flavonol compound. According to the molecular structure, it is a relatively non-polar compound, with strong UV absorption. So, it can be determined by a reversed phase chromatography-PDA method.

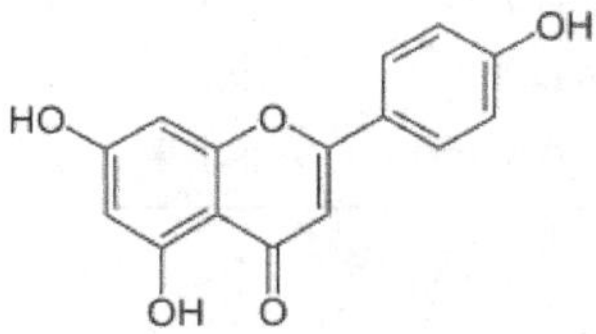

Apigenin

(i) *Test procedure*

Solvent 1 - Water/Methanol (30%/70%)

Preparation of standard solution — Accurately weigh about 5 mg of apigenin standard, transfer it to a 25 ml volumetric flask, add enough solvent 1 to dissolve the standard, fill to the mark with the same solvent, then mix well. Transfer 1 ml of the above solution to a 25 ml volumetric flask, fill with solvent 1 to mark, and shake well. The standard solution can be injected.

Preparation of sample solution — Weigh a certain amount of ground sample containing about 1 mg of apigenin, transfer it to a 100 ml volumetric flask, add 30 ml of solvent 1, and sonicate for 10 min. Then cool to room temperature, add solvent 1 to the mark, and shake and mix well. Centrifuge for 5 min (10,000 rpm). The clear solution can be injected.

(ii) *UPLC conditions*

Column: Acquity UPLC®, BEH C18, 1.7 μm, 2.1 × 150 mm
Flow rate: 0.4 mL/min

Injection volume: 2 μL
UV wavelength: 338 nm
Mobile phase A: 0.1% phosphoric acid in water
Mobile phase B: Acetonitrile
Column temperature: 45°C

Gradient:

Time (min)	A%	B%
0	80	20
0–6.0	40	60
6.0–6.8	40	60
6.8–7.0	80	20
7.0–9.0	80	20

(iii) *Results and calculation*

$$Apigenin\ (\%) = \frac{Aa \times Wstand \times Vsam \times 100\%}{As \times Vstd \times Wsam}$$

or

$$Apigenin\ (mg/unit) = \frac{Aa \times Wsand \times Vsam \times UW}{As \times Vstd \times Wsam}$$

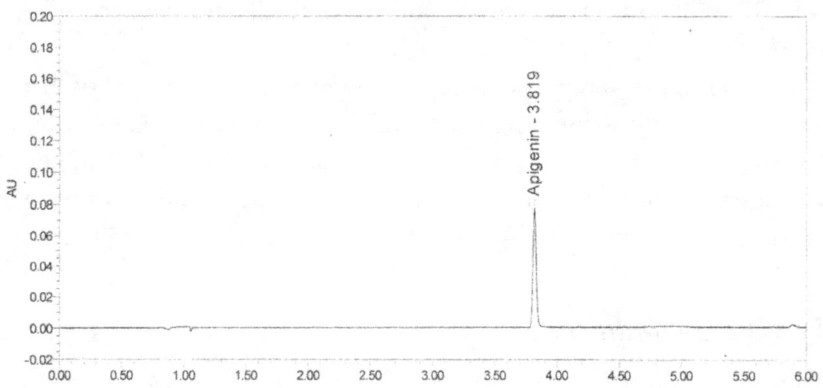

Figure 4.21: UPLC chromatogram of apigenin.

Here
Aa = Peak area of apigenin in sample solution
As = Peak area of apigenin in standard solution
Wsand = Weight of apigenin standard (mg)
Wsam = Weight of sample (mg)
Vstd = Total volume of standard solution (ml)
Vsam = Total volume of sample solution (ml)
UW= Unit weight (mg/unit)

4.26 Maca Test Method

Maca contains two sets of active ingredients: macaenes and macamides. It is difficult to get all of the individual standards of macaene and macamide. This method uses a known maca powder as a standard. The total peak area of macaenes in the sample is compared with the total area of macaenes in the standard material to calculate the content of macaene in the sample. The total peak area of the macamides in the sample is compared to the total area of macamides in the standard material to calculate the content of macamides in the sample.

Macamide has two groups, one is measured at 275 nm and the other at 315 nm. The sum of these two groups of macamides is the amount of total macamides in the sample. Macaene is measured at 210 nm. Generally, the total content of macaenes and macamides in maca powder will not exceed 1%.

The following shows one of the macaene molecules and one of the macamide molecules.

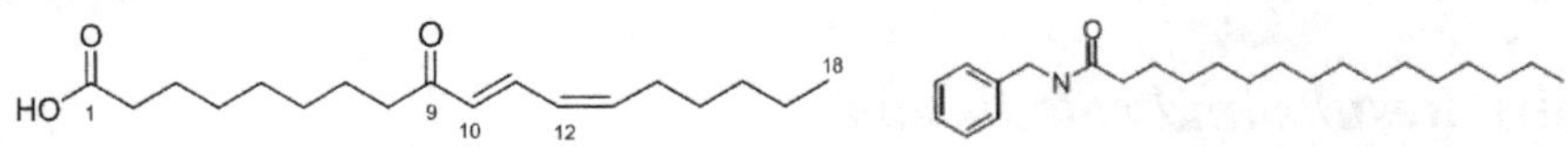

Macaene Macamide

(i) *Test procedure*

Preparation of standard solution — Accurately weigh about 2 g of known content maca standard powder, transfer it to a 100 ml volumetric flask. Accurately transfer 50 ml of methanol to the flask, and sonicate for 50 min, shaking for 10 sec every 5 min. Shake and mix the slurry well, then centrifuge (10,000 rpm) for 5 min. Take the clear solution for injection.

Preparation of sample solution — Accurately weigh a certain amount of sample equivalent to 2 g of the standard maca, transfer it to a 100 ml volumetric flask. Accurately transfer 50 ml of methanol to the flask, and sonicate for 50 min, shaking for 10 sec every 5 min. After sonication, shake and mix the sample slurry well, then centrifuge (10,000 rpm) for 5 min, and take the clear solution for injection.

(ii) *UPLC conditions*

Column: Acquity UPLC®, BEH C18, 1.7 μm, 2.1 × 150 mm
Flow rate: 0.4 mL/min
Injection volume: 2 μL
UV wavelength: 210 nm (macaene); 275 nm, 315 nm (macamide)
Mobile phase A: 0.1% phosphoric acid in water
Mobile phase B: Acetonitrile
Column temperature: 45°C

Gradient:

Time (min)	A%	B%
0	75	25
0–15	5	95
15–17.5	5	95
17.5–18	75	25
18–20	75	25

(iii) *Results and calculation*

$$Macamide(275nm)(\%) = \frac{Aa^1 \times Wstand \times Vsam \times 100\%}{As^1 \times Vstd \times Wsam}$$

$$macamide(310nm)\% = \frac{Aa^2 \times Wstand \times Vsam \times 100\%}{As^2 \times Vstd \times Wsam}$$

$$macaene\ \% = \frac{Aa^3 \times Wsand \times Vsam \times UW}{As^3 \times Vstd \times Wsam}$$

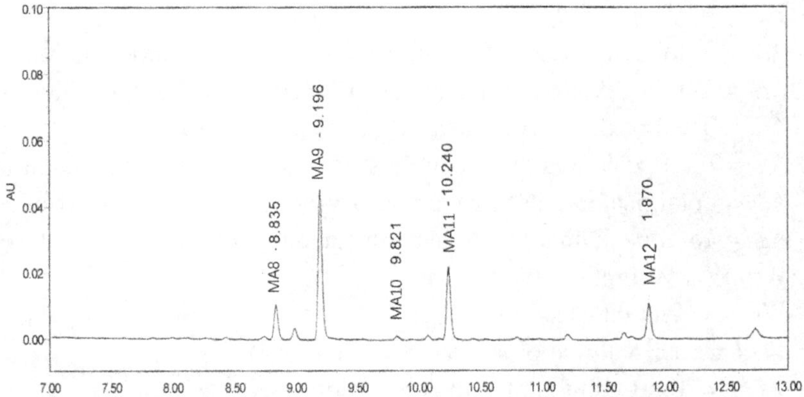

Figure 4.22: Chromatogram of macamide at 275 nm.

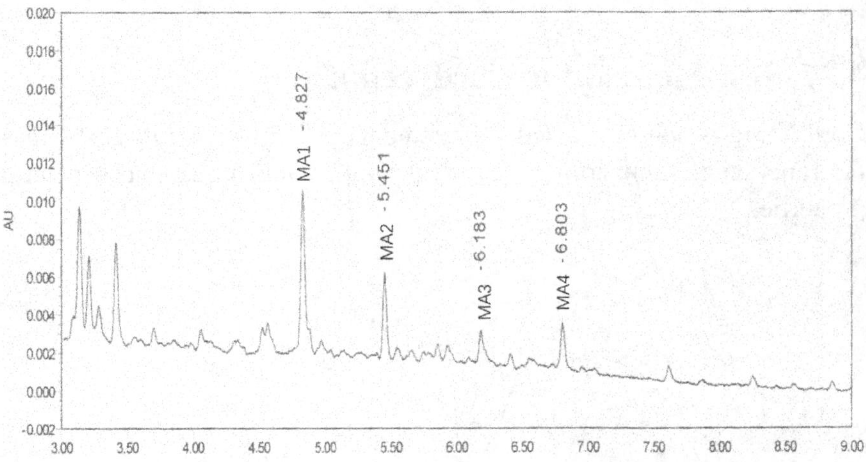

Figure 4.23: Chromatogram of macamide at 315 nm.

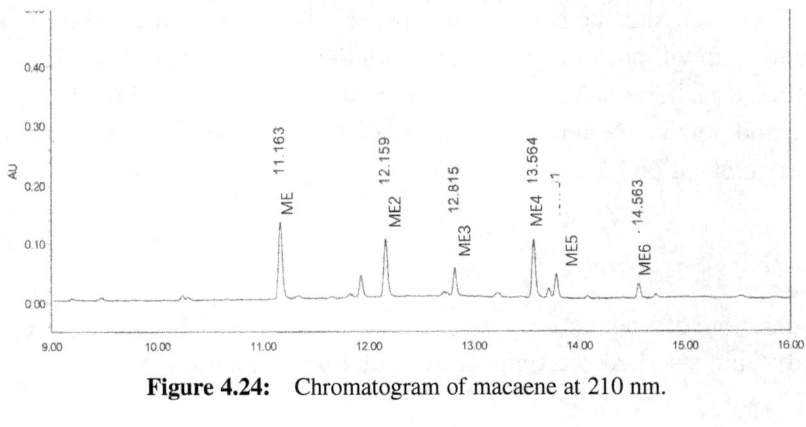

Figure 4.24: Chromatogram of macaene at 210 nm.

Here
Aa^1 = Total peak area of macamides (@275 nm) in sample solution
Aa^2 = Total peak area of macamides (@310 nm) in sample solution
Aa^3 = Total peak area of macaene in sample solution
As^1 = Total peak area of macamides (@275 nm) in standard solution
As^2 = Total peak area of macamides (@310 nm) in standard solution
As^3 = Total peak area of macaene in standard solution
Wsand = Weight of standard (mg)
Wsam = Weight of sample (mg)
Vstd = Total volume of standard solution (ml)
Vsam = Total volume of sample solution (ml)

Total Content = Macaminde content + macaene content

4.27 Test Method for Cordycepin

Cordycepin is one of the active ingredients of *cordyceps sinensis*. It has the function of immunomodulation, as well as anti-fungal and anti-viral properties.

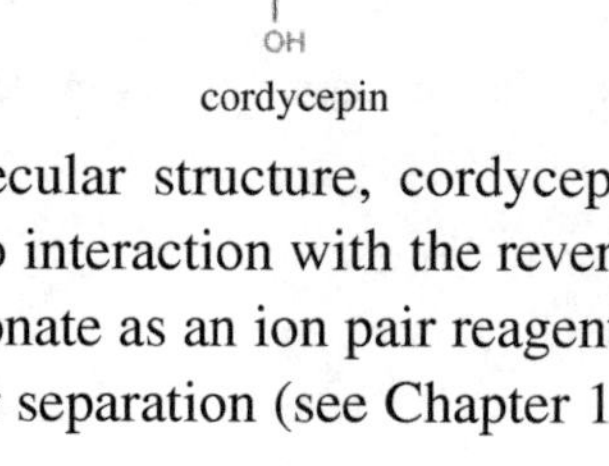

cordycepin

Based on the molecular structure, cordycepin is an alkaline compound, and will have no interaction with the reversed phase column. This method uses hexansulfonate as an ion pair reagent to extend the retention time and obtain a better separation (see Chapter 1, Section 1.1.2 "Mobile phase application").

(i) *Test procedure*

Preparation of standard solution — Accurately weigh about 5 mg of cordycepin standard and transfer to a 100 ml volumetric Flask. Add 60 ml water, shake and vortex until all the standard is dissolved, and then add water to the mark, then shake well. The standard solution is ready for injection.

Preparation of sample solution — Weigh a certain amount of ground sample containing about 2–3 mg of cordycepin, and transfer to 100 ml volumetric flask. Add exactly 50 ml of water and sonicate 10 min for cordyceps extract materials or sonicate for 40 min for cordyceps powder. Shake well, centrifuge for 5 min (10,000 rpm), then draw the clear solution for injection.

(ii) *UPLC conditions*

Column: Acquity UPLC HSS T3 C18, 2.1 × 150 mm, 1.8 μm
Column temperature: 45°C
Flow rate: 0.4 ml/min
Injection volume: 2 μL
UV wavelength: 258 nm
Mobile phase A: 10 mM hexansulfonic acid sodium salt in Water, pH 2.0
Mobile phase B: Acetonitrile

Gradient:

Time (min)	A%	B%
0	95	5
0–4.0	85	15
4.0–4.5	70	30
4.5–5.0	70	30
5.0–5.5	95	5
5.5–8.0	95	5

(iii) *Results and calculation*

$$Cordycepin\ (\%) = \frac{Aa \times Wstand \times Vsam \times 100\%}{As \times Vstd \times Wsam}$$

or

$$Cordycepin\ (mg/unit) = \frac{Aa \times Wsand \times Vsam \times UW}{As \times Vstd \times Wsam}$$

Here
Aa = Peak area of sample
As = Peak area of standard
Wsand = Weight of standard (mg)
Wsam = Weight of sample (mg)
Vstd = Total volume of standard solution (ml)
Vsam = Total volume of sample solution (ml)
UW = Unit weight (mg/unit)

4.28 Fisetin Test Method

Fisetin can be extracted from *rhus succedanea L.* It can function as an antioxidant and an anti-spasming agent. There are some bioactivities that are still under study.

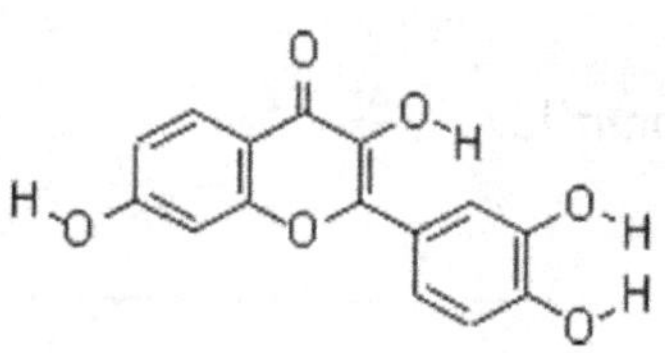

Fisetin

(i) *Test procedure*

Preparation of standard solution — Accurately weigh about 5 mg of fisetin standard and transfer to a 100 ml volumetric flask. Add 60 ml methanol, shake and vortex until standard completely dissolved, then add methanol to the mark. After shaking well, it is ready for injection.

Preparation of sample solution — Weigh a certain amount of ground sample containing about 5 mg of fisetin and transfer it to a 100 ml volumetric flask. Add 10 ml water, sonicate for 10 min, then add 60 ml ethanol. Sonicate for another 10 min for extract materials or sonicate for 40 min when testing herbs. Cool to room temperature and fill with methanol to volume. Shake well, centrifuge (10,000 rpm) for 5 min. The clear solution can be injected.

(ii) *HPLC conditions*

Column: Suplcosil Discovery C18, 4.6 × 15 mm
Column temperature: Room temperature
Flow rate: 1.1 ml/min
Injection volume: 10 μL
UV wavelength: 335 nm
Mobile phase A: Nano pure water
Mobile phase B: Methanol

Gradient:

Time (min)	**A%**	**B%**
0	95	5
0–7.0	85	15
7.0–9.0	70	30
9.0–9.5	70	30
9.5–10	95	5
10–15.0	95	5

(iii) *Results and calculation*

$$Fisetin\ (\%) = \frac{Aa \times Wstand \times Vsam \times 100\%}{As \times Vstd \times Wsam}$$

or

$$Fisetin\ (mg/unit) = \frac{Aa \times Wsand \times Vsam \times UW}{As \times Vstd \times Wsam}$$

Here
Aa = Peak area of sample
As = Peak area of standard
Wsand = Weight of standard (mg)
Wsam = Weight of sample (mg)

Vstd = Total volume of standard solution (ml)
Vsam = Total volume of sample solution (ml)
UW = Unit weight (mg/unit)

4.29 St. John's Wort Extract Test Method

St. John's wort, known as *Hypericum perforatum*, is a flowering plant in the family Hypericaceaehas. It has been used as a medicinal herb for its antidepressant and anti-inflammatory properties. The main active compounds of the St. John's wort are hypericin, hyperforin, and pseudo-hyperforin.

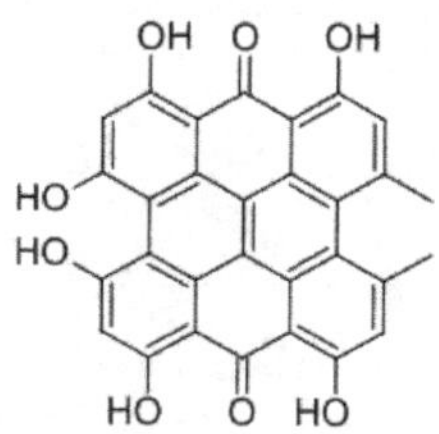

Hypericin

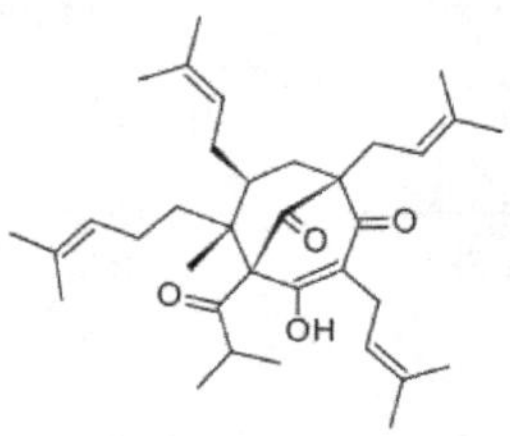

Hyperforin

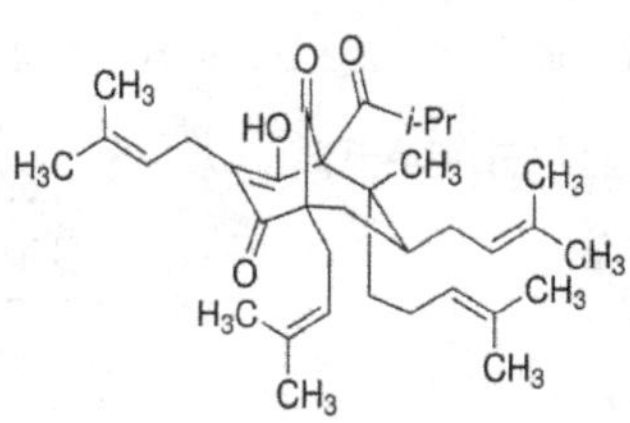

Pseudo-hyperforin

The above three compounds are non-polar compounds, therefore a reversed phase HPLC column can be used to perform the test.

(i) *Test procedure*

Hypericin, hyperforin and pseudo-hyperforin levels in St. John's wort extracts are very low in concentration (less than 0.3%). In order to avoid using a large mass of sample resulting in an increase in the concentration of interferences, causing separation difficulties, and affecting the column lifetime, this method reduces the concentration of the standard solution to 1 ppm, or even lower.

Preparation of standard solution — Accurately weigh about 5 mg of each hypericin, hyperforin and pseudo-hyperforin standards, and transfer it to a 50 ml volumetric flask. Add 30 ml of methanol, shake and vortex until standards are completely dissolved. Then add methanol to the mark, and shake well. Transfer 1 ml of this solution to a 100 ml volumetric flask, dilute to volume with methanol, and mix well. The standard solution is ready to inject.

Preparation of sample solution — Weigh a certain amount of St. John's wort extract sample containing about 0.1 mg of hypericin, or hyperforin, and transfer to a 100 ml volumetric flask. Add 20 ml of DMSO, sonicate for 5 min, add 60 ml of ethanol, sonicate for another 10 min. Cool to room temperature, fill with methanol to volume, and shake well. Then centrifuge (10,000 rpm) for 5 min, the clear solution can be injected.

(ii) *HPLC conditions*

Column: WATERS Symmetry C18, 3.5 μm, 4.6 × 150 mm
Column temperature: Room temperature
Flow rate: 1.0 ml/min
Injection volunme: 10 μL
UV wavelength: 270 nm for hyperforin and Pseudo-hyperforin; 590 nm for Hypericin.
Mobile phase A: 0.5% TFA in nano pure water
Mobile phase B: Methanol
Mobile phase C: Acetonitrile

Gradient:

Time (min)	A%	B%	C%
0	90	0	10
5	80	0	20
7	62	20	18
10	45	25	30
20	1	60	39
30	1	60	39
30.5	90	0	10
36.0	90	0	10 Finish

(iii) *Result and calculation*

$$Hypericin/hyperforin/Pseudohyperforin\ (\%) = \frac{Aa \times Wstand \times Vsam \times 100\%}{As \times Vstd \times Wsam}$$

or

$$Hypericin/hyperforin/Pseudohyperforin(mg/unit) = \frac{Aa \times Wsand \times Vsam \times UW}{As \times Vstd \times Wsam}$$

Here
Aa = Peak area of corresponding compound in sample solution
As = Peak area of corresponding standard in standard solution
$Wsand$ = Weight of corresponding standard (mg)
$Wsam$ = Weight of sample (mg)
$Vstd$ = Total volume of standard solution (ml)
$Vsam$ = Total volume of sample solution (ml)
UW = Unit weight (mg/unit)

4.30 Test Method for Sesamin and Sesamolin

Sesamin and sesamolin are the major lignans found in sesame seeds. They can help reduce cholesterol, support liver function and help maintain healthy lipid profiles. Studies have also shown that sesamin can help accelerate fat loss and help prevent the body from storing fat by helping to break down fatty acids.

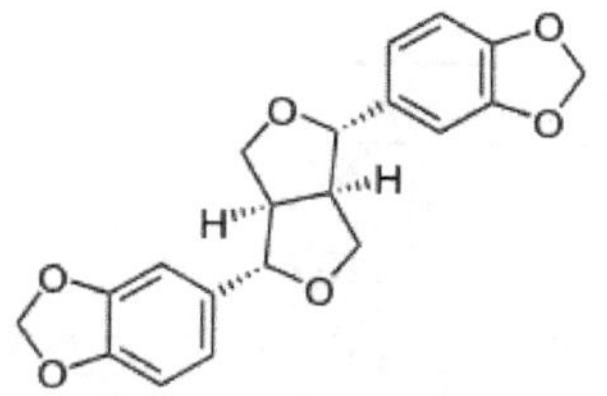

Sesamin

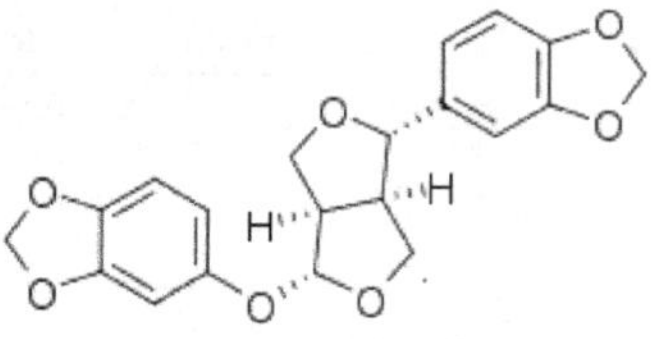

Sesamolin

Both sesamin and sesamolin are non-polar compounds and thus A C18 column is a good choice for this test.

(i) *Test procedure*

Preparation of standard solution — Accurately weigh about 10 mg of sesamin and 2 mg of sesamolin, transfer it to a 100 ml volumetric flask, and add 60 ml of methanol. Shake and vortex until the standards are completely dissolved, and add methanol to the mark. Shake well, the standard solution is ready for injection.

Preparation of sample solution — Weigh a certain amount of ground sample containing about 10 mg of sesamin, or 2 mg of sasemolin, and transfer it to a 100 ml volumetric flask. Add 10 ml of water, and sonicate for 5 min. Add 60 ml of ethanol, sonicate for 10 min for sesame extract powder or sonicate for 40 min for raw sesame seed powder. Cool to room temperature, add methanol to the mark, shake and mix well. Centrifuge 5 for min (10,000 rpm), and the clear solution can be injected.

(ii) *UPLC conditions*

Column: Acquity BEH C18 1.7 μm, 2.1 × 150 mm
Flow rate: 0.4 ml/min
Injection volume: 1.0 μL
UV Wavelength: 286 nm
Mobile phase A: 0.1% phosphoric acid in nano pure water
Mobile phase B: Acetonitrile

Gradient:

Time (min)	A%	B%
0	85	15
7	30	70
7.8	30	70
8.0	85	15
10	85	15

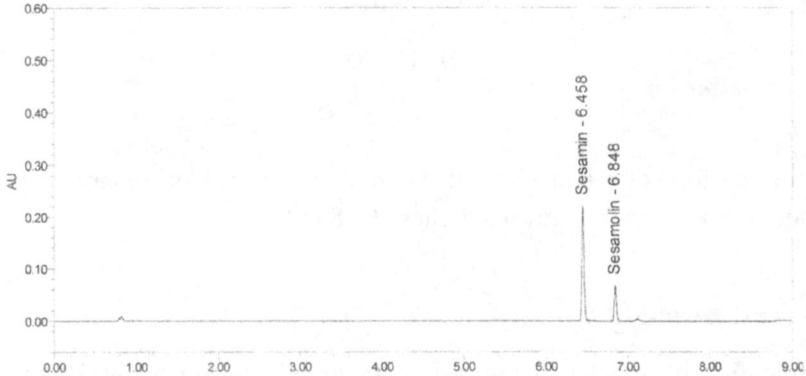

Figure 4.25: UPLC chromatogram of sesamin and sesamolid.

(iii) *Results and calculation*

$$\text{Sesamin and sesamolin}(\%) = \frac{Aa \times Wstand \times Vsam \times 100\%}{As \times Vstd \times Wsam}$$

or

$$\text{Sesamin and sesamolin } (mg/unit) = \frac{Aa \times Wsand \times Vsam \times UW}{As \times Vstd \times Wsam}$$

Here
Aa = Peak area of sesamin/sesamolin in sample solution
As = Peak area of sesamin/sesamolin in standard solution
Wsand = Weight of sesamin/sesamolin standard (mg)
Wsam = Weight of sample (mg)
Vstd = Total volume of standard solution (ml)
Vsam = Total volume of sample solution (ml)
UW = Unit weight (mg/unit)

4.31 Test for Forskolin in Plectranthus Barbatus

Forskolin is derived from Indian *Plectranthus Barbatus*. As a dietary supplement, forskolin may help lower blood pressure, lower eye pressure, and assist in weight loss and other functions.

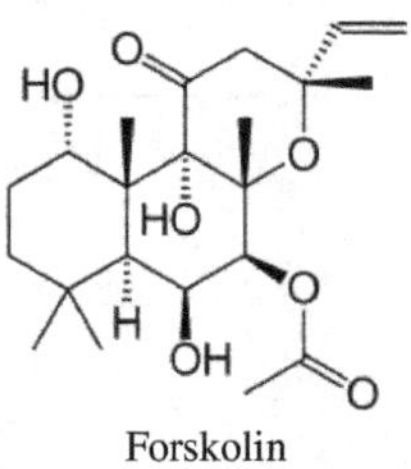

Forskolin

Since forskolin is a non-polar compound, it can be separated from other components by a reversed phase C18 column.

(i) *Test procedure*

Preparation of standard solution — Accurately weigh about 10 mg of forskolin standard. Transfer it to a 50 ml volumetric flask, add about

30 ml methanol. Sonicate until the standard is dissolved, add methanol to mark, and shake well. The standard is ready for injection.

Preparation of sample solution — Weigh a certain amount of ground sample containing about 10 mg of forskolin. Transfer it to a 50 volumetric flask and add 10 ml DMSO of water. Sonicate for 5 min, then add 30 ml of methanol. Sonicate for 10 min when testing extract powders or sonicate for 50 min when analyzing *plectranthus barbatus* powder. Cool to room temperature, add methanol to mark, shake and mix well. Centrifuge (10,000 rpm) for 5 min, and take the clear solution for injection.

(ii) *UPLC conditions*

Column: Waters Acquity BEH Phenyl 1.7 μm, 2.1 × 150 mm
Flow rate: 0.4 ml/min
Injection volume: 2.0 μL
UV wavelength: 210 nm
Mobile phase A: 0.1% phosphoric acid in water
Mobile phase B: Acetonitrile

Gradient:

Time (min)	A%	B%
0	70	30
5.5	40	60
6.0	40	60
6.5	70	30
9.0	70	30

(iii) *Results and calculation*

$$Forskolin\ (\%) = \frac{Aa \times Wstand \times Vsam \times 100\%}{As \times Vstd \times Wsam}$$

or

$$Forskolin\ (mg/unit) = \frac{Aa \times Wsand \times Vsam \times UW}{As \times Vstd \times Wsam}$$

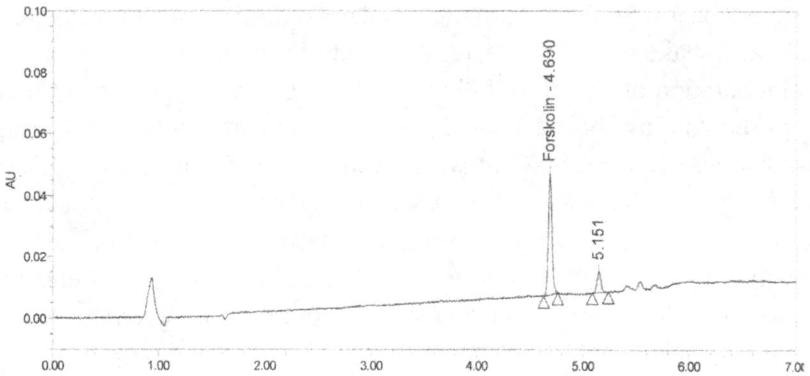

Figure 4.26: UPLC chromatogram of forskolin.

Here
Aa = Peak area of sample
As = Peak area of standard
Wsand = Weight of standard (mg)
Wsam = Weight of sample (mg)
Vstd = Total volume of standard solution (ml)
Vsam = Total volume of sample solution (ml)
UW = Unit weight (mg/unit)

4.32 Test Method for Glycyrrhizic Acid

Glycyrrhizic acid is a natural sweetener, extracted from licorice.

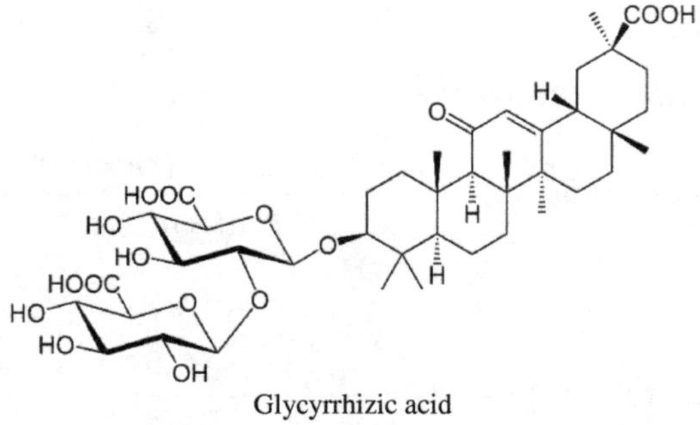

Glycyrrhizic acid

(i) *Test procedure*

Preparation of standard solution — Accurately weigh about 10 mg of a glycyrrhizic acid standard, transfer it to a 100 ml volumetric flask, and add 60 ml of methanol. Sonicate until completely dissolved, add methanol to the volume, then shake and mix well.

Preparation of sample solution — Accurately weigh a certain amount of ground sample containing about 10 mg of glycyrrhizic acid, and transfer it to a 100 ml volumetric flask. Add 10 ml of water, sonicate for 5 min, then add 60 ml ethanol. Sonicate again for 10 min when testing licorice extract; or 40 min for licorice powder. Cool to room temperature, fill methanol to the mark, shake and mix well. Centrifuge (10,000 rpm) for 5 min, draw the clear solution to a 2 ml injection vial, it is ready for injection.

(ii) *HPLC conditions*

Column: Phenomenex LUNA C18 (2) 5 μm, 4.6 × 150 mm 100A
Flow rate: 1.0 ml/min
Injection volume: 10 μL
UV Wavelength: 220 nm
Mobile phase A: 0.1% phosphoric acid in water
Mobile phase B: Acetonitrile

Gradient:

Time (min)	A%	B%
0	95	5
20	35	65
21.0	35	65
21.5	95	5
25.0	95	5

(iii) *Results and calculation*

$$Glycyrrhizic\ acid\ (\%) = \frac{Aa \times Wstand \times Vsam \times 100\%}{As \times Vstd \times Wsam}$$

or

$$Glycyrrhizic\ acid\ (mg/unit) = \frac{Aa \times Wsand \times Vsam \times UW}{As \times Vstd \times Wsam}$$

Here
Aa = Peak area of sample
As = Peak area of standard
Wsand = Weight of standard (mg)
Wsam = Weight of sample (mg)
Vstd = Total volume of standard solution (ml)
Vsam = Total volume of sample solution (ml)
UW = Unit weight (mg/unit)

4.33 Rosemary Test Method

Rosemary is used as flavor additive for various foods. It has also shown health benefits. Rosemary is considered functional as an antioxidant, anti-inflammatory and also as a memory-enhancing material. The chemical composition of rosemary includes these compounds: rosmarinic acid, carnosic acid, carlnosol and ursolic acid.

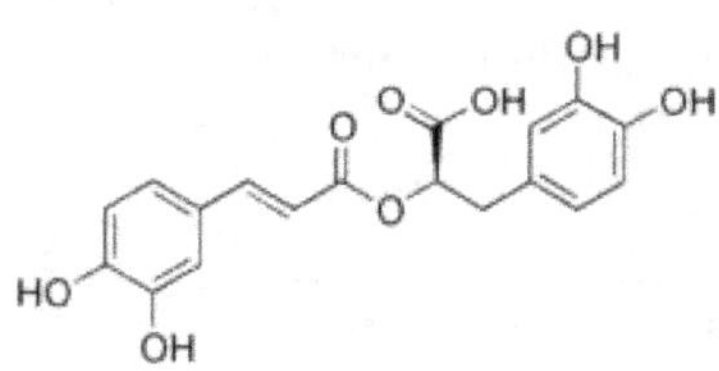

Rosmarinic acid

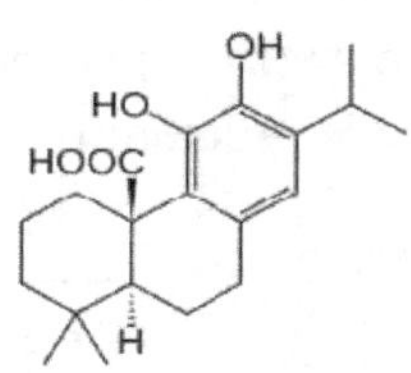

Carnosic acid

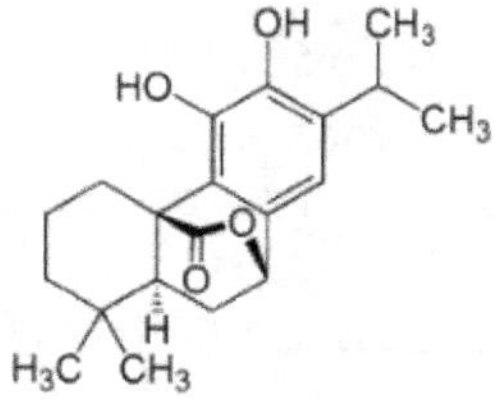

Carlnosol

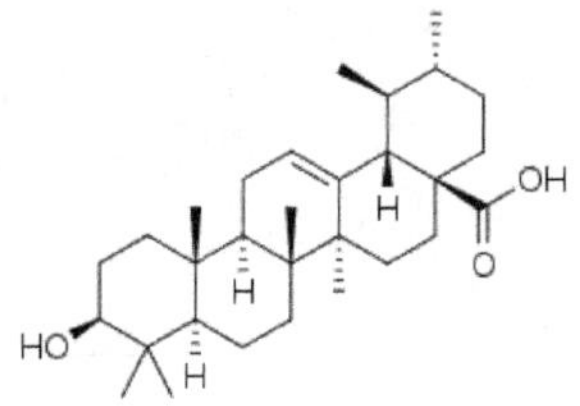

Ursolic acid

(i) *Test procedure*

According to their molecular structure, all the four analytes are non-polar compounds, three of them contain aromatic π electrons which can create

π–π interactions with phenyl column, improving the column separation (see Chapter 1, Section 1.1.1 "Types of stationary phases").

Preparation of standard solution — Accurately weigh about 5 mg of rosmarinic acid, carnosic acid, carlnosol and ursolic acid, and transfer it to a 50 ml volumetric flask. Add 30 ml methanol, and sonicate for 5 min. After cooling, add methanol to the volume. The standard solution is ready to inject.

Preparation of sample solution — Accurately weigh a certain amount of ground sample containing about 5 mg of any above compounds, and transfer it to a 50 ml volumetric flask. Add 30 ml of methanol, and sonicate for 10 min for rosemary extracts or sonicate for 40 min when testing rosemary powder. After cooling, add methanol to the volume, shake and mix well. Then centrifuge (10,000 rpm) for 5 min, and draw the upper clear solution to a 2 ml injection vail. The sample extract is ready to inject.

(ii) *UPLC conditions*

Column: Waters Acquity BEH Phenyl, 1.7 μm, 4.6 × 150 mm
Flow rate: 0.4 ml/min
Inject volume: 2.0 μL
UV wavelength: 215 nm
Mobile phase A: 0.1% phosphoric acid in nano pure water
Mobile phase B: Acetonitrile

Gradient:

Time (min)	A%	B%
0	90	10
5.0	65	35
8.0	0	100
8.8	0	100
9.0	90	10
11.0	90	10

(iii) *Results and calculation*

$$Individual\ compound\ (\%) = \frac{Aa \times Wstand \times Vsam \times 100\%}{As \times Vstd \times Wsam}$$

or

$$Individual\ compound\ (mg/unit) = \frac{Aa \times Wsand \times Vsam \times UW}{As \times Vstd \times Wsam}$$

Here
Aa = Peak area of corresponding compound in sample solution
As = Peak area of corresponding compound in standard solution
$Wsand$ = Weight of corresponding standard compound (mg)
$Wsam$ = Weight of sample (mg)
$Vstd$ = Total volume of standard solution (ml)
$Vsam$ = Total volume of sample solution (ml)
UW = Unit weight (mg/unit)

4.34 Test method for Gymnemagenin in Gymnenic acid

Gymnenic acid is a group of compounds (see the molecular structure below). R could be acetyl, acparagine or methylbutyl, coupled with a variety of different glycosides, so it is a larger group of compounds. It is not possible to quantitatively test each compound in this group. This method is used to obtain a single aglycon (gymnemagenin) by using acid and alkali hydrolysis. The hydrolysates then separated and quantified it by reversed phase chromatography.

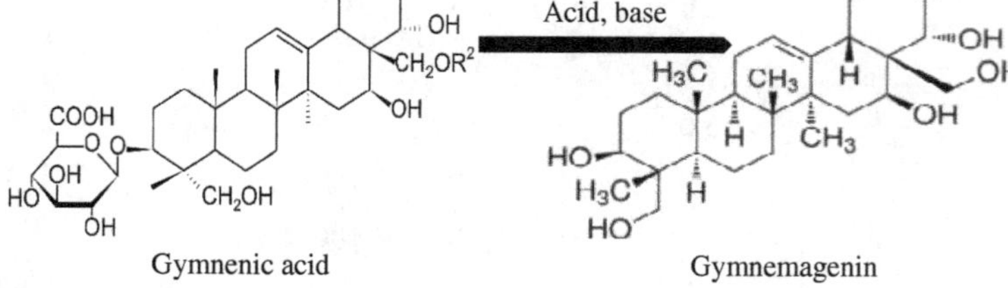

Gymnenic acid   Gymnemagenin

(i) *Test procedure*

Preparation of standard solution — Accurately weigh about 5 mg of gymnemagenin standard, and transfer to 25 ml volumetric flask. Add 15 ml methanol/water (60:40), sonicate until completely dissolved, then fill with methanol/water (60:40) to the volume. Shake this solution well, the solution is ready to inject.

Preparation of sample solution — Accurately weigh a certain amount of ground sample containing about 5 mg of gymnemagenin equivalent. Transfer to 10 ml test tube with screw cap, add 5 ml of 0.5 N potassium hydroxide water/methanol (1:1) solution, cap the test tube, and shake vigorously for 1 min. Put the test tube in 95°C water bath for 1 h. Remove from the water bath and cool. Add 1 ml of concentrated hydrochloric acid, cap again, shake vigorously for 1 min, and then put in 95°C water bath for 1 h again. After cooling, add potassium hydroxide solution to neutralize the solution, and transfer the solution from test tube to a 25 ml volumetric flask. Rinse the tube with 5 ml of methanol/water (80:20) two times, combining the rinses in the 25 ml volumetric flask. Fill the flask with methanol/water (80:20) to mark, and shake vigorously. Centrifuge (10,000 rpm) for 5 min, draw the clear solution into a 2 ml injection vail. It is ready for injection.

(ii) *UPLC conditions*

Column: Acquity UPLC® BEH Phenyl 1.7 μm, 2.1 × 150 mm
Flow rate: 0.4 ml/min
Injection volume: 2.0 μL
UV wavelength: 210 nm
Mobile phase A: 0.1% phosphoric acid in water
Mobile phase B: Acetonitrile
Column temperature: 45°C

Gradient:

Time (min)	A%	B%
0	85	15
6.0	60	40
6.8	60	40
7.0	85	15
9.0	85	15

(iii) *Results and calculation*

$$Gymnemagenin\ (\%) = \frac{Aa \times Wstand \times Vsam \times 100\%}{As \times Vstd \times Wsam}$$

or

$$Gymnemagenin\ (mg/unit) = \frac{Aa \times Wsand \times Vsam \times UW}{As \times Vstd \times Wsam}$$

Here
Aa = Peak area of sample
As = Peak area of standard
Wsand = Weight of standard (mg)
Wsam = Weight of sample (mg)
Vstd = Total volume of standard solution (ml)
Vsam = Total volume of sample solution (ml)
UW = Unit weight (mg/unit)

4.35 Test Method for Withaferin A in Ashwaganda

Withaferin A is one of the withnaolides, a group of active compounds found in ashwaganda. It may have anti-inflammatory and anti-cancer bioactivity.

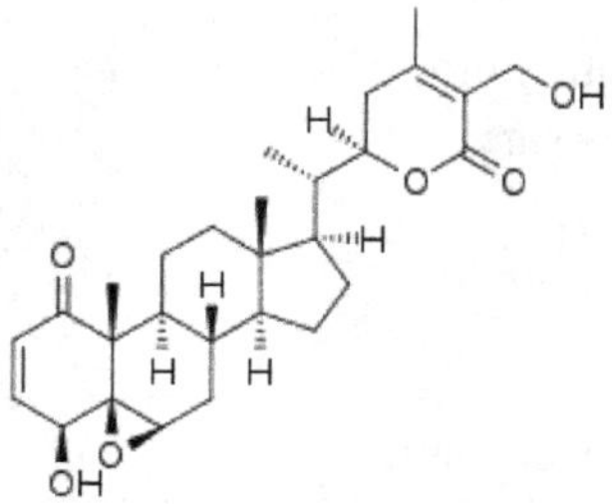

Withaferin A

(i) *Test procedure*

Preparation of standard solution — Accurately weigh about 5 mg of withaferin A standard, and transfer to a 50 ml volumetric flask. Add 30 ml of methanol, shake, and sonicate until the standard fully dissolved. After cooling, add methanol to the volume, and shake well. The solution is ready for injection.

Preparation of sample solution — Weigh a certain amount of ground sample containing about 5 mg of withaferin A, and transfer to a 50 ml volumetric flask. Add 5 ml of water, and sonicate for 5 min. Then add 30 ml of ethanol, sonicate 10 min for extract materials or sonicate 40 min when testing ashwaganda powder. Cool to room temperature, then add methanol to the volume, and shake vigorously. Centrifuge (10,000 rpm) for 5 min, and take the clear solution for injection.

(ii) *UPLC conditions*

Column: Acquity UPLC® BEH Phenyl, 1.7 μm, 2.1 × 150 mm
Flow rate: 0.4 ml/min
Injection volume: 2.0 μL
UV wavelength: 215 nm
Mobile phase A: 0.1% phosphoric acid in water
Mobile phase B: Methanol
Column temperature: 45°C

Gradient:

Time (min)	A%	B%
0	80	20
7	55	45
8.0	20	80
8.8	20	80
9.0	80	20
11.0	80	20

(iii) *Results and calculation*

$$Withaferin\ A\ (\%) = \frac{Aa \times Wstand \times Vsam \times 100\%}{As \times Vstd \times Wsam}$$

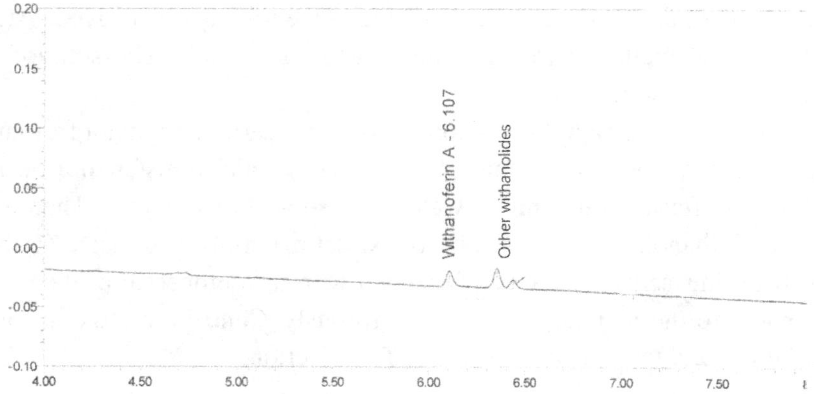

Figure 4.27: Chromatogram of ashwaganda, containing withaferin A and other withanolides.

or

$$Withaferin\ A\ (mg/unit) = \frac{Aa \times Wsand \times Vsam \times UW}{As \times Vstd \times Wsam}$$

Here
Aa = Peak area of sample
As = Peak area of standard
Wsand = Weight of standard (mg)
Wsam = Weight of sample (mg)
Vstd = Total volume of standard solution (ml)
Vsam = Total volume of sample solution (ml)
UW =Unit weight (mg/unit)

4.36 Test Method for Evodiamine

Evodiamine, a chemical compound extracted from the *Evodia spp* family plants, has been shown to reduce fat uptake in mouse studies. It can be dissolved and extracted with methanol and can be separated by a reversed phase UPLC column, HSS T3 C18. By comparing the chromatogram with a known concentration reference standard, evodiamine can be quantified.

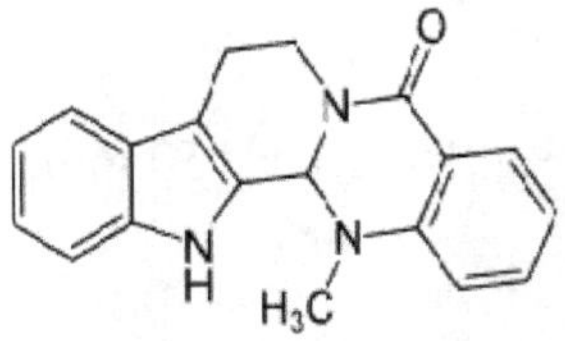

Evodiamine

(i) *Test procedure*

Preparation of standard solution — Accurately weigh about 5 mg of evodiamine standard, and transfer it to a 100 ml volumetric flask. Add 60 ml of methanol, shake, and sonicate until the standard is fully dissolved. After cooling add methanol to volume, and shake well. The solution is ready for injection.

Preparation of sample solution — Accurately weigh a certain amount of ground sample containing about 5 mg of evodiamine, and transfer it to a 100 ml volumetric flask. Add 10 ml water, sonicate for 5 min, and then add 50 ml of ethanol. Sonicate again for 10 min for extract materials or sonicate for 40 min when testing *evodia spp* powder. Cool to room temperature, then add methanol to volume, and shake vigorously. Centrifuge (10,000 rpm) for 5 min, and take the clear solution for injection.

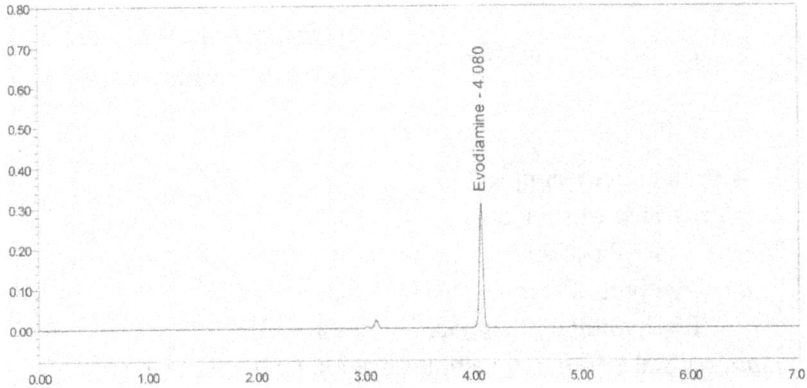

Figure 4.28: UPLC chromatogram of evodiamine.

(ii) *UPLC conditions*

Column: Acquity HSS T3, C18, 2.1 × 150 mm, 1.8 μm
Flow rate: 0.4 ml/min
Injection volume: 1.0 μL
UV 波长: 268 nm
Mobile phase A: 0.1% phosphoric acid in water
Mobile phase B: 0.1% phosphoric acid in acetonitrile
Column temperature: 45°C

Gradient:

Time (min)	A%	B%
0	60	40
5	35	65
5.8	35	65
6.0	60	40
8.0	60	40

(iii) *Results and calculation*

$$Evodiamine\ (\%) = \frac{Aa \times Wstand \times Vsam \times 100\%}{As \times Vstd \times Wsam}$$

or

$$Evodiamine\ (mg/unit) = \frac{Aa \times Wsand \times Vsam \times UW}{As \times Vstd \times Wsam}$$

Here
Aa = Peak area of sample
As = Peak area of standard
Wsand = Weight of standard (mg)
Wsam = Weight of sample (mg)
Vstd = Total volume of standard solution (ml)
Vsam = Total volume of sample solution (ml)
UW = Unit weight (mg/unit)

4.37 Test Method for Huperzine A

Huperzine A is a naturally occurring sesquiterpene alkaloid compound found in the firmoss *Huperzia serrata*. It can be dissolved and extracted using methanol. The main function of this compound is to help improve memory, which may help Alzheimer's disease.

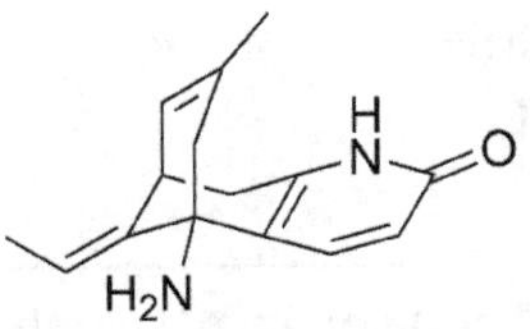

Huperzine A

From the molecular structure it can be seen that the huperzine A is an alkaline molecule. In order to extend the chromatographic retention time, and to improve the peak separation, this method uses an ion pair mobile phase, coupled with the reversed phase column and PDA detector. This is used to quantify huperzine A in the sample (see Chapter 1, Section 1.1.2 "Mobile phase application").

(i) *Test procedure*

Preparation of standard solution — Accurately weigh about 10 mg of huperzine A standard, and transfer it to a 100 ml volumetric flask. Add 60 ml methanol, and sonicate until the standard fully dissolved. After cooling add methanol to mark, and shake well. The solution is ready for injection.

Preparation of sample solution — Weigh a certain amount of ground sample containing about 10 mg of huperzine A, and transfer it to 100 ml volumetric flask. Add 10 ml of water, and sonicate for 5 min. Add 60 ml of methanol, and shake 2 min. Sonicate for 10 min for extract material or sonicate 40 min when testing firmoss Huperzia powder. After cooling add methanol to volume and shake vigorously. Centrifuge (10,000 rpm) for 5 min, and draw the clear liquid to a 2 ml injection vail. This solution is ready for injection.

(ii) *UPLC conditions*

Column: Acquity UPLC® BEH Phenyl 1.7 μm, 2.1 × 150 mm
Flow rate: 0.4 ml/min
Injection volume: 1.0 μL
UV wavelength: 312 nm
Mobile phase A: 10 mM hexansulfonic acid in water, pH 3.0
Mobile phase B: Acetonitrile
Column temperature: 45°C

Gradient:

Time (min)	A%	B%
0	95	5
4.0	75	25
5.0	50	50
5.8	50	50
6.0	95	5
8.0	95	5

(iii) *Results and calculation*

$$Huperzine\ A\ (\%) = \frac{Aa \times Wstand \times Vsam \times 100\%}{As \times Vstd \times Wsam}$$

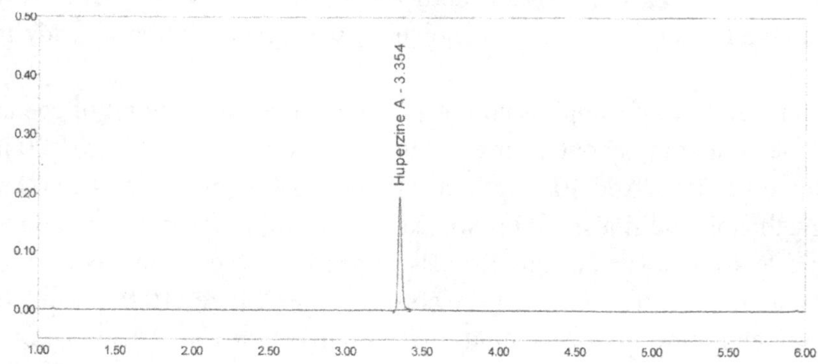

Figure 4.29: Huperzine A chromatogram.

or

$$Huperzine\ A\ (mg/unit) = \frac{Aa \times Wsand \times Vsam \times UW}{As \times Vstd \times Wsam}$$

Here
Aa = Peak area of sample
As = Peak area of standard
Wsand = Weight of standard (mg)
Wsam = Weight of sample (mg)
Vstd = Total volume of standard solution (ml)
Vsam = Total volume of sample solution (ml)
UW = Unit weight (mg/unit)

4.38 L-theanine Test Method

L-theanine is a natural amino acid found in tea. L-theanine is

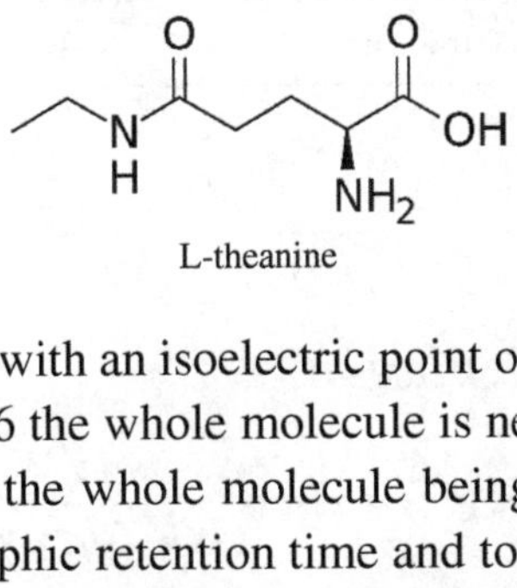

L-theanine

a multipolar compound with an isoelectric point of about 5.6. This means, that when the pH is >5.6 the whole molecule is negatively charged, while a pH of <5.6 results in the whole molecule being positively charged. To extend the chromatographic retention time and to improve the peak separation, this method uses decanesulfonate as an ion pair reagent in to the mobile phase. The mobile phase is adjusted to pH 2.0 (see Chapter 1, Section, Section 1.1.2"Mobile phase application").

(i) *Test procedure*

Preparation of standard solution — Accurately weigh about 20 mg of L-theanine standard, and transfer to a 50 ml volumetric flask. Add 30 ml of water, vortex until the standard is fully dissolved, then add water to the mark, and shake well. The standard solution is ready for injection.

Preparation of sample solution — Weigh a certain amount of ground sample containing about 20 mg of L-theanine, and transfer it to a 50 ml volumetric flask. Add 30 ml of water, and shake with a wrist action shaker for 15 min. Add water to the mark, shake well, then centrifuge (10,000 rpm) for 5 min. Take the clear solution for injection.

(ii) *UPLC conditions*

Column: Acquity UPLC® BEH C18 1.7 μm, 2.1 × 150 mm
Flow rate: 0.4 ml/min
Injection volume: 2.0 μL
UV wavelength: 210 nm
Mobile phase A: 10 mM decanesulfonate in water, pH 2.0
Mobile phase B: Acetonitrile
Column temperature: 45°C

Gradient: (isocratic)

Time (min)	A%	B%
0	80	20
6	80	20

(iii) *Results and calculation*

$$L-theanine\,(\%) = \frac{Aa \times Wstand \times Vsam \times 100\%}{As \times Vstd \times Wsam}$$

or

$$L-theanine\ (mg/unit) = \frac{Aa \times Wsand \times Vsam \times UW}{As \times Vstd \times Wsam}$$

Here
Aa = Peak area of sample
As = Peak area of standard
Wsand = Weight of standard (mg)
Wsam = Weight of sample (mg)

Vstd = Total volume of standard solution (ml)
Vsam = Total volume of sample solution (ml)
UW = Unit weight (mg/unit)

4.39 Limonene Test Method

Limonene can be extracted from orange peels. It is widely used in food, beverages and dietary supplements.

Limonene is a non-polar compound, soluble in methanol and it can be separated and quantified by UPLC with a reversed phase column (HSS T3 C18).

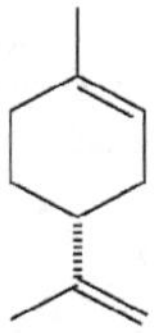

Limonene

(i) *Test procedure*

Preparation of standard solution — Accurately weigh about 20 mg of a limonene standard, and transfer it to a 100 ml volumetric flask. Add 60 ml methanol, and vortex until the standard is fully dissolved. Fill with methanol to the volume, and shake well. The standard solution is ready for injection.

Preparation of sample solution — Weigh a certain amount of ground sample containing about 20 mg of limonene, and transfer it to a 100 ml volumetric flask. Add 20 ml DMSO and sonicate for 5 min. Add 60 ml ethanol, and sonicate for 10 min. After cooling add methanol to volume, and centrifuge (10,000 rpm) for 5 min. The clear solution can be injected.

(ii) *UPLC conditions*

Column: Acquity UPLC® HSS T3, C18 1.8 μm, 2.1 × 100 mm
Flow rate: 0.4 ml/min
Injection volume: 1.0 μL

UV wavelength: 210 nm
Mobile phase A: 0.1% phosphoric acid in water
Mobile phase B: Acetonitrile
Column temperature: 45°C

Gradient:

Time (min)	A%	B%
0	40	60
5	10	90
5.8	10	90
6.0	40	60
8.0	40	60

(iii) *Results and calculation*

$$Limonene\ (\%) = \frac{Aa \times Wstand \times Vsam \times 100\%}{As \times Vstd \times Wsam}$$

or

$$Limonene\ (mg/unit) = \frac{Aa \times Wsand \times Vsam \times UW}{As \times Vstd \times Wsam}$$

Here
Aa = Peak area of sample
As = Peak area of standard
Wsand = Weight of standard (mg)
Wsam = Weight of sample (mg)
Vstd = Total volume of standard solution (ml)
Vsam = Total volume of sample solution (ml)
UW = Unit weight (mg/unit)

4.40 Test Method for Oleuropein

Oleuropein is found in olive leaves. Its metabolite hydroxytyrosol, has powerful antioxidant activity, and oleuropein preparations have been claimed to strengthen the immune system. Oleuropein can be dissolved and extracted with methanol and can be separated by a reversed phase UPLC column, BEH C18. By comparing with a known concentration reference standard, oleuropein can be quantified.

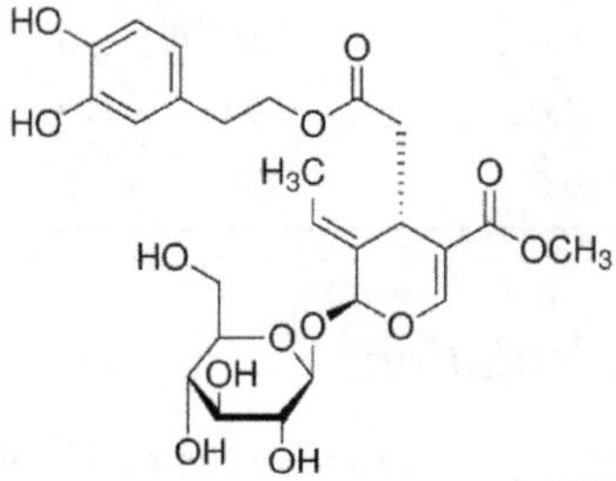

Oleuropein

(i) *Test procedure*

Preparation of standard solution — Accurately weigh about 10 mg of an Oleuropein standard, and transfer it to a 100 ml volumetric flask. Add 60 ml methanol, vortex until the standard is fully dissolved, fill with methanol to the volume, and shake well. The standard solution can be injected.

Preparation of sample solution — Weigh a certain amount of ground sample which contains about 10 mg of oleuropein, and transfer it to a 100 ml volumetric flask. Add 10 ml of water, sonicate for 5 min, add 50 ml ethanol, and sonicate for another 10 min. After cooling, add methanol to volume, and centrifuge (10,000 rpm) for 5 min. The clear solution can be injected.

(ii) *UPLC conditions*

Column: Acquity UPLC® BEH C18, 1.7 μm, 2.1 × 150 mm
Flow rate: 0.4 ml/min
Injection volume: 1.0 μL
UV wavelength: 230 nm
Mobile phase A: 0.1% phosphoric acid in nano pure water
Mobile phase B: Acetonitrile
Column temperature: 45°C

Gradient:

Time (min)	A%	B%
0	90	10
6	60	40
6.8	60	40
7.0	90	10
9.0	90	10

(iii) *Results and calculation*

$$Oleuropein\ (\%) = \frac{Aa \times Wstand \times Vsam \times 100\%}{As \times Vstd \times Wsam}$$

or

$$Oleuropein\ (mg/unit) = \frac{Aa \times Wsand \times Vsam \times UW}{As \times Vstd \times Wsam}$$

Here
Aa = Peak area of sample
As = Peak area of standard
Wsand = Weight of standard (mg)
Wsam = Weight of sample (mg)
Vstd = Total volume of standard solution (ml)
Vsam = Total volume of sample solution (ml)
UW = Unit weight (mg/unit)

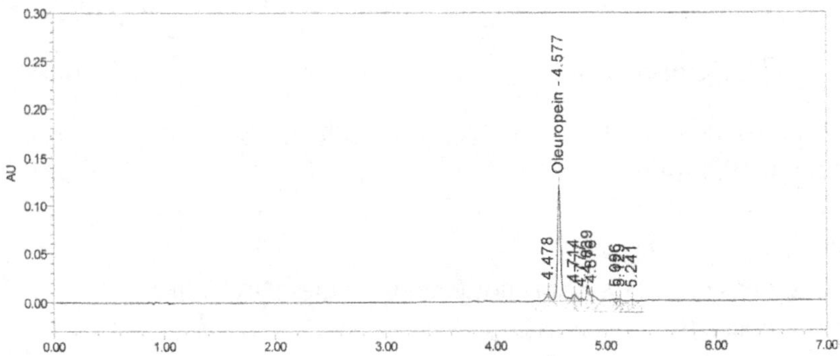

Figure 4.30: UPLC chromatogram of oleuropein.

4.41 Ellagic Acid Test Method

Many plants contain ellagic acid, which has antioxidant properties and is commonly used as raw material for dietary supplement products.

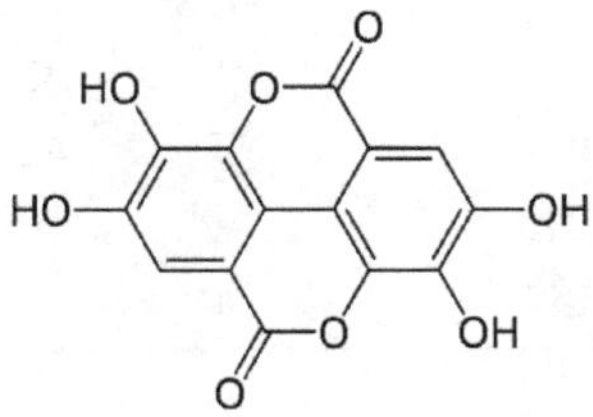

Ellagic acid

(i) *Test procedure*

Preparation of standard solution — Accurately weigh about 20 mg of an ellagic acid standard, and transfer it to a 100 ml volumetric flask. Add 60 ml 0.05 N sodium hydroxide, and vortex until the standard is fully dissolved. Fill with 0.05 N sodium hydroxide to the volume, and shake well. Transfer 1 ml of the aforementioned solution to a 50 ml volumetric flask, dilute to volume with 0.05 N sodium hydroxide. The standard solution can be injected.

Preparation of sample solution — Weigh a certain amount of ground sample that contains about 5 mg of ellagic acid, and transfer it to a 100 ml volumetric flask. Add 60 ml 0.05 N sodium hydroxide, and sonicate for 5 min. Then add 0.05 N sodium hydroxide to volume, shake well, and centrifuge (10,000 rpm) for 5 min. Transfer 1 ml of the clear solution to a 10 ml volumetric flask, add 0.05 N sodium hydroxide to the mark, and shake well. The solution is ready for injection.

(ii) *HPLC conditions*

Column: Agilent ZORBAX SB-C8 5 μm 4.60 × 150 mm
Flow rate: 1.2 ml/min
Injection volume: 10.0 μL
UV wavelength: 366 nm
Mobile phase A: 0.1% phosphoric acid in water
Mobile phase B: 0.1% phosphoric acid in acetonitrile
Column temperature: Room temperature

Gradient:

Time (min)	A%	B%
0	90	10
1	90	10
9.0	58	42
10.0	58	42
10.2	90	10
15.0	90	10

(iii) *Results and calculation*

$$Ellagic\,acid\,(\%) = \frac{Aa \times Wstand \times Vsam \times 100\%}{As \times Vstd \times Wsam}$$

or

$$Ellagic\,acid\ (mg/unit) = \frac{Aa \times Wsand \times Vsam \times UW}{As \times Vstd \times Wsam}$$

Here
Aa = Peak area of sample
As = Peak area of standard
Wsand = Weight of standard (mg)
Wsam = Weight of sample (mg)
Vstd = Total volume of standard solution (ml)
Vsam = Total volume of sample solution (ml)
UW = Unit weight (mg/unit)

4.42 Yohimbine Test Method

Yuhenbine alkali is extracted from the bark of the Yuhenbin tree in Africa and is thought to increase sexual function.

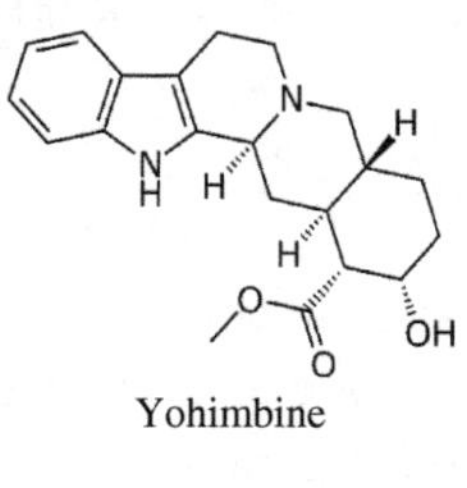

Yohimbine

(i) *Test procedure*

Preparation of standard solution — Accurately weigh about 5 mg of a yohimbine standard into 50 ml volumetric flask, then add 30 ml methanol, and sonicate until the standard is completely dissolved. Then add methanol to the volume, and shake well. The solution is ready for injection.

Preparation of sample solution — Accurately weigh a certain amount of ground sample that contains about 5 mg of yohimbine, and transfer to 50 ml volumetric flask. Add 10 ml DMSO and sonicate for 5 min. Then add 30 ml ethanol, and sonicate for 10 min for extract materials or 50 min for samples of Yuhenbin tree bark. After the solution is cooled, add methanol to the mark, shake well, and centrifuge (10,000 rpm) for 5 min. Take the clear solution for injection.

(ii) *HPLC conditions*

Column: Agilent ZORBAX SB-C8 5μm 4.60 × 150mm
Flow rate: 1.2 ml/min
Injection volume: 10.0 μL
UV wavelength: 280 nm
Mobile phase A: 0.1% phosphoric acid in water
Mobile phase B: Acetonitrile
Column temperature: Room temperature

Gradient:

Time (min)	A%	B%
0	90	10
1	90	10
8	60	40
8.8	60	40
9.0	90	10
12.0	90	10

(iii) *Results and calculation*

$$Yohimbine\ (\%) = \frac{Aa \times Wstand \times Vsam \times 100\%}{As \times Vstd \times Wsam}$$

or

$$Yohimbine\ (mg/unit) = \frac{Aa \times Wsand \times Vsam \times UW}{As \times Vstd \times Wsam}$$

Here
Aa = Peak area of sample
As = Peak area of standard
Wsand = Weight of standard (mg)
Wsam = Weight of sample (mg)
Vstd = Total volume of standard solution (ml)
Vsam = Total volume of sample solution (ml)
UW = Unit weight (mg/unit)

4.43 Guto Kola Test Method

Gotu Kola and its extracts contain four triterpenes, asiatic acid, asiaticoside, madecassic acid and madecassoside.

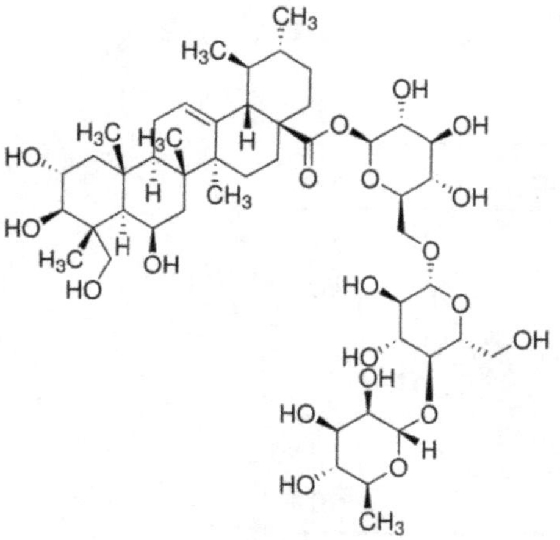

Asiaticoside

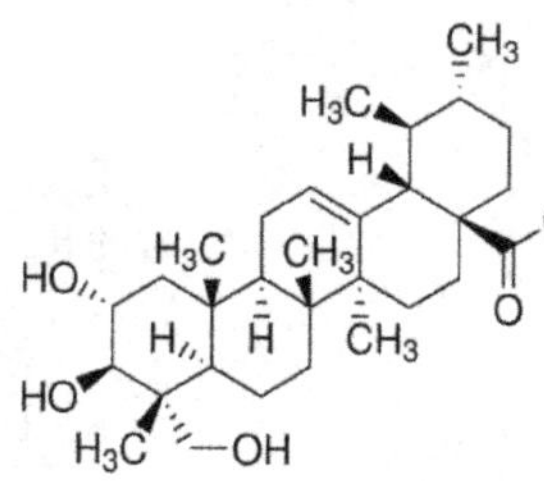

Asiatic acid

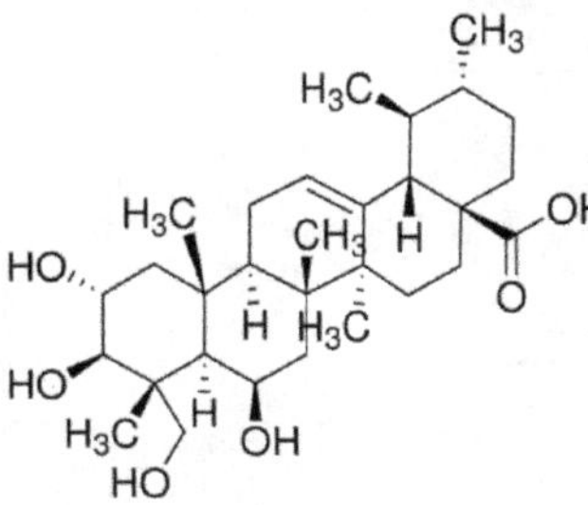

Madecassic acid

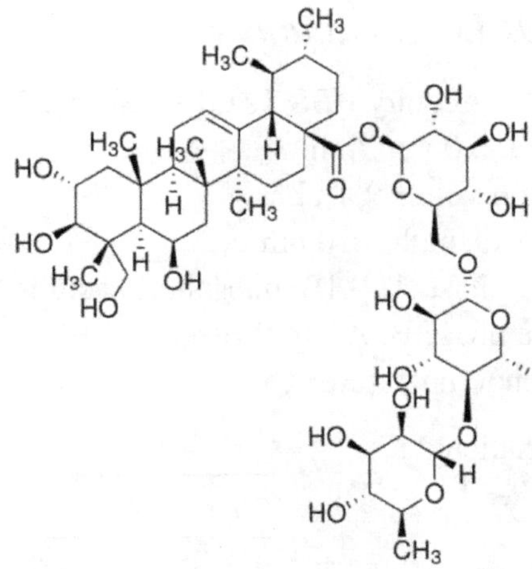

Madecassoside

(i) *Test procedure*

Preparation of standard solution — Accurately weigh about 10 mg of each of the aforementioned standard, and transfer it to a 50 ml volumetric flask. Add 30 ml of methanol, vortex until the standards are dissolved, and then add methanol to the mark, and shake well. This standard can be injected.

Preparation of sample solution (raw plant sample) — Weigh about 2 g of ground samples, and transfer it to a 100 ml of round bottom flask. Add 20 ml ethanol/water (70:30), reflux for 15 min, cool, and transfer the reflux fluid to a 50 ml volumetric flask. Repeat the reflux extraction again with 20 ml of ethanol/water (70:30). After cooling, the reflux liquid is combined with the first reflux solution. Then add ethanol/water (70:30) to the mark, shake well and centrifuge (10,000 rpm) for 5 min. Take the clear solution to inject.

Preparation of sample solution for extract materials — Accurately weigh a certain amount of the samples so that the content of the above-mentioned compounds are similar to the standard solution, and transfer it to a 50 ml volumetric flask. Add 30 ml of methanol, sonicate for 10 min, and cool to room temperature. Fill with methanol to volume, shake well, and centrifuge (10,000 rpm) for 5 min. Take the upper clear solution for injection.

(ii) *UPLC conditions*

Column: Acquity HSS Ts C18, 1.8 μm, 2.1 × 150 mm
Flow rate: 0.4 ml/min
Injection volume: 1 μL
UV wavelength: 210 nm
Mobile phase A: 0.1% phosphoric acid in water
Mobile phase B: Acetonitrile
Column temperature: 45°C

Gradient:

Time (min)	A%	B%
0	95	5
6	40	60
6.8	40	60
7.0	95	5
9.0	95	5

(iii) *Results and calculation*

$$Individual\,triterpene\ (\%) = \frac{Aa \times Wstand \times Vsam \times 100\%}{As \times Vstd \times Wsam}$$

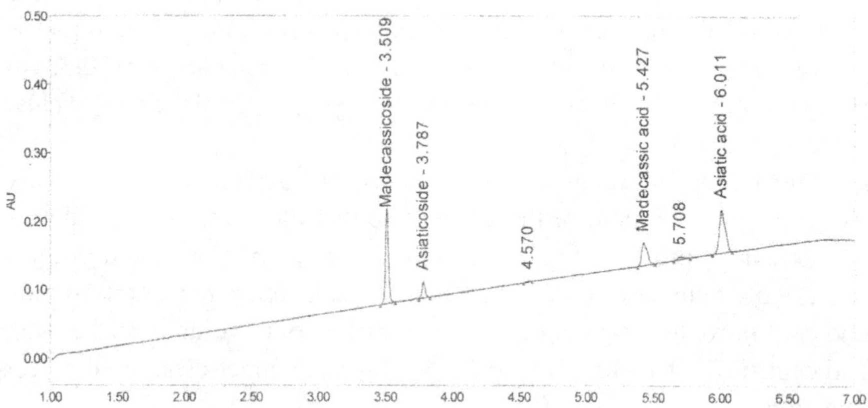

Figure 4.31: UPLC chromatogram of Guto Kola standard solution.

or

$$Individual\ triterpene\ (mg/unit) = \frac{Aa \times Wsand \times Vsam \times UW}{As \times Vstd \times Wsam}$$

Here
Aa = Peak area of corresponding triterpene in sample solution
As = Peak area of corresponding triterpene in standard solution
Wsand = Weight of corresponding triterpene standard (mg)
Wsam = Weight of sample (mg)
Vstd = Total volume of standard solution (ml)
Vsam= Total volume of sample solution (ml)
UW = Unit weight (mg/unit)
Total triterpenes = Sum of individual triterpenes

4.44 Test Method for Punicalagin

Punicalagin is the main active compound in pomegranate and has antioxidant properties. Punicalagin A and B are just α and β forms of punicalagin.

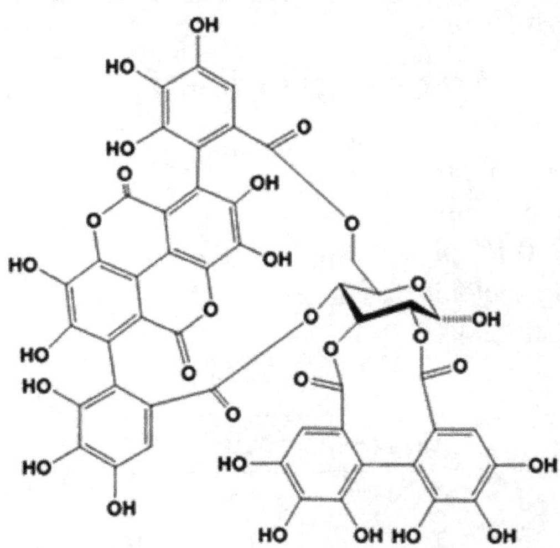

Punicalagin

(i) *Test procedure*

Preparation of standard solution — Accurately weigh about 10 mg of a punicalagin standard, and transfer it to a 100 ml volumetric flask. Add

60 ml of methanol, and sonicate for 5 min. Then add methanol/water (50:50) to the final volume, and shake well. This standard is ready to be injected.

Preparation of sample solution (raw plant sample) — Accurately weigh a certain amount of pomegranate sample which contains about 5 mg of punicalagin, and transfer it to a 100 ml volumetric flask. Add exactly 30 ml of ethanol/water (70:30), cap the flask, and sonicate for 30 min. Cool to room temperature, then add exactly 20 ml of methanol /water (50:50), and shake well. Centrifuge (10,000 rpm) for 5 min, and then take the upper clear solution for injection.

Preparation of sample solution (extract sample) — Accurately weigh a certain amount of sample which contains 10 mg of punicalagin, and transfer it to 100 ml volumetric flask. Add 60 ml of methanol/water (70:30), and sonicate for 10 min. Cool to room temperature, add methanol/water (50:50) to the final volume, shake well, and centrifuge (10,000 rpm) for 5 min. Take the upper clear solution for injection.

(ii) *UPLC conditions*

Column: Acquity UPLC® BEH C18 1.7 μm, 2.1 × 150 mm
Flow rate: 0.4 ml/min
Injection volume: 1.0 μl
UV wavelength: 346 nm
Mobile phase A: 0.1% phosphoric acid in water
Mobile phase B: Acetonitrile
Column temperature: 45°C

Gradient:

Time (min)	A%	B%
0	98	2
3	80	20
4	50	50
4.8	50	50
5.0	98	2
7.0	98	2

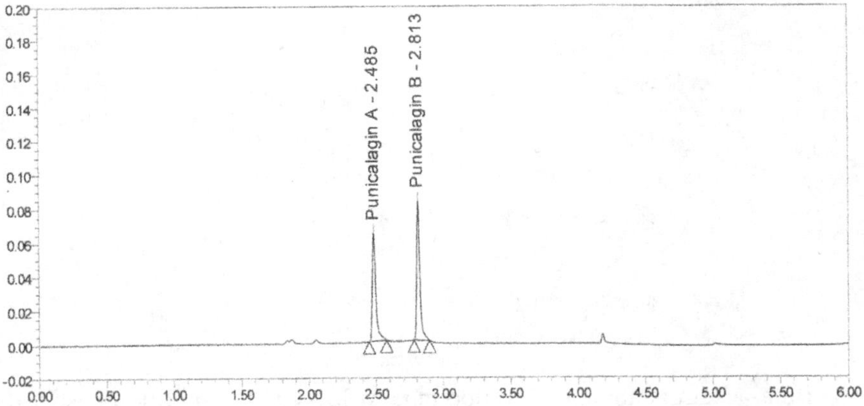

Figure 4.32: UPLC chromatogram of α and β forms of punicalagin.

(iii) *Results and calculation*

$$Punicalagin\ A/B\ (\%) = \frac{Aa \times Wstand \times Vsam \times 100\%}{As \times Vstd \times Wsam}$$

or

$$Punicalagin\ A/B\ (mg/unit) = \frac{Aa \times Wsand \times Vsam \times UW}{As \times Vstd \times Wsam}$$

Here
Aa = Total peak area of punicalagin A/B in sample solution
As = Total peak area of punicalagin A/B in standard solution
Wsand = Weight of punicalagin standard (mg)
Wsam = Weight of sample (mg)
Vstd = Total volume of standard solution (ml)
Vsam = Total volume of sample solution (ml)
UW = Unit weight (mg/unit)

4.45 Beta-Aescin Test Method

Beta-aescin is extracted from horse chestnut. It has anti-inflammatory and vaso-protective functions.

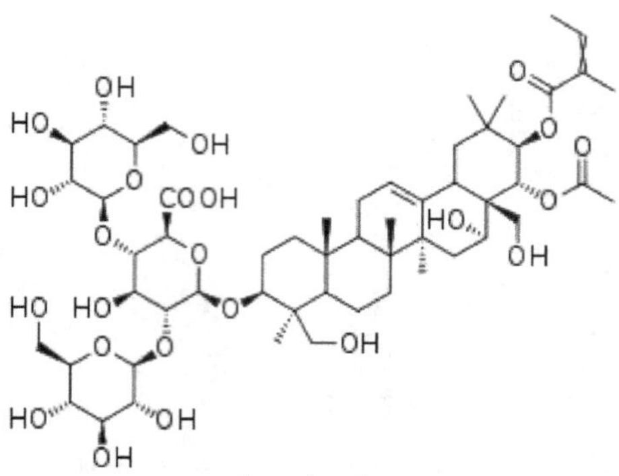

beta-Aescin

Beta-aescin is an acidic compound. At low pH the mobile phase will be neutralized, then it can be retained on revered phase C18 column. See Chapter 1, Section 1.1.2 "Mobile phase application".

(i) *Test procedure*

Preparation of standard solution — Accurately weigh about 10 mg of beta-aescin standard, and transfer it to a 50 ml volumetric flask. Add 30 ml methanol, and vortex until the standard is dissolved. Then add methanol to the mark, and shake well. This solution can be injected.

Preparation of sample solution (for extract powder) — Accurately weigh a certain amount of ground sample that contains about 10 mg of beta-aescin, and transfer to a 50 ml volumetric flask. Add 10 ml of water, and sonicate for 5 min. Then add 30 ml ethanol, and sonicate for another 10 min. Cool to room temperature, add methanol to the volume, shake well, and centrifuge (10,000 rpm) for 5 min. The clear solution can be injected.

Preparation of sample solution (for horse chestnut powder) — Weigh a certain amount of grinded sample containing about 10 mg of beta-aescin, transfer it to a 100 ml volumetric flask, add exact 50 ml of methanol, sonicate for 40 min, shake well, cool to room temperature, centrifuge (10,000 rpm) for 5 min. The clear solution can then be injected.

(ii) *HPLC conditions*

Column: Phenomenex LUNA C18 (2) 5 μm, 4.6 × 150 mm 100A
Flow rate: 1.0 ml/min

Injection volume: 10.0 μL
UV wavelength: 210 nm
Mobile phase A: 0.1% TFA in water
Mobile phase B: 0.1% TFA in acetonitrile
Column temperature: Room temperature

Gradient:

Time (min)	A%	B%
0	70	30
22	44	56
22.7	44	56
23.0	70	30
28.0	70	30

(iii) *Results and calculation*

$$Beta-aescin\ (\%) = \frac{Aa \times Wstand \times Vsam \times 100\%}{As \times Vstd \times Wsam}$$

or

$$Beta-aescin\ (mg/unit) = \frac{Aa \times Wsand \times Vsam \times UW}{As \times Vstd \times Wsam}$$

Here
Aa = Total peak area of beta-aescin in sample solution
As = Total peak area of beta-aescin in standard solution
Wsand = Weight of beta-aescin standard (mg)
Wsam = Weight of sample (mg)
Vstd = Total volume of standard solution (ml)
Vsam = Total volume of sample solution (ml)
UW = Unit weight (mg/unit)

4.46 Resveratrol Test Method

Resveratrol is found in a variety of food sources, such as blueberry, raspberry and in the skin of grapes. Resveratrol is commonly used in dietary supplements. Resveratrol is an antioxidant and may reduce oxidant-induced apoptosis and low-density lipoprotein (LDL). Resveratrol may be responsible, in part, for the correlation between increased wine consumption and decreased risk of coronary heart disease.

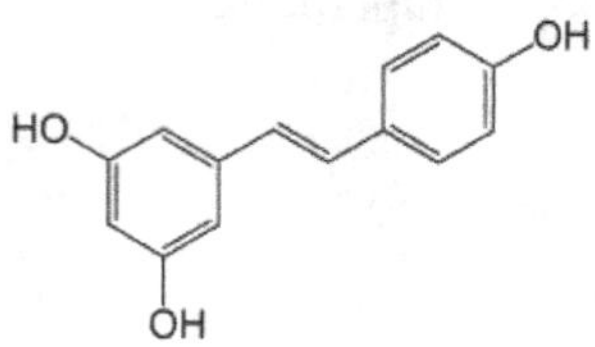

Resveratrol

(i) *Test procedure*

Preparation of standard solution — Accurately weigh about 5 mg resveratrol standard, and transfer it to a 50 ml volumetric flask. Add 30 ml methanol/water (50:50), and vortex until the standard is dissolved completely. Then fill with methanol/water (50:50) to the volume, and shake well. Accurately transfer 5 ml of this solution into a 50 ml volumetric flask, dilute to the volume with methanol/water (50:50), and shake well. The standard solution is ready for injection.

Preparation of sample solution — Accurately weigh a certain amount of sample which contains about 5 mg of resveratrol, and transfer it to a 50 ml volumetric flask. Add 10 ml of water, sonicate for 5 min, add 20 ml methanol, and sonicate for another 15 min. Cool the solution to room temperature, and fill with methanol/water (50:50) to the mark. Shake well, and then centrifuge (10,000 rpm) for 5 min. Take the clear solution and make a 10-fold dilution with methanol/water (50:50), and shake well. This final solution is ready for injection.

(ii) *HPLC conditions*

Column: Phenomenex Prodigy 5 μm, 4.6 × 250 mm, 100A
Flow rate: 1.1 ml/min
Injection volume: 10 μL
UV wavelength: 315 nm

Mobile phase A: 0.1% phosphoric acid in water
Mobile phase B: 0.1% phosphoric acid in acetonitrile
Column temperature: Room temperature

Gradient:

Time (min)	A%	B%
0	85	15
15	5	95
16.5	5	95
17.0	85	15
25.0	85	15

(iii) *Results and calculation*

$$Resveratrol\ (\%) = \frac{Aa \times Wstand \times Vsam \times 100\%}{As \times Vstd \times Wsam}$$

or

$$Resveratrol\ (mg/unit) = \frac{Aa \times Wsand \times Vsam \times UW}{As \times Vstd \times Wsam}$$

Here
Aa = Peak area of resveratrol in sample solution
As = Peak area of resveratrol in standard solution
Wsand = Weight of resveratrol standard (mg)
Wsam = Weight of sample (mg)
Vstd = Total volume of standard solution (ml)
Vsam = Total volume of sample solution (ml)
UW = Unit weight (mg/unit)

4.47 Goldenseal Test Method

Berberine and hydrastine are the main active compounds of goldenseal.

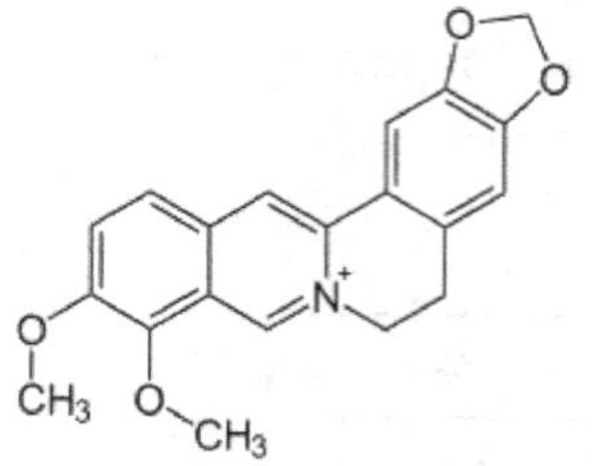

Berberine

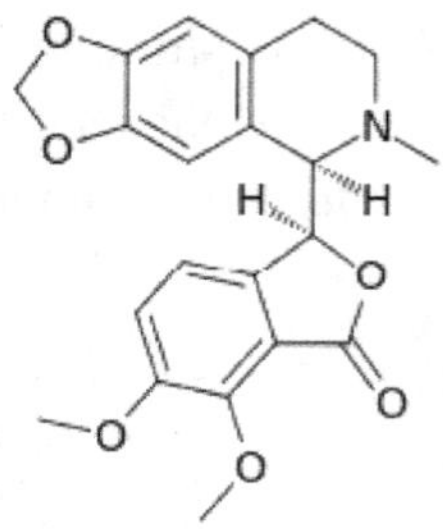

hydrastine

Berberine and hydrastine are alkaline compounds, to extend the chromatography retention time, and to get better separation, this method adds hexane sulfonate as an ion pair reagent in mobile phase. See Chapter 1, Section 1.1.2 "Mobile phase application".

(i) *Test procedure*

Preparation of standard solution — Accurately weigh about 5 mg of berberine and 5 mg of hydrastine standards, and transfer it to a 100 ml volumetric flask. Add 60 ml methanol, sonicate until the standards are completely dissolved, then add methanol to the volume. After shaking well, the solution is ready for injection.

Preparation of sample solution — Accurately weigh a certain amount of ground sample that contains about 5 mg of berberine and/or hydrastine, and transfer it to a 100 ml volumetric flask. Add 10 ml water, sonicate for 5 min, and then add 50 ml ethanol. Sonicate for 10 min for extract powders and sonicate for 40 min for goldenseal powder. Cool to room temperature and then add methanol to the mark, and shake well. Centrifuge (10,000 rpm) for 5 min, and take the clear solution for injection.

(ii) *HPLC conditions*

Column: Supecol Discovery Amide C16, 150 × 4.6 mm, 5 um
Flow rate: 1.1 ml/min
Injection volume: 10μL
UV wavelength: 338 nm
Mobile phase A: 10 mM hexansulfonic acid sodium salt, pH 3.0
Mobile phase B: Acetonitrile
Column temperature: Room temperature

Gradient:

Time (min)	A%	B%
0	85	15
9.0	45	55
10.0	45	55
10.5	85	15
15.0	85	15

(iii) *Results and calculation*

$$Berberine/hydrastine\,(\%) = \frac{Aa \times Wstand \times Vsam \times 100\%}{As \times Vstd \times Wsam}$$

or

$$Berberine/hydrastine\ (mg/unit) = \frac{Aa \times Wsand \times Vsam \times UW}{As \times Vstd \times Wsam}$$

Here
Aa = Peak area of Berberine/hydrastine in sample solution
As = Peak area of Berberine/hydrastine in standard solution
Wsand = Weight of Berberine/hydrastine standard (mg)
Wsam = Weight of sample (mg)
Vstd = Total volume of standard solution (ml)
Vsam = Total volume of sample solution (ml)
UW = Unit weight (mg/unit)

4.48 Test Parthenolide in Feverfew

Feverfew or feverfew extracts can be used to prevent and treat migraine headaches, fever, dizziness and nausea. The active compound is parthenolide.

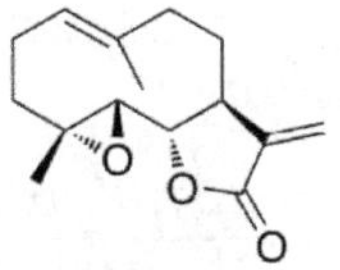

Parthenolide

(i) *Test procedure*

Preparation of standard solution — Accurately weigh about 5 mg of a parthenolide standard, and transfer it to a 100 ml volumetric flask. Add 60 ml methanol, sonicate until the standard is completely dissolved, and then add methanol to the volume. After shaking well, the solution is ready for injection.

Preparation of sample solution — Accurately weigh a certain amount of ground sample that contains about 5 mg of parthenolide, and transfer it to a 100 ml volumetric flask. Add 10 ml water, sonicate 5 min, and then add 60 ml ethanol. Sonicate 10 min for extract powders; or sonicate 40 min for feverfew powder. Cool to room temperature and then add methanol to the mark, and shake well. Centrifuge (10,000 rpm) for 5 min, and take the clear solution for injection.

(ii) *UPLC conditions*

Column: Acquity UPLC® HSS Ts C18, 1.8 μm, 2.1 × 100 mm
Flow rate: 0.4 ml/min
Injection volume: 2.0 μL
UV wavelength: 210 nm
Mobile phase A: 0.1% phosphoric acid in water
Mobile phase B: Acetonitrile
Column temperature: 45°C

Gradient:

Time (min)	A%	B%
0	70	30
5	57	43
5.8	57	43
6.0	70	30
8.0	70	30

(iii) *Results and calculation*

$$Parthenolide\,(\%) = \frac{Aa \times Wstand \times Vsam \times 100\%}{As \times Vstd \times Wsam}$$

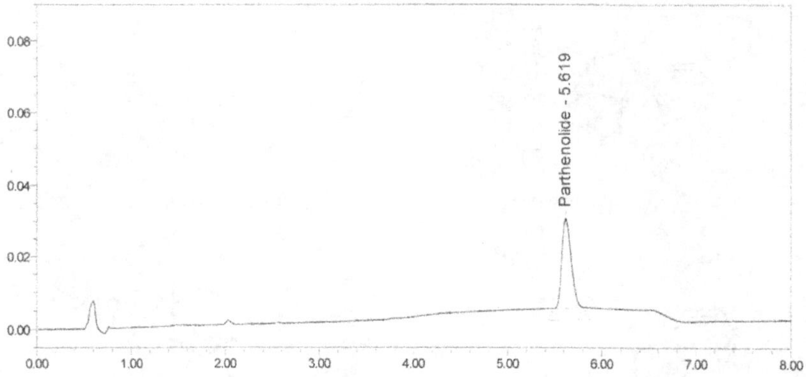

Figure 4.33: Chromatogram of parthenolide.

or

$$Parthenolide\ (mg/unit) = \frac{Aa \times Wsand \times Vsam \times UW}{As \times Vstd \times Wsam}$$

Here

Aa = Peak area of parthenolide in sample solution
As = Peak area of parthenolide in standard solution
Wsand = Weight of parthenolide standard (mg)
Wsam = Weight of sample (mg)
Vstd = Total volume of standard solution (ml)
Vsam = Total volume of sample solution (ml)
UW = Unit weight (mg/unit)

4.49 Determination of Oxindole Alkaloids in Cat's Claw by HPLC

Cat's claw is a woody vine plant found in South and Central America. Its root bark has been used as a traditional medicine to treat arthritis, stomach ulcers, inflammation and fever. The active compounds of cat's claw are composed of oxindole alkaloids, including mitraphylline, isomitraphylline, pteropodine and isopteropodine.

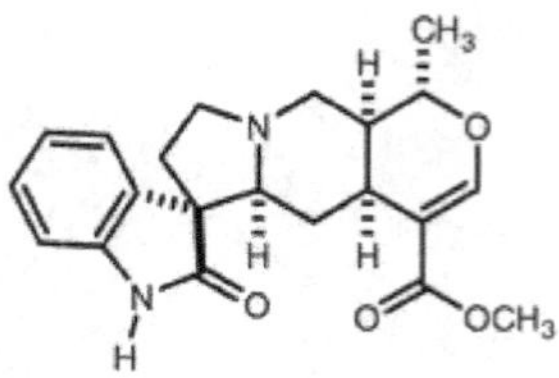

Pteropodine

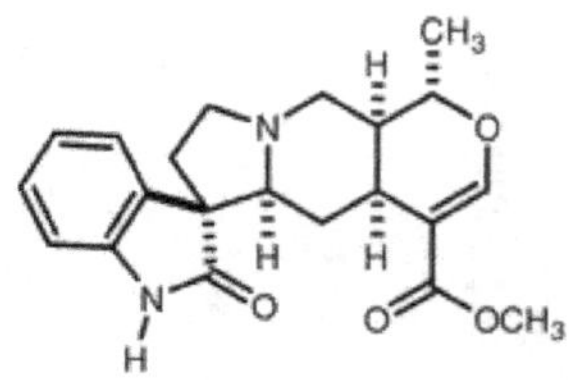

Isopteropodine

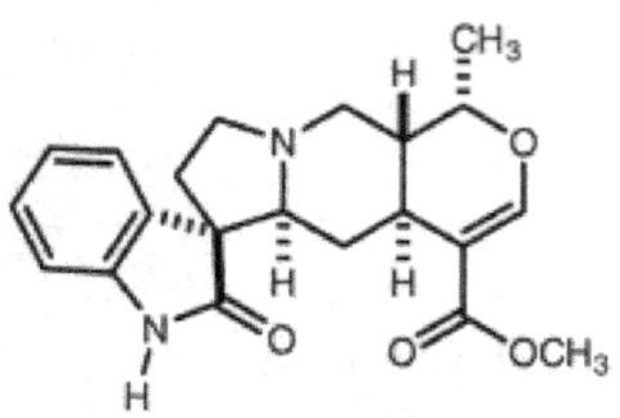

Mitraphylline

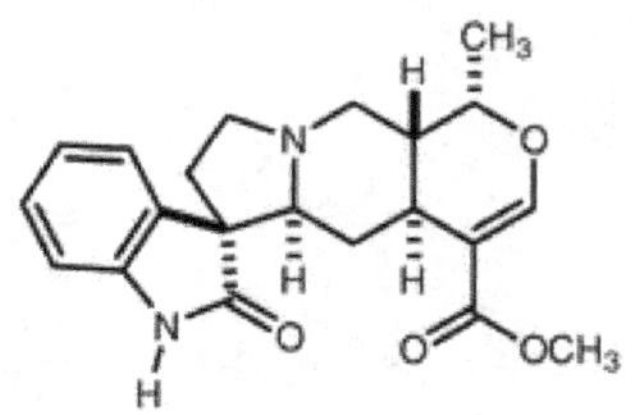

Isomitraphylline

From the aforementioned molecular structures it can been seen that these compounds have the same molecular formula $C_{2}1H_{2}4N_{2}O_{4}$ with same molecular weights 368.4. Their UV spectrum is the same, the maximum absorption is at 245 nm. Therefore, this method only uses mitraphylline as a standard, the other compounds are calculated according to the mitraphylline standard.

(i) *Test procedure*

Preparation of standard solution — Accurately weigh about 5 mg of mitraphylline standard, and transfer it to a 100 ml volumetric flask. Add 60 ml methanol, sonicate until the standard is completely dissolved. After the solution is cooled, add methanol to the volume, and shake well. The solution can be injected.

Preparation of sample solution — Accurately weigh a certain amount of ground sample that contains about 5 mg of mitraphylline, and transfer it to a 100 ml volumetric flask. Add 10 ml of water, sonicate for 5 min, and then add 60 ml of ethanol. Sonicate for 10 min for extract materials or sonicate for 50 min for cat's claw bark powder. Cool to room temperature, then add methanol to the volume, and shake and mix well. Centrifuge (10,000 rpm) for 5 min, and take the upper-level clear solution for injection.

(ii) *HPLC conditions*

Column: Phenomenex Luna C18 (2) 5 μm 4.6 × 150 mm 100A
Flow rate: 1.0 ml/min
Injection volume: 10 μL
UV wavelength: 245 nm
Mobile phase A: pH 7.0 buffer (1,000 ml water add 480 mg sodium phosphate dibasic and 900 mg of sodium phosphate monobasic)
Mobile phase B: Methanol
Mobile phase C: Acetonitrile
Column temperature: room temperature

Gradient:

Time	A	B	C
0	60	20	20
30.0	30	35	35
30.1	60	20	20
40.0	60	20	20

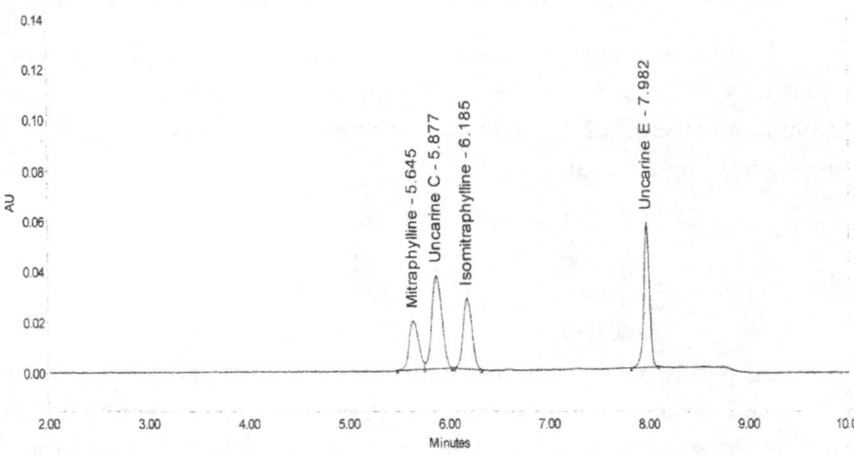

Figure 4.34: HPLC chromatogram of cat's claw (uncarine C is pteropodine, uncarine E is isopteropodine).

(iii) *Results and calculation*

$$Individual\ oxindole\ alkaloid\ (\%) = \frac{Aa \times Wstand \times Vsam \times 100\%}{As \times Vstd \times Wsam}$$

or

$$Individual\ oxindole\ alkaloid\ (mg/unit) = \frac{Aa \times Wsand \times Vsam \times UW}{As \times Vstd \times Wsam}$$

Here
Aa = Peak area of corresponding oxindole alkaloid in sample solution
As = Peak area of mitraphylline in standard solution
Wsand = Weight of mitraphylline standard (mg)
Wsam = Weight of sample (mg)
Vstd = Total volume of standard solution (ml)
Vsam = Total volume of sample solution (ml)
UW = Unit weight (mg/unit)

Total of oxindole alkaloids = Sum of all individual oxindole alkaloids measured.

4.50 Determination of Synephrine and N-methlytyroamine in Bitter Orange by HPLC

Bitter orange contains synephrine and n-methyltyroamine. These compounds may be beneficial by regulating the fat levels in blood and lowering blood glcouse levels. It may help individuals who have lower blood pressure level by increasing it.

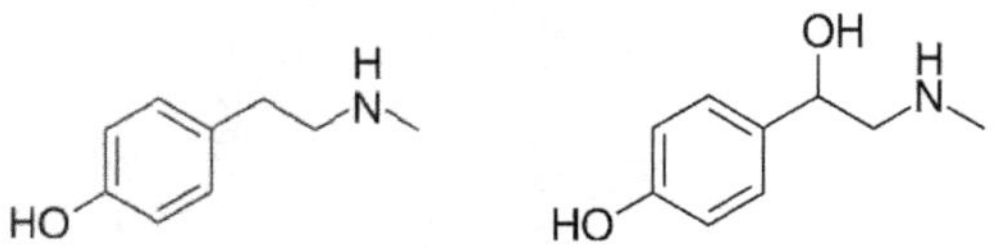

N-methlytyroamine Synephrine

Based on the aforementioned molecular structures, both compounds are alkaline. To extend the retention time and to get a good separation with reversed phase column, this method uses the addition of hexansulfonic acid to the mobile phase as an ion pairing reagent. By polarity, synephrine has one more hydroxyl group in the molecule, so it will be eluted earlier than n-methlytyroamine.

(i) *Test procedure*

Preparation of standard solution — Accurately weigh about 10 mg of synephrine and 10 mg of N-methlytyroamine standard, and transfer it to a 100 ml volumetric flask. Add 60 ml methanol, vortex until the standards are fully dissolved, and then add methanol to the mark. Shake well, and the standard solution is ready for injection.

Preparation of sample solution — Accurately weigh a certain amount of ground sample that contains about 10 mg of synephrine or N-methlytyroamine, and transfer it to a 100 ml volumetric flask. Add 10 ml of water, sonicate for 5 min, and then add 50 ml of ethanol. Sonicate for 10 min for extract samples or sonicate for 40 min for bitter orange powder. Cool to room temperature, fill methanol to mark, and shake well. Centrifuge (10,000 rpm) for 5 min, and the upper clear solution can be injected.

(ii) *UPLC conditions*

Column: Acquity UPLC® BEH C18, 1.7 μm, 2.1 × 150 mm
Flow rate: 0.4 ml/min
Injection volume: 1.0 μL
UV wavelength: 270 nm
Mobile phase A: 10 mM hexansulfonic acid sodium in water, pH 3.0
Mobile phase B: Acetonitrile
Column temperature: 45°C

Gradient:

Time (min)	A%	B%
0	95	5
4	80	20
5	65	35
5.5	65	35
6.0	95	5
8.0	95	5

(iii) *Results and calculation*

$$Synephrine/methyltyroamine\,(\%) = \frac{Aa \times Wstand \times Vsam \times 100\%}{As \times Vstd \times Wsam}$$

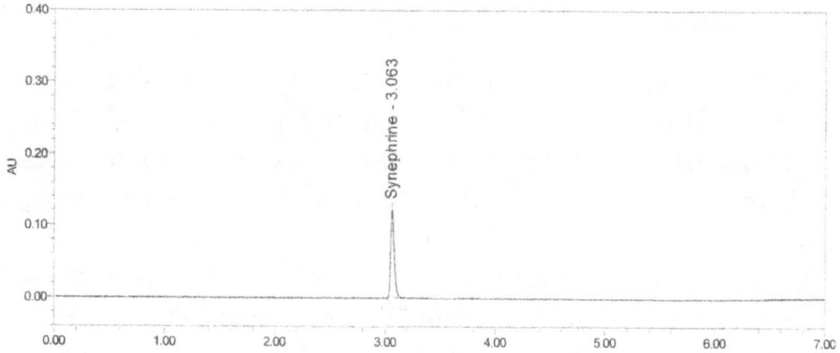

Figure 4.35: UPLC chromatogram of synephrine.

or

$$Synephrine/methyltyroamine\ (mg/unit) = \frac{Aa \times Wsand \times Vsam \times UW}{As \times Vstd \times Wsam}$$

Here
Aa = Peak area of synephrine/methyltyroamine in sample solution
As = Peak area of synephrine/methyltyroamine in standard solution
Wsand = Weight of synephrine/methyltyroamine standard (mg)
Wsam = Weight of sample (mg)
Vstd = Total volume of standard solution (ml)
Vsam = Total volume of sample solution (ml)
UW = Unit weight (mg/unit)

4.51 Test Method for 4′-Hydroxy-3′-Methoxyisoflavone-7-sug, from Astragalus

4′-Hydroxy-3′-Methoxyisoflavone-7-sug is extracted from astragalus. Its main function is that it has an alleviating effect on osteoarthritis, and it is antimicrobial.

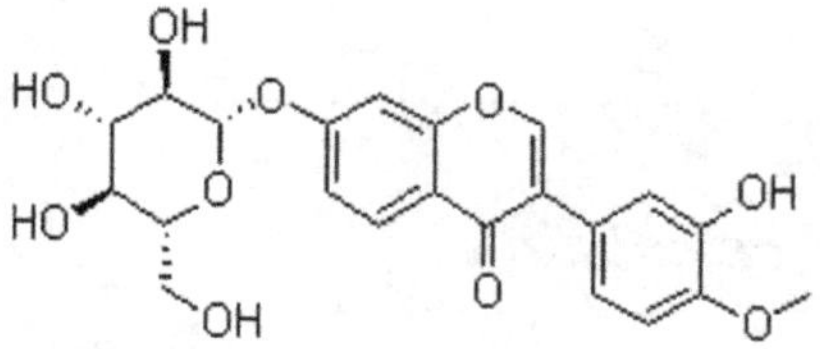

4’-Hydroxy-3’-Methoxyisoflavone-7-sug

(i) *Test procedure*

Preparation of standard solution — Accurately weigh approximately 5 mg of a 4′-Hydroxy-3′-Methoxyisoflavone-7-sug standard, and transfer it to a 100 ml volumetric flask. Add 60 ml methanol, and sonicate until all standard dissolved. Then add methanol to the mark, and shake well. This standard solution can be injected.

Preparation of sample solution — Accurately weigh a certain amount of ground sample containing about 5 mg of 4′-Hydroxy-3′-Methoxyisoflavone-7-sug, and transfer it to a 100 ml volumetric flask. Add 20 ml of water, and sonicate for 5 min. Add 50 ml ethanol, and sonicate for 10 min for extract materials or 50 min for astragalus powder. Cool to room temperature, fill with methanol to the mark, and shake well. Centrifuge (10,000 rpm) for 5 min, and the upper-level clear solution can be injected.

(ii) *HPLC conditions*

Column: Phenomenex LUNA C18 (2) 5 μm 4.6 × 250 mm 100A
Flow rate: 1.0 ml/min
Injection volume: 10μL
UV wavelength: 254 nm
Mobile phase A: 0.1% phosphoric acid in water
Mobile phase B: Acetonitrile
Column temperature: Room temperature

Gradient:

Time (min)	A%	B%
0	85	15
25	70	30
28	55	45
29	55	45
29.5	85	15
35	85	15

(iii) *Results and calculation*

$$Hydroxy'\text{-}Methoxyisoflavonesug\ (\%) = \frac{Aa \times Wstand \times Vsam \times 100\%}{As \times Vstd \times Wsam}$$

or

$$Hydroxy'\text{-}Methoxyisoflavonesug\ (mg/unit) = \frac{Aa \times Wsand \times Vsam \times UW}{As \times Vstd \times Wsam}$$

Here
Aa = Peak area of sample
As = Peak area of standard
Wsand = Weight of standard (mg)
Wsam = Weight of sample (mg)
Vstd = Total volume of standard solution (ml)
Vsam = Total volume of sample solution (ml)
UW = Unit weight (mg/unit)

4.52 Test Method for Glucoraphanin in Broccoli

According to current scientific research, broccoli contains glucoraphanin, which may have anti-cancer activity, or help low-cholesterol and other functions.

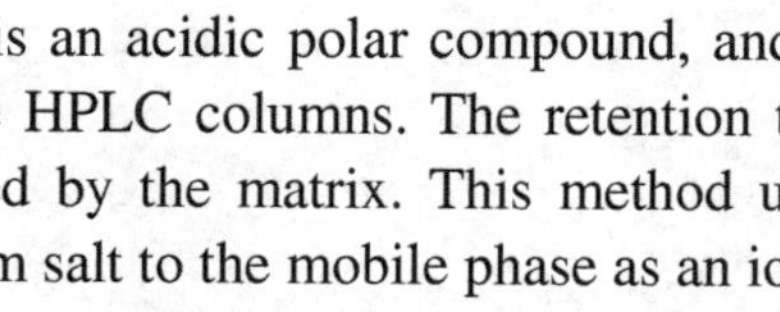

Glucoraphanin

Glucoraphanin is an acidic polar compound, and has no interaction with reversed phase HPLC columns. The retention time is short and is easy to be interfered by the matrix. This method uses the addition of tetrabutyl ammonium salt to the mobile phase as an ion pair reagent. This attracts the glucoraphanin anion to form a neutral ion pair, which extends the retention time and obtains better separation with a reversed phase column. See Chapter 1, Section 1.1.2 "Mobile Phase Applications".

(i) *Test procedure*

Preparation of solvent A — Equally mix the following four reagents: water, DMSO, DMF and acetonitrile, shake and mix well.

Preparation of standard solution — Accurately weigh about 10 mg of a glucoraphanin standard, and transfer it to a 50 ml volumetric flask. Add 30 ml of water, and vortex until all standard dissolved. Fill with water to volume, then shake and mix well. This standard solution is ready for injection.

Preparation of sample solution (for free glucoraphanin sample) — Accurately weigh a certain amount of sample that contains about 10 mg of glucoraphanin, and transfer it to a 50 ml volumetric flask. Add 30 ml of water, and shake with wrist action shaker for 15 min. Then fill with water to volume, mix well, and centrifuge (10,000 rpm) for 5 min. The clear solution is ready for injection.

Preparation of sample solution (for broccoli and other plants) — Accurately weigh a certain amount of sample that contains about 10 mg of glucoraphanin, mix with 50 ml of solvent A. Transfer the sludge to a blender and homogenize the sample for at least five minutes. Let it stand for 5 min, then centrifuge (10,000 rpm) for 5 min. The a clear solution can be injected.

(ii) *UPLC conditions*

Column: Acquity UPLC® HSS T3 C18, 1.8 μm, 2.1 × 150 mm
Flow rate: 0.4 ml/min
Injection volume: 2 μl
Column temperature: 45°C
Mobile phase A: 2 mM Tetrabutylammonium Hydrogen Sulfate, pH 3.5.
Mobile phase B: Acetonitrile

Gradient:

Time (min)	A%	B%
0	95	5
6	70	30
6.8	70	30
7.0	95	5
9.0	95	5

(iii) *Results and calculation*

$$Glucoraphanin(\%) = \frac{Aa \times Wstand \times Vsam \times 100\%}{As \times Vstd \times Wsam}$$

or

$$Glucoraphanin\ (mg/unit) = \frac{Aa \times Wsand \times Vsam \times UW}{As \times Vstd \times Wsam}$$

Here
Aa = Peak area of sample
As = Peak area of standard
Wsand = Weight of standard (mg)
Wsam = Weight of sample (mg)
Vstd = Total volume of standard solution (ml)
Vsam = Total volume of sample solution (ml)
UW = Unit weight (mg/unit)

4.53 Test Method for Harpagoside

Harpagoside is extracted from Devil's claw that is native to South Africa. It has been used as a medicine for hundreds of years and helps to treat cold, high blood pressure and other ailments.

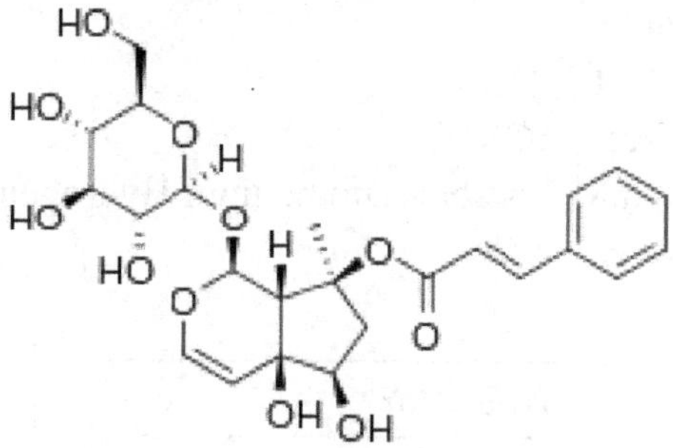

Harpagoside

(i) *Test procedure*

Preparation of standard solution — Accurately weigh about 5 mg of harpagoside standard, and transfer it to a 100 ml volumetric flask. Add 60 ml methanol, and sonicate until all standards are dissolved. Then add methanol to the 100 ml mark, and shake well. This standard solution is ready for injection.

Preparation of sample solution — Weigh a certain amount of ground sample that contains about 5 mg of harpagoside, and transfer it to a 100 ml volumetric flask. Add 10 ml of water, and sonicate for 5 min. Then add 60 ml methanol, and sonicate for 10 min for extract materials or sonicate 40 min for Devil's claw powder. Cool to room temperature, add methanol to the volume, shake and mix well. Centrifuge for 5 min (10,000 rpm), and draw the abovementioned clear solution for injection.

(ii) *UPLC conditions*

Column: Acquity UPLC® HSS T3 1.8 μm, 2.1 × 150 mm
Flow rate: 0.4 ml/min
Injection volume: 1.0 μL
UV wavelength: 275 nm
Mobile phase A: 0.1% phosphoric acid in water
Mobile phase B: Acetonitrile
Column temperature: 45°C

Gradient:

Time (min)	A%	B%
0	95	5
8.0	50	50
9.5	50	50
10.0	95	5
12.0	95	5

(iii) *Results and calculation*

$$Harpagoside\ (\%) = \frac{Aa \times Wstand \times Vsam \times 100\%}{As \times Vstd \times Wsam}$$

or

$$Harpagoside\ (mg/unit) = \frac{Aa \times Wsand \times Vsam \times UW}{As \times Vstd \times Wsam}$$

Here
Aa = Peak area of sample
As = Peak area of standard
Wsand = Weight of standard (mg)
Wsam = Weight of sample (mg)
Vstd = Total volume of standard solution (ml)
Vsam = Total volume of sample solution (ml)
UW = Unit weight (mg/unit)

4.54 Determination of Ligustilide in Dong Quai by HPLC

Ligustilide can be extracted from Dong Quai, a traditional Chinese medicine, used to treat Alzheimer's disease increased antioxidants and decreased oxidation levels in the brain.

Ligustilide is a highly non-polar compound. To dissolve it you must use chloroform and other non-polar strong organic solvents. With reversed phase-C18 column it is not easy to be eluded. This method uses C8 columns to make the ligustilide elute faster and easier.

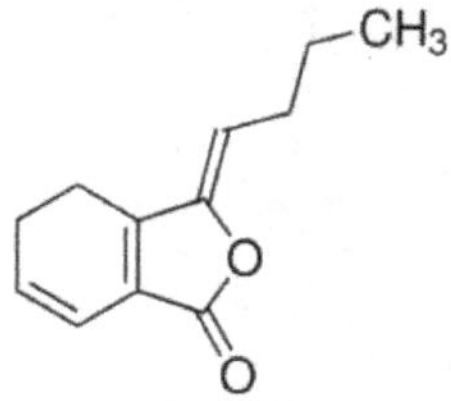

Ligustilide

(i) *Test procedure*

Preparation of standard solution — Accurately weigh about 5 mg of ligustilide standard, and transfer it to a 100 ml volumetric flask. Add 20 ml of chloroform, sonicate until the standard completely dissolved, then add ethanol to 100 ml volume. Shake and mix well, the standard solution is now ready for injection.

Preparation of sample solution — Weigh a certain amount of ground sample that contains about 5 mg of ligustilide, and transfer it to a 100 ml volumetric flask. Add 15 ml of water, and sonicate for 5 min. Centrifuge for 5 min (10,000 r/min), remove all the water then add 20 ml of isopropanol and 30 ml of chloroform. Sonicate for 40 min for Dong Quai powder or 10 min for extract powders. After cooling add ethanol to mark, shake and mix well. Centrifuge (10,000 rpm) for 5 min, the clear solution can be injected.

(ii) *UPLC conditions*

Column: Acquity BEH C8, 1.7 μm, 2.1 × 100 mm
Flowrate: 0.4 ml/min
Injection volume: 1.0 μL
UV wavelength: 254 nm
Mobile phase A: Nano pure water
Mobile phase B: Acetonitrile
Column temperature: 45°C

Gradient:

Time (min)	A%	B%
0	30	70
5	0	100
8.0	0	100
8.5	30	70
12.0	30	70

(iii) *Results and calculation*

$$Ligustilide\ (\%) = \frac{Aa \times Wstand \times Vsam \times 100\%}{As \times Vstd \times Wsam}$$

or

$$Ligustilide\ (mg/unit) = \frac{Aa \times Wsand \times Vsam \times UW}{As \times Vstd \times Wsam}$$

Here
Aa = Peak area of sample
As = Peak area of standard
Wsand = Weight of standard (mg)
Wsam = Weight of sample (mg)
Vstd = Total volume of standard solution (ml)
Vsam = Total volume of sample solution (ml)
UW = Unit weight (mg/unit)

4.55 Sennoside A and B Test Method

Sennoside can be extrcated from *Folium Sennae*. This compound has laxative properties.

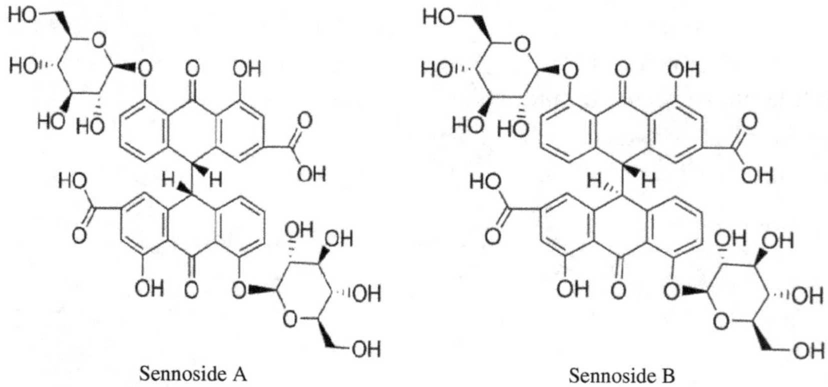

Sennoside A Sennoside B

(i) *Test procedure*

Preparation of standard solution — Accurately weigh about 5 mg of sennoside A and 5 mg sennoside B standards, and transfer both to 100 ml volumetric flask. Add 60 ml acetonitrile/water (50:50), vortex until all standards dissolved, then add methanol to 100 ml mark. After shaking well, the standard solution is ready to inject.

Preparation of sample solution (raw plant) — Weigh a certain amount of ground sample that contains about 5 mg of sennoside A or B, and transfer it to a 100 ml volumetric flask. Add 60 ml of water at 80°C.

Shake for 10 sec every 2 min, for a total of 10 min. Cool to room temperature, add methanol slowly with frequent shaking to the volume. Shake well, centrifuge (10,000 rpm) for 5 min, and draw the clear solution for injection.

Preparation of sample solution (extract powder) — Accurately weigh a certain amount of ground sample that contains about 5 mg of sennoside A or B, and transfer it to a 100 ml volumetric flask. Add 10 ml water and vortex for 5 min. Add 50 ml of acetonitrile/water (50:50), and sonicate for 5 min. After the solution is cooled, fill to volume with acetonitrile/water (50:50). Shake well, centrifuge (10,000 rpm) for 5 min, and take the clear solution for injection.

(ii) *UPLC conditions*

Column: Acquity UPLC® HSS T3, C18, 1.8 μm, 2.1 × 150 mm
Floe rate: 0.4 ml/min
Injection volume: 1.0 μL
UV wavelength: 270 nm
Mobile phase A: 0.1% phosphoric acid in water
Mobile phase B: Acetonitrile
Column temperature: 45°C

Gradient:

Time (min)	A%	B%
0	95	5
7.0	70	30
8.5	50	50
9.5	50	50
10.0	95	5
12.0	95	5

(iii) *Results and calculation*

$$Sennoside\ A/B\,(\%) = \frac{Aa \times Wstand \times Vsam \times 100\%}{As \times Vstd \times Wsam}$$

or

$$Sennoside\ A/B\ (mg/unit) = \frac{Aa \times Wsand \times Vsam \times UW}{As \times Vstd \times Wsam}$$

Here
Aa = Peak area of sennoside A/B in sample solution
As = Peak area of sennoside A/B in standard solution
Wsand = Weight of sennoside A/B standards (mg)
Wsam = Weight of sample (mg)
Vstd = Total volume of standard solution (ml)
Vsam = Total volume of sample solution (ml)
UW = Unit weight (mg/unit)

Total sennosides = Sennoside A + sennoside B

4.56 Guggulsterone E and Z Test Method

Guggulsterone is a plant steroid found in the resin of the guggul plant. Guggulsterones can exist as either of two isomers: E-guggulsterone and Z-guggulsterone. The guggulsterones can be dissolved and extracted with methanol and can be separated by a reversed phase UPLC column, BEH C18. By comparing with a known concentration reference standard, guggulsterones can be quantified.

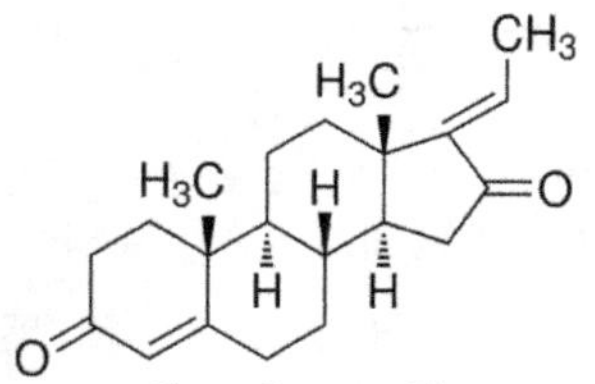

Guggulsterone E

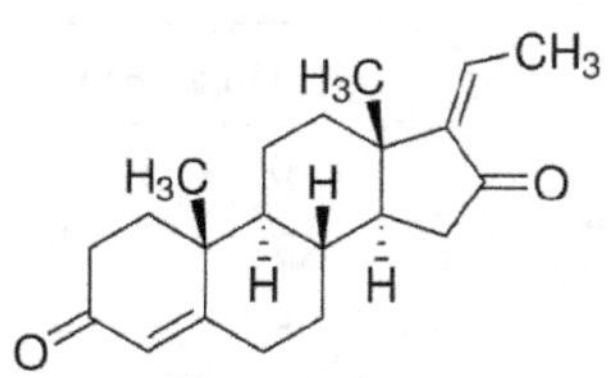

Guggulsterone Z

(i) *Test procedure*

Preparation of standard solution — Accurately weight about 10 mg of guggulsterone E and 10 mg guggulsterone Z standard, and transfer it to a 100 ml volumetric flask. Add 60 ml of methanol and vortex until all standards dissolved. Then add methanol to the mark, shake well, and the standard is ready for injection.

Preparation of sample solution — Accurately weigh a certain amount of ground sample that contains about 10 mg of guggulsterone E or Z, and transfer it to a 100 ml volumetric flask. Add 10 of water, and sonicate for 5 min. Add 60 ml of ethanol, and sonicate raw plants for 45 min or extract powders for 10 min. After the solution is cooled add methanol to the mark. Shake well, centrifuge (10,000 rpm) for 5 min, and take the clear solution for injection.

(ii) *UPLC conditions*

Column: Acquity HSS T3 C18, 1.8 μm, 2.1 × 150 mm
Flow Rate: 0.4 ml/min
Injection volume: 2.0 μL
UV wavelength: 243 nm
Mobile phase A: 0.1% phosphoric acid in water
Mobile phase B: Acetonitrile
Column temperature: 45°C

Gradient:

Time (min)	A%	B%
0	65	45
8.0	35	80
8.8	35	80
9.0	65	45
11.0	65	45

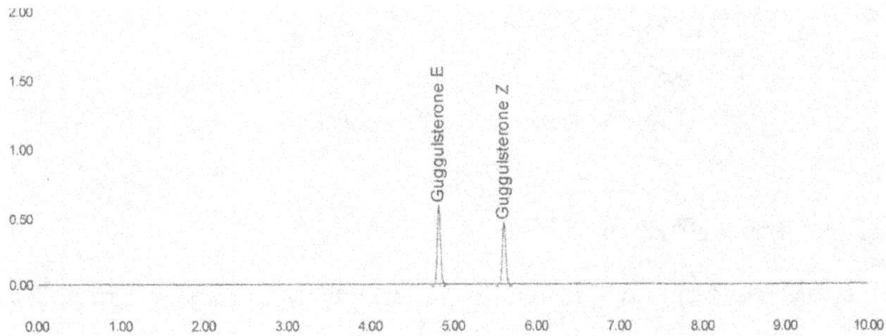

Figure 4.36: UPLC chromatogram of guggulsterone E and Z.

(iii) *Results and calculation*

$$Guggulsterone\ E/Z\ (\%) = \frac{Aa \times Wstand \times Vsam \times 100\%}{As \times Vstd \times Wsam}$$

or

$$Guggulsterone\ E/Z\ (mg/unit) = \frac{Aa \times Wsand \times Vsam \times UW}{As \times Vstd \times Wsam}$$

Here
Aa = Peak area of guggulsterone E/Z in sample solution
As = Peak area of guggulsterone E/Z in standard solution
Wsand = Weight of guggulsterone E/Z standards (mg)
Wsam = Weight of sample (mg)
Vstd = Total volume of standard solution (ml)
Vsam = Total volume of sample solution (ml)
UW = Unit weight (mg/unit)

Total Guggulsterones = Guggulsterone E + Guggulsterone Z

4.57 Test Method for Aristolochic Acid I and II

Aristolochic acids are carcinogens, and they are found in some Chinese herbs, especially in plants of the *aristolochiaceae* family.

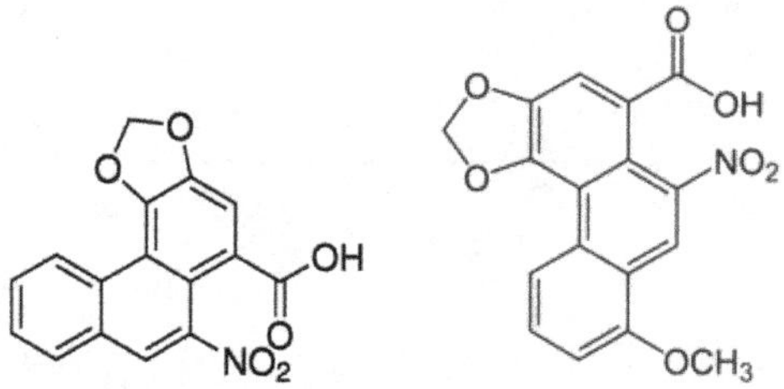

Aristolochic acid I   Aristolochic acid II

(i) *Test procedure*

Preparation of standard solution — Accurately weigh about 2 mg of aristolochic acid I and 2 mg of aristolochic acid II standards, and transfer it to a 100 ml volumetric flask. Add 60 ml of methanol, and vortex until all the standards gets dissolved. Add methanol to 100 ml mark, and shake well. Transfer 0.5 ml of the original solution to 100 ml volumetric flask, add methanol dilution to 100 ml, and shake well. The standard solution is ready for injection.

Preparation of sample solution — Accurately weigh about 3 g of sample, and transfer it to a 100 ml volumetric flask. Add exactly 50 ml of water/acetonitrile (50:50), cap the flask, and vortex for 5 min. Sonicate for 40 min, and then centrifuge the solution (10,000 rpm) for 5 min. Draw the clear solution to injection vail, it is ready for injection.

The sample amount taken will depend on the sensitivity of the instrument and the nature of the sample. It can be adjusted according to the actual situation. The concentration of the standard solution of this method is 0.1 ppm, and the final method detection limit is about 1 ppm.

(ii) *HPLC conditions*

Column: Phenomenex PRODIGY ODS3 5 μm, 4.6 × 250 mm, 100A
Flow rate: 1.1 ml/min
Injection volume: 20 μL
UV wavelength: 390 nm
Mobile phase A: 0.1% phosphoric acid in water
Mobile phase B: Acetonitrile
Column temperature: Room temperature

Gradient:

Time (min)	A%	B%
0	65	35
12	10	90
15.5	10	90
16.0	65	35
20.0	65	35

(iii) *Results and calculation*

$$Aristolochic\,acid\,I/II\,(\%) = \frac{Aa \times Wstand \times Vsam \times 100\%}{As \times Vstd \times Wsam}$$

or

$$Aristolochic\,acid\,I/II\ (mg/unit) = \frac{Aa \times Wsand \times Vsam \times UW}{As \times Vstd \times Wsam}$$

Here
Aa = Peak area of aristolochic acid I/II in sample solution
As = Peak area of aristolochic acid I/II in standard solution
Wsand = Weight of aristolochic acid I/II standards (mg)
Wsam = Weight of sample (mg)
Vstd = Total volume of standard solution (ml)
Vsam = Total volume of sample solution (ml)
UW = Unit weight (mg/unit)

4.58 Saw Palmetto Fatty Acids Assay by GC/FID

Saw palmetto generally is used to decrease the symptoms of an enlarged prostate. Fatty acids, especially short-chain fatty acids (C4–C10), may be the active components. The 11 fatty acids are extracted using Hexane, then they are methylated, and quantified using Gas Chromatography with Flame Ionization detection.

(i) *Test procedure*

Internal standard solution — Accurately weigh 100 mg of nonadecane and transfer it to a 100 ml volumetric flask. Add hexane to dissolve, fill with hexane to the mark. This results in a solution of 1.0 mg per ml.

Preparation of standard solution — Accurately weigh 250 mg of methyl laurate and methyl oleate; 50 mg of methyl linoleate; 20 mg of methyl caproate, methyl caprylate, methyl caprate, methyl palmitoleate, methyl stearate, and methyl linolenate in a 50 ml volumetric flask. Add 30 ml of internal standard solution, and sonicate for 5 min. Then add internal standard solution to mark, and shake and mix well. This standard is ready for injection.

Some methyl esters are air and light sensitive and should be prepared freshly on the test day.

Sample preparation — Accurately weigh 100 mg of pulverized powder of saw palmetto samples and transfer into a 100 mL round bottom flask fitted with a water-cooled reflux condenser and a magnetic bar. Add 10 mL of 0.5 N methanolic sodium hydroxide solution and heat the flask with stirring under reflux conditions for 15 min. Add 5 mL of Boron Trifluoride (BF_3) solution through the reflux condenser into the flask and continue to boil for 3 more min. Add 5.0 mL of internal standard solution, boil for another 1 min. Cool the flask, remove the condenser, and add 15 mL of saturated sodium chloride solution into the flask. Insert a stopper into the flask and shake vigorously. Wait for levels to separate, and transfer 1 mL of the hexane layer into a GC injection vail. It ready for injection.

(ii) *GC conditions*

FID temperature: maintain at 300°C
Injector temperature: 250°C
Garry gas: N_2
Flow rate: 1 ml/min
Column: Restek low temperature GC column, Restek Stabil Wax, 30 m × 0.25 mm id, 0.25 μm
Oven temperature: 120°C for 3 min. Then increase to 220°C at a rate of 5°C/min. Hold at 220°C for 12 min.
Injection Volume: 1 μL

(iii) *Results and calculation*

$$Individual\ fatty\ acid\ (\%) = \frac{Cs \times PARu \times 5 \times Ma \times 100\%}{PARs \times Wu \times Me}$$

or

$$Individual\ fatty\ acid(mg/unit) = \frac{Cs \times PARu \times 5 \times Ma \times UW}{PARs \times Wu \times Me}$$

Here

Cs = Concentration of corresponding fatty acid methyl ester in standard solution (mg/ml)

PARu = The peak area ratio of corresponding fatty acid methyl ester/internal standard in sample solution

PARs = The peak area ratio of corresponding fatty acid methyl ester/internal standard in standard solution

Vu = Total volume of sample solution (5.0 ml)

Wu = Sample weigh (mg)

Ma = MW of corresponding fatty acid

Me = MW of corresponding fatty acid methyl ester

UW = Unit weight (mg/unit)

5 = Sample volume (5ml)

Total fatty acids = Sum of individual fatty acid measured

4.59 Emodin Test Method

Emodin is an active component of several plants used in traditional Chinese medicine such as *Rheum almatum*, *Polygonum cuspidatum* and *Polygonum multiflorum*. It has various activities including as a laxative, an anti-bacterial and an anti-inflammatory agent. It has also been identified as having potential antiviral activity.

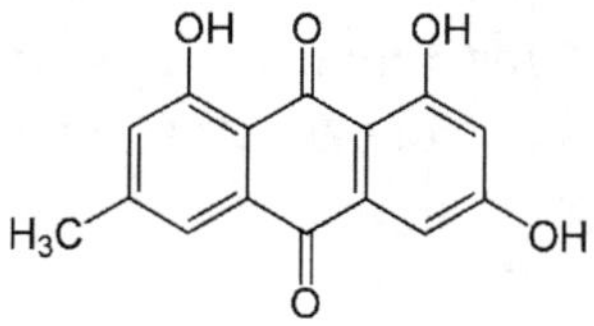

Emodin

(i) *Test procedure*

Preparation of standard solution — Accurately weigh about 10 mg of emodin standard, and transfer it to a 100 ml volumetric flask. Add 60 ml methanol, and sonicate until all standard dissolved. Then add methanol to 100 ml volume, and shake well. The standard solution can be injected.

Preparation of sample solution — Weigh a certain amount of ground samples containing about 10 mg of emodin, and transfer it to a 100 ml volumetric flask. Add 10 ml of water, and sonicate for 5 min. Add 60 ml of ethanol, and sonicate for 10 min when analyzing extract material or 40 min for raw herbs. Cool to room temperature, add methanol to the mark, and shake well. Centrifuge (10,000 rpm) for 5 min, and draw the clear solution into a 2 ml injection vail. It is ready for injection.

(ii) *UPLC conditions*

Column: Acquity UPLC® BEH C18, 1.7 μm, 2.1 × 150 mm
Flow rate: 0.4 ml/min
Injection volume: 1.0 μL
UV wavelength: 288 nm
Mobile phase A: 0.1% phosphoric acid in water
Mobile phase B: Acetonitrile
Column temperature: 45°C

Gradient:

Time (min)	A%	B%
0	60	40
6.0	25	75
7.0	25	75
7.5	60	40
10.0	60	40

(iii) *Results and calculation*

$$Emodin\ (\%) = \frac{Aa \times Wstand \times Vsam \times 100\%}{As \times Vstd \times Wsam}$$

or

$$Emodin\ (mg/unit) = \frac{Aa \times Wsand \times Vsam \times UW}{As \times Vstd \times Wsam}$$

Here
Aa = Peak area of sample
As = Peak area of standard

Wsand = Weight of standard (mg)
Wsam = Weight of sample (mg)
Vstd = Total volume of standard solution (ml)
Vsam = Total volume of sample solution (ml)
UW = Unit weight (mg/unit)

4.60 Andrographolide Test Method

Andrographolide is extracted from *andrographis paniculata*. The main function of this compound is improved immunity and anti-inflammatory effects.

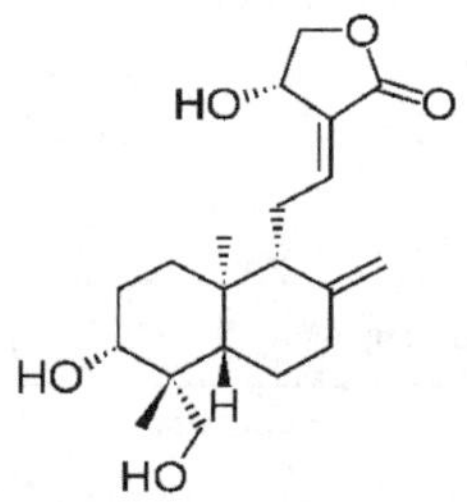

Andrographolide

(i) *Test procedure*

Preparation of standard solution — Accurately weigh about 10 mg of andrographolide, and transfer it to a 50 ml volumetric flask. Add 30 ml of ethanol, sonicate until all of the standards are dissolved. Add ethanol to 50 ml volume, and shake well. The standard solution is ready to inject.

Preparation of sample solution — Accurately weigh a certain amount of ground sample which contains about 10 mg of andrographolide, and transfer it to a 50 ml volumetric flask. Add 5 ml of water, and sonicate for 5 min. Next, add 30 ml of ethanol, and sonicate 45 min for raw herb powder or 10 min for extract powders. Cool to room temperature, add ethanol to mark, and shake well. Centrifuge (10,000 rpm) for 5 min, take the clear solution to inject.

(ii) *UPLC conditions*

Column: Acquity UPLC® HSS Ts C18, 1.8 μm, 2.1 × 150 mm
Flow rate: 0.4 ml/min
Injection volume: 2.0 μL
UV wavelength: 225 nm
Mobile phase A: 0.1% phosphoric acid in water
Mobile phase B: Acetonitrile
Column temperature: 45°C

Gradient:

Time (min)	A%	B%
0	80	20
5	50	50
5.6	50	50
6.0	80	20
8.0	80	20

(iii) *Results and calculation*

$$Andrographolide\ (\%) = \frac{Aa \times Wstand \times Vsam \times 100\%}{As \times Vstd \times Wsam}$$

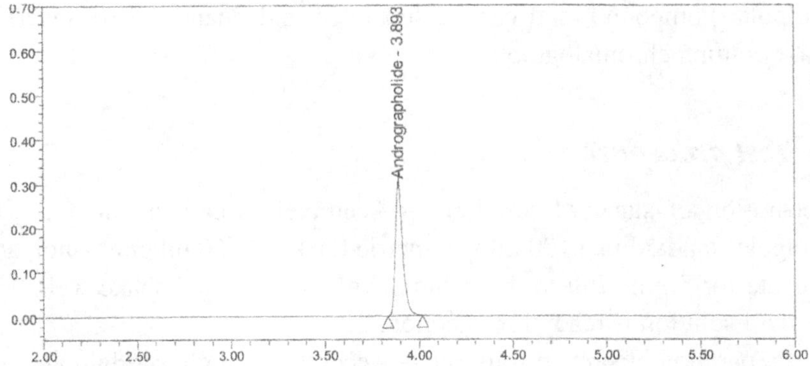

Figure 4.37: UPLC chromatogram of andrographolide.

or

$$Andrographolide\ (mg/unit) = \frac{Aa \times Wsand \times Vsam \times UW}{As \times Vstd \times Wsam}$$

Here
Aa = Peak area of sample
As = Peak area of standard
Wsand = Weight of standard (mg)
Wsam = Weight of sample (mg)
Vstd = Total volume of standard solution (ml)
Vsam = Total volume of sample solution (ml)
UW = Unit weight (mg/unit)

4.61 Test Method for Estragole

Estragole is a colorless liquid, although impure samples can appear yellow. It is a component of various trees and plants, including turpentine (pine oil), anise, fennel, bay, tarragon, and basil. It is used in the preparation of fragrances.

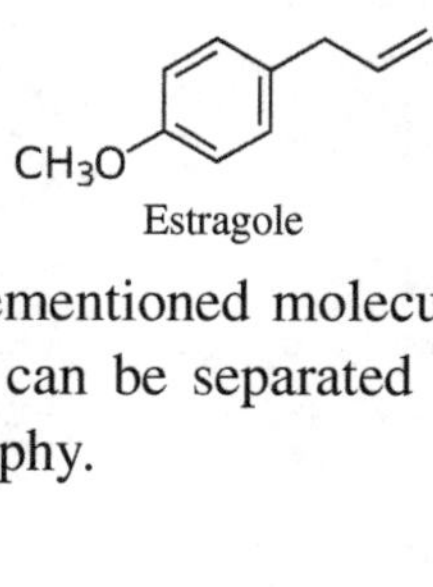

Estragole

According to the aforementioned molecular structure, estragole is a non-polar compound, and can be separated and quantified by reversed phase column chromatography.

(i) *Test procedure*

Preparation of standard solution — Accurately weigh about 5 mg of estragole standard in a 100 ml volumetric flask, add 60 ml of ethanol, and sonicate for 5 min. Fill to the volume with ethanol, and shake well. The standard solution is ready for injection.

Preparation of sample solution — Accurately weigh a certain amount of sample that contains about 5 mg of estragole in a 100 ml volumetric flask. Add 10 ml of water, and sonicate for 5 min. Then add 60 ml of isopropanol, and sonicate for 40 min when testing raw plant material or 10 min for extract materials. After the solution is cooled, add ethanol to the mark, and shake well. Centrifuge (10,000 rpm) for 5 min, and take the clear solution for injection.

(ii) *UPLC conditions*

Column: Acquity UPLC® HSS Ts C18, 1.8 μm, 2.1 × 150 mm
Flow rate: 0.4 ml/min
Injection volume: 1.0 μL
UV wavelength: 277 nm
Mobile phase A: 0.1% phosphoric acid in water
Mobile phase B: Acetonitrile
Column temperature: 45°C

Gradient:

Time (min)	A%	B%
0	55	45
5	20	80
5.6	20	80
6.0	55	45
8.0	55	45

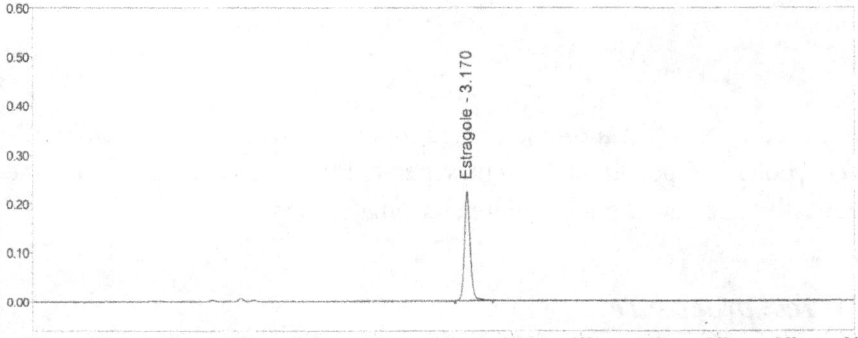

Figure 4.38: Chromatogram of estragole.

(iii) *Results and calculation*

$$Estragole\ (\%) = \frac{Aa \times Wstand \times Vsam \times 100\%}{As \times Vstd \times Wsam}$$

or

$$Estragole\ (mg/unit) = \frac{Aa \times Wsand \times Vsam \times UW}{As \times Vstd \times Wsam}$$

Here
Aa = Peak area of sample
As = Peak area of standard
Wsand = Weight of standard (mg)
Wsam = Weight of sample (mg)
Vstd = Total volume of standard solution (ml)
Vsam = Total volume of sample solution (ml)
UW = Unit weight (mg/unit)

4.62 α-Bisabolol Test Method

α-Bisabolol is the principal component of chamomiile. It has a sweet floral aroma and is used in various fragrances. It has also been used for cosmetics because of its perceived skin healing properties. Bisabolol is known to have anti-irritant, anti-inflammatory and anti-microbial properties.

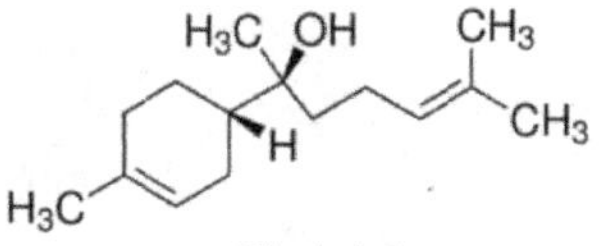

α-Bisabolol

According to the aforementioned molecular structure, α-Bisabolol is a non-polar compound, and can be separated from other ingredients in the matrix by a reversed phase column chromatography.

(i) *Test procedure*

Preparation of standard solution — Accurately weigh about 10 mg of α-bisabolol standard in a 50 ml volumetric flask, and add 30 ml of ethanol.

Sonicate for 5 min, fill with ethanol to mark, and shake well. The standard is ready for injection.

Preparation of sample solution — Accurately weigh a certain amount of ground sample, which contains 10 mg of α-bisabolol, and place in a 50 ml volumetric flask. Add 5 ml of water, and sonicate for 5 min. Then add 30 ml isopropyl alcohol and sonicate for 45 min when testing plant powder or 10 min for extract material samples. Cool to room temperature, add ethanol to volume, and shake well. Centrifuge (10,000 rpm) for 5 min, and take the clear solution for injection.

(ii) *UPLC conditions*

Column: Acquity UPLC® BEH C18, 1.7 μm, 2.1 × 150 mm
Flow rate: 0.4 ml/min
Injection volume: 2.0 μL
UV wavelength: 210 nm
Mobile phase A: 0.1% phosphoric acid in water
Mobile phase B: Acetonitrile
Column temperature: 45°C

Gradient:

Time (min)	A%	B%
0	40	60
5	10	90
5.6	10	90
6.0	40	60
8.0	40	60

(iii) *Results and calculation*

$$\alpha - Bisabolol\,(\%) = \frac{Aa \times Wstand \times Vsam \times 100\%}{As \times Vstd \times Wsam}$$

or

$$\alpha - Bisabolol\ (mg/unit) = \frac{Aa \times Wsand \times Vsam \times UW}{As \times Vstd \times Wsam}$$

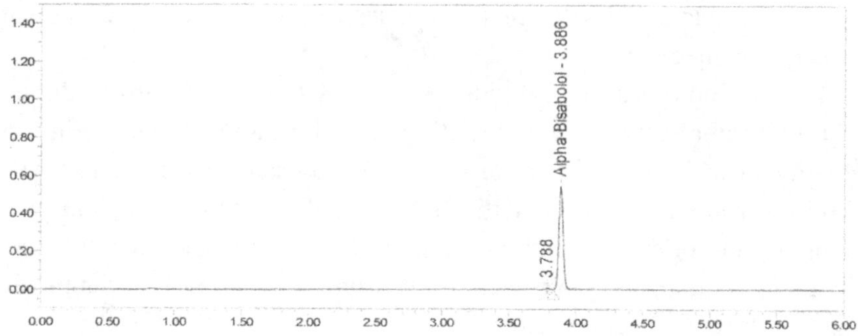

Figure 4.39: Chromatogram of α-bisabolol.

Here
Aa = Peak area of sample
As = Peak area of standard
Wsand = Weight of standard (mg)
Wsam = Weight of sample (mg)
Vstd = Total volume of standard solution (ml)
Vsam = Total volume of sample solution (ml)
UW = Unit weight (mg/unit)

4.63 Test Method for Honokiol and Magnolol

Honokiol and magnolol are extracted from *Magnolia officinalis*. The biological activities include anti-microbial effects, anti-inflammatory effect and as an antioxidant. Honokiol and magnolol can be separated and quantified by reversed phase chromatography.

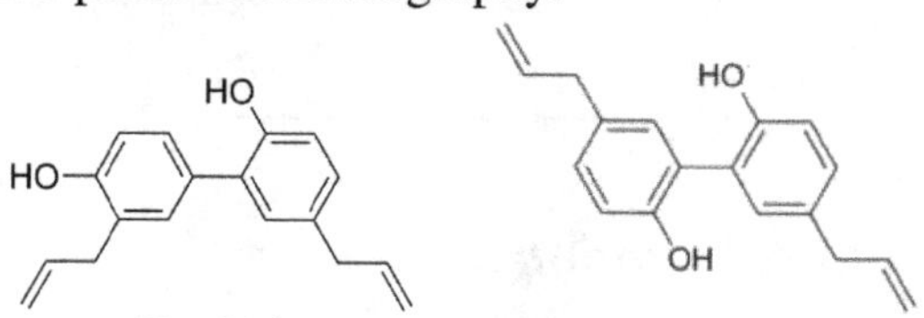

Honokiol Magnolol

(i) *Test procedure*

Preparation of standard solution — Accurately weigh about 10 mg of honokiol and 10 mg of magnolol standards, and transfer it to a 100 ml volumetric flask. Add 60 ml methanol, and sonicate until all standards are dissolved. After cooling, fill with methanol to the mark, and shake well. The standard solution can be injected.

Preparation of sample solution — Accurately weigh a certain amount of ground sample containing about 10 mg of honokiol or magnolol, and transfer it to a 100 ml volumetric flask. Add 20 ml of water, and sonicate for 5 min. Then add 50 ml ethanol, and sonicate for 45 min for *magnolia officinalis* powder or 10 min for extract powder samples. Cool to room temperature, fill methanol to mark, and shake well. Centrifuge (10,000 rpm) for 5 min, and take the clear solution to inject.

(ii) *UPLC conditions*

Column: Acquity UPLC® BEH C18 1.7 μm, 2.1 × 150 mm
Flow rate: 0.4 ml/min
Injection volume: 1 μL
UV wavelength: 293 nm
Mobile phase A: 0.1% phosphoric acid in water
Mobile phase B: 0.1% phosphoric acid in acetonitrile
Column temperature: 45°C

Gradient:

Time (min)	A%	B%
0	75	25
2.5	65	35
7	30	70
7.8	30	70
8	75	25
10	75	25

(iii) *Results and calculation for Honokiol*

$$Honokiol/magnolol\ (\%) = \frac{Aa \times Wstand \times Vsam \times 100\%}{As \times Vstd \times Wsam}$$

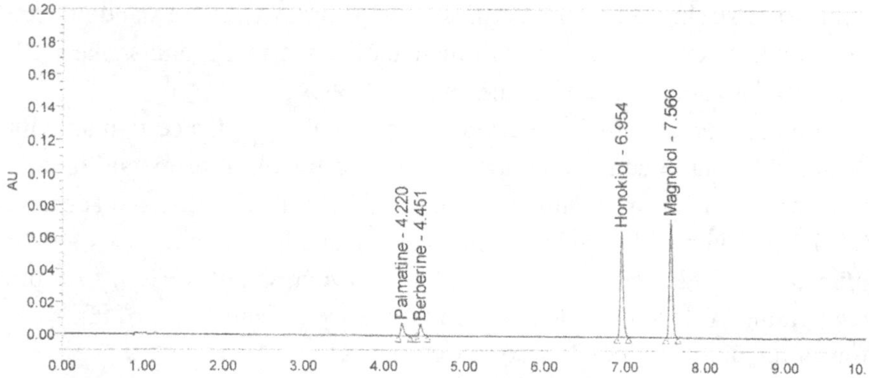

Figure 4.40: Chromatogram of honokiol and magnolol combine with palmatine and berberine.

or

$$Honokiol/magnolol\ (mg/unit) = \frac{Aa \times Wsand \times Vsam \times UW}{As \times Vstd \times Wsam}$$

Here

Aa = Peak area of honokiol/magnolol in sample solution
As = Peak area of honokiol/magnolol in standard solution
Wsand = Weight of honokiol/magnolol standards (mg)
Wsam = Weight of sample (mg)
Vstd = Total volume of standard solution (ml)
Vsam = Total volume of sample solution (ml)
UW = Unit weight (mg/unit)

4.64 Carvacrol Test Method

Carvacrol exists in *origanum vulgare* and other plants. It has a characteristic pungent, and a warm odor of oregano. Carvacrol possesses a wide range of bioactivities. It is potentially useful for clinical applications such as antimicrobial, antioxidant and anticancer activities. Carvacrol can be dissolved and extracted using methanol and can be separated by a reverse phase UPLC column, HSS T3. By comparing with a known concentration reference standard, unknown samples can be quantified.

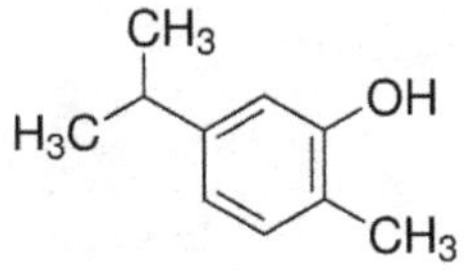

Carvacrol

(i) *Test procedure*

Preparation of standard solution — Accurately weigh about 10 mg of carvacrol in a 100 ml volumetric flask, and add 60 ml methanol. Sonicate for 2 min, fill methanol to mark, and shake well. The standard is ready for injection.

Preparation of sample solution — Accurately weigh a certain amount of ground sample that contains about 10 mg of carvacrol, and transfer it to a 100 ml volumetric flask. Add 10 ml of water, and sonicate for 5 min. Then add 50 ml of ethanol, and sonicate for 15 min. After the solution is cooled, add methanol to the mark, and shake well. Centrifuge (10,000 rpm) for 5 min, and draw clear solution for injection.

(ii) *UPLC conditions*

Column: Acquity UPLC® HSS T3, C18, 1.8 μm, 2.1 × 150 mm
Flow rate: 0.4 ml/min
Injection volume: 1 μL
UV wavelength: 275 nm
Mobile phase A: 0.1% phosphoric acid in water
Mobile phase B: 0.1% phosphoric acid in acetonitrile
Column temperature: 45°C

Gradient:

Time (min)	A%	B%
0	60	40
4.0	35	65
4.8	35	65
5.2	60	40
8.0	60	40

(iii) *Results and calculation*

$$Carvacrol\ (\%) = \frac{Aa \times Wstand \times Vsam \times 100\%}{As \times Vstd \times Wsam}$$

or

$$Carvacrol\ (mg/unit) = \frac{Aa \times Wsand \times Vsam \times UW}{As \times Vstd \times Wsam}$$

Here
Aa = Peak area of sample
As = Peak area of standard
Wsand = Weight of standard (mg)
Wsam = Weight of sample (mg)
Vstd = Total volume of standard solution (ml)
Vsam = Total volume of sample solution (ml)
UW = Unit weight (mg/unit)

4.65 Test Method for Eugenol

Eugenol is used in perfumes, flavorings, essential oils and in medicine as a local antiseptic and anesthetic. It is extracted from certain essential oils especially from clove oil, nutmeg, cinnamon, basil and bay leaf. Eugenol can be separated and quantified by a reversed phase UPLC column, BEH C18. By comparing with a known concentration reference standard, eugenol can be quantified.

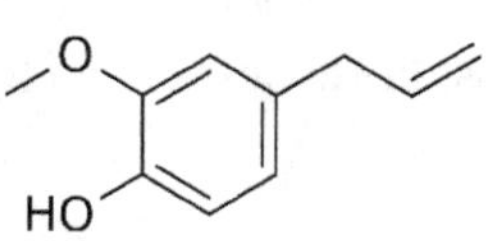

Eugenol

(i) *Test procedure*

Preparation of standard solution — Accurately weigh about 5 mg eugenol in a 100 ml volumetric flask. Add 60 ml of ethanol and sonicate for 2 min. Then add ethanol to 100 ml volume, shake well, and the standard is ready for injection.

Preparation of sample solution — Accurately weigh a certain amount of ground sample containing about 5 mg of eugenol, and transfer it to a 100 ml volumetric flask. Add 10 ml of water, and sonicate for 5 min. Then add 60 ml of isopropyl alcohol, and sonicate for 10 min when analyzing extract materials or 40 min for raw plants. After the solution is cooled add ethanol to the mark, and shake well. Centrifuge (10,000 rpm) for 5 min, and draw the clear solution for injection.

(ii) *UPLC conditions*

Column: Acquity UPLC® BEH C18, 1.7 μm, 2.1 × 150 mm
Flow rate: 0.4 ml/min
Injection volume: 1.0 μL
UV wavelength: 280 nm
Mobile phase A: 0.1% phosphoric acid in water
Mobile phase B: Acetonitrile
Column temperature: 45°C

Gradient:

Time (min)	A%	B%
0	80	20
4	40	60
4.8	40	60
5.2	80	20
8.0	80	20

(iii) *Results and calculation*

$$Eugenol\ (\%) = \frac{Aa \times Wstand \times Vsam \times 100\%}{As \times Vstd \times Wsam}$$

or

$$Eugenol\ (mg/unit) = \frac{Aa \times Wsand \times Vsam \times UW}{As \times Vstd \times Wsam}$$

Here
Aa = Peak area of sample
As = Peak area of standard

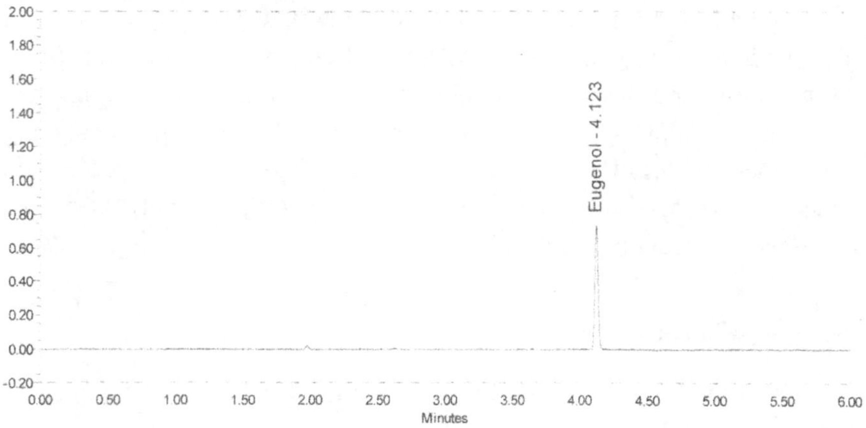

Figure 4.41: Chromatogram of eugenol.

Wsand = Weight of standard (mg)
Wsam = Weight of sample (mg)
Vstd = Total volume of standard solution (ml)
Vsam = Total volume of sample solution (ml)
UW = Unit weight (mg/unit)

4.66 Jujuboside A Test Method

Jujuboside A is extracted from *Semen Ziziphus spinose*. It has sedation and hypnotic effects.

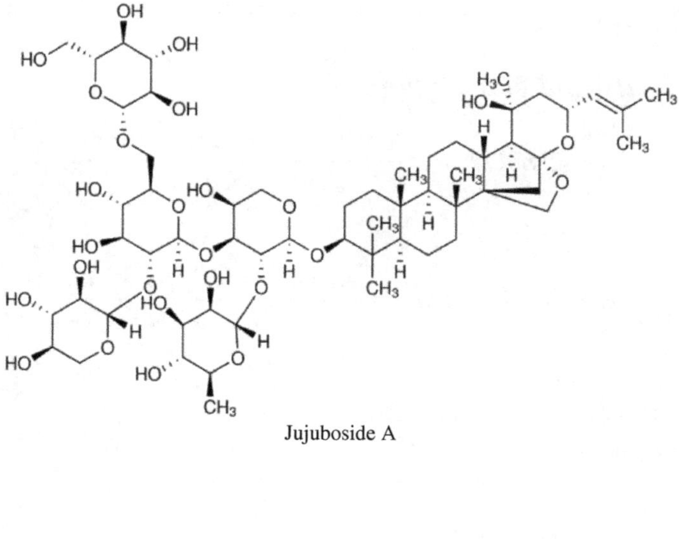

Jujuboside A

(i) *Test procedure*

Preparation of standard solution — Accurately weigh about 10 mg jujuboside A, and transfer it to a 50 ml volumetric flask. Add 30 ml of water, and sonicate until the standard is dissolved. Then add water to 50 ml volume, shake well, and the standard solution is ready for injection.

Preparation of sample solution — Accurately weigh a certain amount of ground sample that contains about 10 mg of jujuboside A, and transfer it to a 50 ml volumetric flask. Add 30 ml of water, and sonicate for 40 min for raw *Ziziphus spinosa* or sonicate 10 min for extract powders. Cool to room temperature, and fill with water to volume. Shake well, and centrifuge (10,000 rpm) for 5 min. The clear solution is ready for injection.

(ii) *UPLC conditions*

Column: Acquity UPLC® BEH C18, 1.7 μm, 2.1 × 150 mm
Flow rate: 0.4 ml/min
Injection volume: 2.0 μL
UV wavelength: 210 nm
Mobile phase A: 0.1% phosphoric acid in water
Mobile phase B: Acetonitrile
Column temperature: 45°C

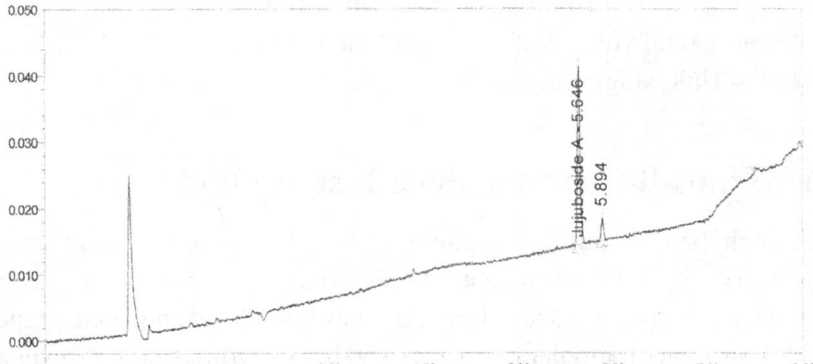

Figure 4.42: Chromatogram of jujuboside A.

Gradient:

Time (min)	A%	B%
0	85	15
6	50	50
7	20	80
7.8	20	80
8.0	85	15
10.0	85	15

(iii) *Results and calculation*

$$Jujuboside\ A\ (\%) = \frac{Aa \times Wstand \times Vsam \times 100\%}{As \times Vstd \times Wsam}$$

or

$$Jujuboside\ A\ (mg/unit) = \frac{Aa \times Wsand \times Vsam \times UW}{As \times Vstd \times Wsam}$$

Here
Aa = Peak area of jujuboside A in sample solution
As = Peak area of jujuboside A in standard solution
Wsand = Weight of jujuboside A standard (mg)
Wsam = Weight of sample (mg)
Vstd = Total volume of standard solution (ml)
Vsam = Total volume of sample solution (ml)
UW = Unit weight (mg/unit)

4.67 Trans-β-Caryophyllene Test Method

β-Caryophyllene is most commonly found in black pepper, cinnamon and hops. Caryophyllene is a potent component in anti-inflammatory salves and topicals, and also has anti-bacterial, anti-fungal and antiseptic properties. It is a strong non-polar compound and can be attracted to the reversed phase UPLC column, HSS T3 C18, and can be separated from other ingredients in the matrix. By comparing with a known concentration reference standard, caryophyllene in unknown samples can be quantified by UPLC-UV system.

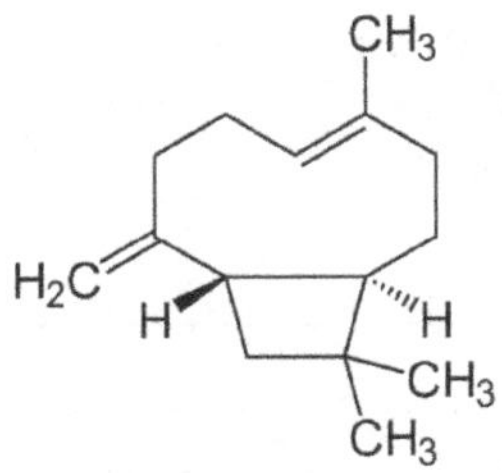

Caryophyllene

(i) *Test procedure*

Preparation of standard solution — Accurately weigh about 10 mg caryophyllene standard, and transfer to a 50 ml volumetric flask. Add 30 ml of ethanol, and sonicate until all the standards are dissolved. Cool to room temperature, add ethanol to 50 ml mark, and shake well. The standard can now be injected.

Preparation of sample solution — Accurately weigh a certain amount of ground sample containing about 10 mg of caryophyllene, and transfer to a 50 ml volumetric flask. Add 30 ml of ethanol, and sonicate for 15 min. After the solution is cooled add ethanol to the mark, and shake well. Centrifuge (10,000 rpm) for 5 min, and draw the clear solution to a 2 ml injection vail, and is ready for injection.

(ii) *UPLC conditions*

Column: Acquity UPLC® HSS Ts C18, 1.8 μm, 2.1 × 100 mm
Flow rate: 0.4 ml/min
Injection volume: 2.0 μL
UV wavelength: 210 nm
Mobile phase A: 0.1% phosphoric acid in water
Mobile phase B: Acetonitrile
Column temperature: 45°C

Gradient:

Time (min)	A%	B%
0	20	80
4	0	100
5.5	0	100
6.0	80	20
8.0	80	20

(iii) *Results and calculation*

$$Caryophyllene\ (\%) = \frac{Aa \times Wstand \times Vsam \times 100\%}{As \times Vstd \times Wsam}$$

or

$$Caryophyllene\ (mg/unit) = \frac{Aa \times Wsand \times Vsam \times UW}{As \times Vstd \times Wsam}$$

Here
Aa = Peak area of caryophyllene in sample solution
As = Peak area of caryophyllene in standard solution
Wsand = Weight of caryophyllene standard (mg)
Wsam = Weight of sample (mg)
Vstd = Total volume of standard solution (ml)
Vsam = Total volume of sample solution (ml)
UW = Unit weight (mg/unit)

4.68 Thymoquinone Test Method

Thymoquinone is an active constituent of *Nigella Sativa* seeds.

Its use can be beneficial in bacterial infections, diabetes, liver disease and joint inflammation. Thymoquinone can be extracted from samples using ethanol. It then can be separated and quantified by reversed phase UPLC column, BEH C18. By comparing with a known concentration of the reference standard, the amount of thymoquinone can be quantified.

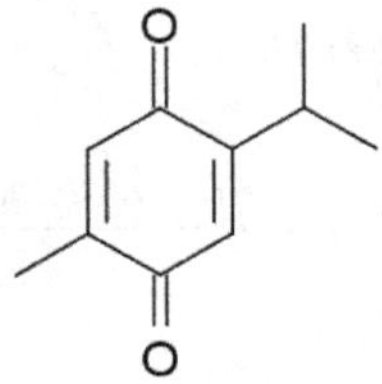

Thymoquinone

(i) *Test procedure*

Preparation of standard solution — Accurately weigh about 10 mg of thymoquinone standard, and transfer it to a 100 ml volumetric flask. Add 60 ml of ethanol, and sonicate until all standards are dissolved. Fill with ethanol to the 100 ml mark, and shake well. The standard solution is ready for injection.

Preparation of sample solution — Accurately weigh a certain amount of ground sample which contains about 10 mg of thymoquinone, and transfer it to a 100 ml volumetric flask. Add 10 ml of water, and sonicate for 5 min. Then add 60 ml isopropyl alcohol, and sonicate for 10 min for extract materials or 40 min for herb powders. Cool to room temperature, then add ethanol to mark, and shake well. Centrifuge (10,000 rpm) for 5 min, and take the clear solution for injection.

(ii) *UPLC conditions*

Column: Acquity UPLC® BEH C18 1.7 μm, 2.1 × 150 mm
Flow rate: 0.4 ml/min
Injection volume: 1 μL
UV wavelength: 255 nm
Mobile phase A: 0.1% phosphoric acid in water
Mobile phase B: Acetonitrile
Column temperature: 45°C

Gradient:

Time (min)	A%	B%
0	75	25
7.0	20	80
8.0	20	80
8.5	75	25
10.0	75	25

(iii) *Results and calculation*

$$Thymoquinone\ (\%) = \frac{Aa \times Wstand \times Vsam \times 100\%}{As \times Vstd \times Wsam}$$

or

$$Thymoquinone\ (mg/unit) = \frac{Aa \times Wsand \times Vsam \times UW}{As \times Vstd \times Wsam}$$

Here
Aa = Peak area of thymoquinone in sample solution
As = Peak area of thymoquinone in standard solution
Wsand = Weight of thymoquinone standard (mg)
Wsam = Weight of sample (mg)
Vstd = Total volume of standard solution (ml)
Vsam = Total volume of sample solution (ml)
UW = Unit weight (mg/unit)

4.69 Test Method for Trans- and Cis-Citral

Citral is either one of or a mixture of a pair of liquid aldehydes; $C_{10}H_{16}O$ isomers. These have a strong lemon-like odor. The E-isomer is known as geranial or Citral A and the Z-isomer is known as neral or citral B. Citral is an aromatic compound used in perfumes for its citrus effect. It can be dissolved and extracted with methanol, and cis- and trans-isomers can be separated by a reversed phase UPLC phenyl column. By comparing with a known concentration reference standard, geranial and neral in unknown samples can be quantified.

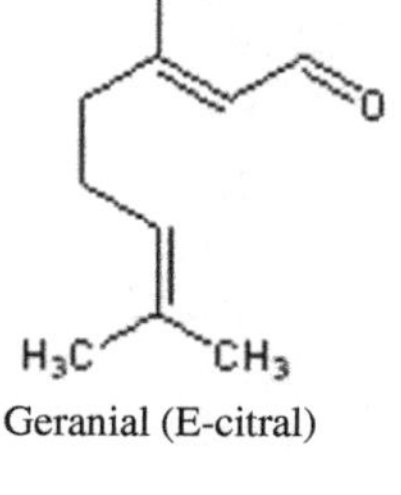

Geranial (E-citral)

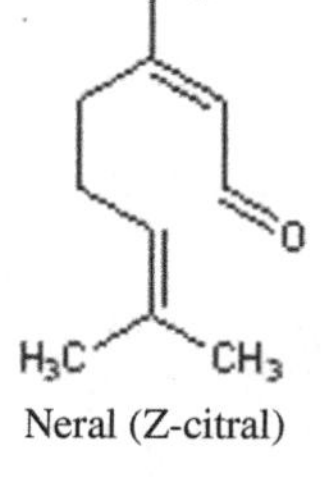

Neral (Z-citral)

(i) *Test procedure*

Preparation of standard solution — Accurately weigh 10 mg of tran-citral and 10 mg of cis-citral, and transfer it to a 100 ml volumetric flask. Add 60 ml of methanol, and vortex until all standards are dissolved. Then add methanol to 100 ml mark, shake well, and the standard solution is ready for injection.

Preparation of sample solution — Accurately weigh a certain amount of ground sample containing about 10 mg of E-citral or Z-citral, and transfer it to a 100 ml volumetric flask. Add 10 ml of water, and sonicate for 5 min. Then add 60 ml of ethanol, sonicate for 10 min, and cool to room temperature. Fill the flask with methanol to the mark, and shake well. Centrifuge for 5 min (10,000 rpm), and take the clear solution for injection.

(ii) *UPLC conditions*

Column: Acquity UPLC® BEH Phenyl, 1.7 μm, 2.1 × 150 mm
Flow rate: 0.4 ml/min
Injection volume: 1.0 μL
UV wavelength: 240 nm
Mobile phase A: 0.1% phosphoric acid in water
Mobile phase B: Acetonitrile
Column temperature: 45°C

Gradient:

Time (min)	A%	B%
0	60	40
4.0	40	60
4.8	40	60
5.0	60	40
8.0	60	40

(iii) *Results and calculation*

$$Citral\ E/Z\ (\%) = \frac{Aa \times Wstand \times Vsam \times 100\%}{As \times Vstd \times Wsam}$$

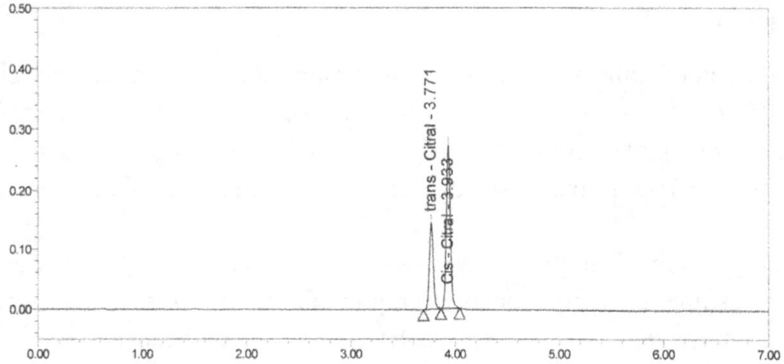

Figure 4.43: Chromatogram of cis and trans citral.

or

$$\text{Citral}\, E/Z\ (mg/unit) = \frac{Aa \times Wsand \times Vsam \times UW}{As \times Vstd \times Wsam}$$

Here
Aa = Peak area of citral E/Z in sample solution
As = Peak area of citral E/Z in standard solution
Wsand = Weight of citral E/Z standard (mg)
Wsam = Weight of sample (mg)
Vstd = Total volume of standard solution (ml)
Vsam = Total volume of sample solution (ml)
UW = Unit weight (mg/unit)

4.70 Test Method for Schisandrin A in Schisandra chinensis

Schisandrin A is found in fruits of several species. It has liver-protective and antioxidant functions.

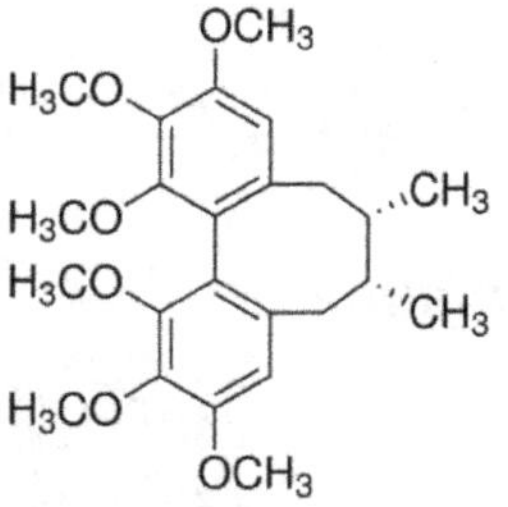

Schisandrin A

Schisandrin A is a non-polar compound, so it will interact with a reversed phase column, and can be separated from other components in the matrix.

(i) *Test procedure*

Preparation of standard solution — Accurately weigh about 10 mg of schisandrin A standard, and transfer it to a 100 ml volumetric flask. Add 60 ml of ethanol, and sonicate until all of the standards are dissolved. After the solution is cooled, add ethanol to 100 ml volume, and shake well. The standard solution is ready to inject.

Preparation of sample solution — Accurately weigh a certain amount of ground sample containing about 10 mg of schisandrin A, and transfer it to a 100 ml volumetric flask. Add 20 ml of DMSO and sonicate for 5 min. Then add 50 ml of ethanol and sonicate for 40 min when testing schisandra raw herb or 10 min for extract materials. Cool to room temperature, add ethanol to the mark, and shake and mix well. Centrifuge (10,000 rpm) for 5 min, and take the clear solution for injection.

(ii) *UPLC conditions*

Column: Acquity UPLC® BEH, C18, 1.7 μm, 2.1 × 150 mm
Flow rate: 0.5 ml/min
Injection volume: 2.0 μL
UV wavelength: 260 nm
Mobile phase A: 0.1% phosphoric acid in water
Mobile phase B: Acetonitrile
Column temperature: 45°C

Gradient:

Time (min)	A%	B%
0	60	40
5	25	75
5.6	25	75
6.0	60	40
8.0	60	40

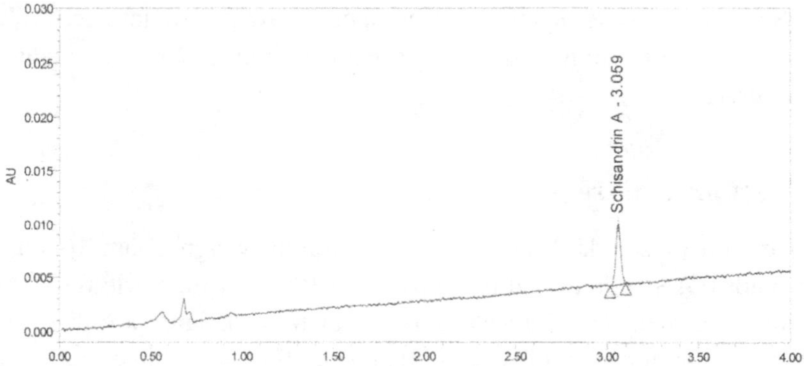

Figure 4.44: Chromatogram of schisandrin A.

(iii) *Results and calculation*

$$Schisandrin\ A\ (\%) = \frac{Aa \times Wstand \times Vsam \times 100\%}{As \times Vstd \times Wsam}$$

or

$$Schisandrin\ A\ (mg/unit) = \frac{Aa \times Wsand \times Vsam \times UW}{As \times Vstd \times Wsam}$$

Here
Aa = Peak area of schisandrin A in sample solution
As = Peak area of schisandrin A in standard solution
Wsand = Weight of schisandrin A standard (mg)
Wsam = Weight of sample (mg)
Vstd = Total volume of standard solution (ml)
Vsam = Total volume of sample solution (ml)
UW = Unit weight (mg/unit)

4.71 Test Method for Diosgenin in Chinese Yam

Diosgenin can be extracted from Chinese yam, and is a precursor to human hormones. It can help regulate human hormones. Diosgenin is a Non-polar compound, and can be separated by a reversed phase UPLC column, BEH Phenyl. By comparing with a known concentration of a reference standard, diosgenin can be quantified.

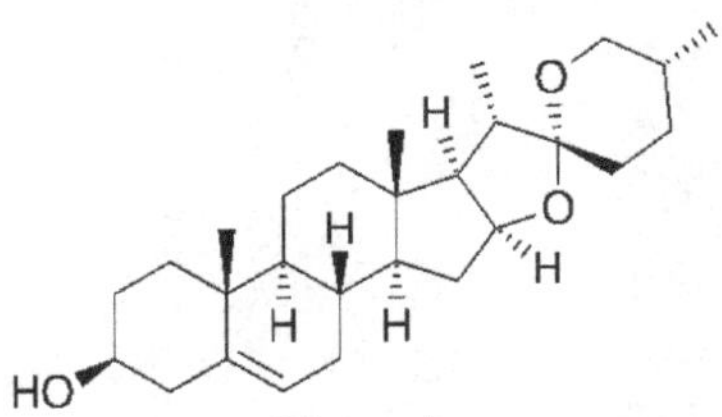

Diosgenin

(i) *Test procedure*

Preparation of standard solution — Accurately weigh 10 mg of diosgenin standard, and transfer it to a 50 ml volumetric flask. Add 30 ml of methanol, and sonicate until all standards are completely dissolved. Then add methanol to 50 ml mark, shake well, and the standard solution is ready to be injected.

Preparation of sample solution — Accurately weigh a certain amount of ground sample containing about 10 mg of diosgenin, and transfer it to a 50 ml of volumetric flask. Add 20 ml of water, and sonicate for 5 min. Centrifuge for 5 min (10,000 r/min), and remove all the water. Then add 30 ml of ethanol, and sonicate 40 min when testing Chinese yam or 10 min for extract materials. Cool to room temperature, add methanol to the mark, and shake well. Centrifuge (10,000 rpm) for 5 min, the clear solution can be injected.

(ii) *UPLC conditions*

Column: Acquity UPLC® BEH, Phenyl, 1.7 μm, 2.1 × 150 mm
Flow rate: 0.4 ml/min
Injection volume: 2.0 μL
UV wavelength: 215 nm
Mobile phase A: 0.1% phosphoric acid in water
Mobile phase B: Acetonitrile
Column temperature: 45°C

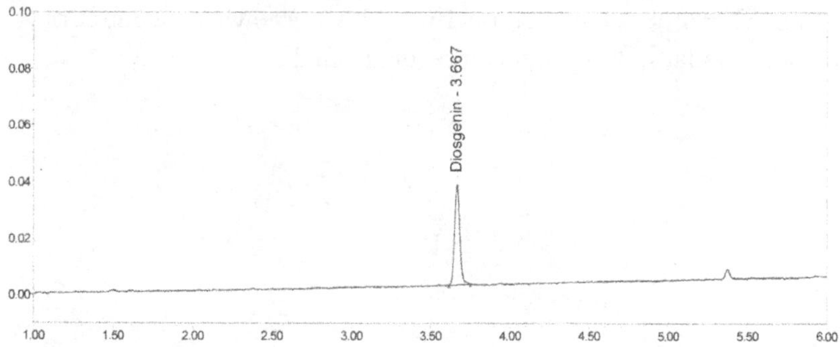

Figure 4.45: UPLC chromatogram of diosgenin.

Gradient:

Time (min)	A%	B%
0	50	50
5.0	5	95
5.6	5	95
6.0	50	50
8.0	50	50

(iii) *Results and calculation*

$$\text{Diosgenin (\%)} = \frac{Aa \times Wstand \times Vsam \times 100\%}{As \times Vstd \times Wsam}$$

or

$$\text{Diosgenin } (mg/unit) = \frac{Aa \times Wsand \times Vsam \times UW}{As \times Vstd \times Wsam}$$

Here
Aa = Peak area of diosmin in sample solution
As = Peak area of diosmin in standard solution
Wsand = Weight of diosmin standard (mg)
Wsam = Weight of sample (mg)

Vstd = Total volume of standard solution (ml)
Vsam = Total volume of sample solution (ml)
UW = Unit weight (mg/unit)

4.72 Test Method for Hydroxytyrosol

Olive oil, and olive leaves contain hydroxytyrosol. Hydroxytyrosol has antioxidant properties and may also help reduce blood lipids. Hydroxytryrosol can be separated and identified by reversed phase UPLC C18 column.

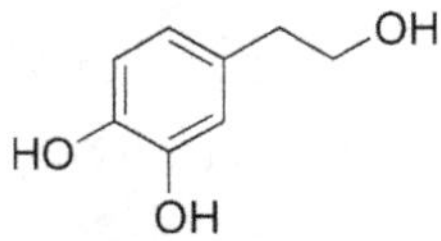

Hydroxytyrosol

(i) *Test procedure*

Preparation of standard solution — Accurately weigh about 10 mg of hydroxytyrosol standard, and transfer it to a 100 ml volumetric flask. Add 60 ml of water, and vortex until all of the standards are dissolved. Then add water to 100 ml mark, and shake well. The standard solution is ready for injection.

Preparation of sample solution — Accurately weigh a certain amount of ground sample containing about 10 mg of hydroxytyrosol, and transfer to a 100 ml volumetric flask. Add 60 ml of water, and sonicate 10 min for extract materials or 40 min when analyzing raw herb powders. Cool to room temperature, fill with water to the mark, and shake well. Centrifuge (10,000 rpm) for 5 min, and the clear solution can be injected.

(ii) *UPLC conditions*

Column: Acquity UPLC® HSS Ts, C18, 1.8 μm, 2.1 × 100 mm
Flow rate: 0.4 ml/min
Injection volume: 1.0 μL
UV wavelength: 280 nm

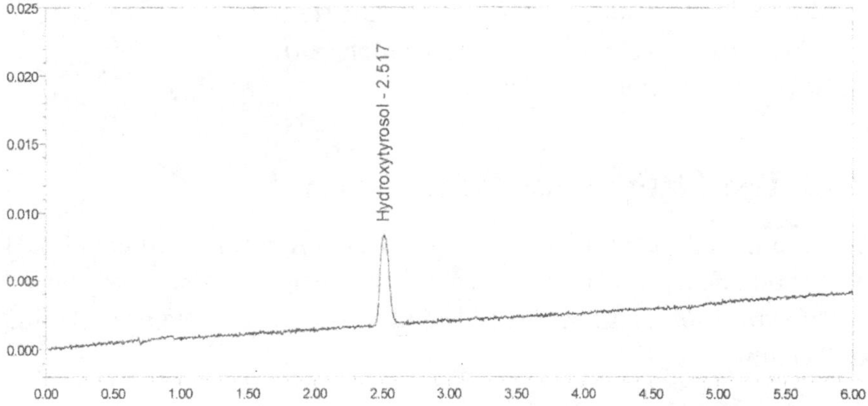

Figure 4.46: Chromatogram of hydroxytyrosol.

Mobile phase A: 0.1% phosphoric acid in water
Mobile phase B: Acetonitrile
Column temperature: 45°C

Gradient:

Time (min)	A%	B%
0	95	5
3.0	90	10
3.8	90	10
4.0	95	5
6.0	95	5

(iii) *Results and calculation*

$$Hydroxytyrosol\ (\%) = \frac{Aa \times Wstand \times Vsam \times 100\%}{As \times Vstd \times Wsam}$$

or

$$Hydroxytyrosol\ (mg/unit) = \frac{Aa \times Wsand \times Vsam \times UW}{As \times Vstd \times Wsam}$$

Here
Aa = Peak area of hydroxytyrosol in sample solution
As = Peak area of hydroxytyrosol in standard solution
Wsand = Weight of hydroxytyrosol standard (mg)
Wsam = Weight of sample (mg)
Vstd = Total volume of standard solution (ml)
Vsam = Total volume of sample solution (ml)
UW = Unit weight (mg/unit)

4.73 Oxymatrine Test Method

Oxymatrine is extracted from *Sophora flavescens*. It has diuretic properties and may improve immunity function. As well, oxymatrine has shown a variety of effects with *in vitro* animal studies, including protection against apoptosis, tumor and fibrotic tissue development and inflammation.

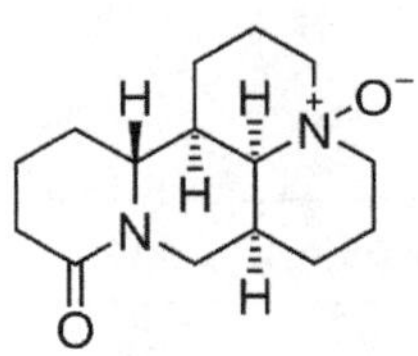

Oxymatrine

According to its molecular structure, oxymatrine is an alkaline compound. In order to extend the chromatographic retention time and improve the separation, this method uses hexansulfonic acid as ion pair reagent. This is added to the mobile phase, to form an ion pair with oxymatrine. See Chapter 1, Section 1.1.2 "Mobile phase application".

(i) *Test procedure*

Preparation of standard solution — Accurately weigh 10 mg of oxymatrine standard, and transfer it to a 50 ml volumetric flask. Add 30 ml methanol, and shake to completely dissolve the standard. Then add methanol to 50 ml mark, and shake well. The standard solution is ready to be injected.

Preparation of sample solution — Accurately weigh a certain amount of ground sample containing about 10 mg of oxymatrine, and transfer it to a 50 ml volumetric flask. Add 10 ml of water, and sonicate for 5 min. Then add 30 ml of ethanol and sonicate for 45 min when testing *Sophora flavescens* powder or 10 min for extract materials. Cool to room temperature, and add methanol to the mark. Shake well, centrifuge (10,000 rpm) for 5 min, and take the clear solution for injection.

(ii) *UPLC conditions*

Column: Acquity UPLC® BEH, C18, 1.7 μm, 2.1 × 150 mm
Flow rate: 0.4 ml/min
Injection volume: 2.0 μL
UV wavelength: 210 nm
Mobile phase A: 10 mM hexansulfonic acid sodium salt, pH 3.0
Mobile phase B: Acetonitrile
Column temperature: 45°C

Gradient:

Time (min)	**A%**	**B%**
0	95	5
5	85	35
7.0	50	45
7.8	50	45
8.0	95	5
10.0	95	5

(iii) *Results and calculation*

$$Oxymatrine\ (\%) = \frac{Aa \times Wstand \times Vsam \times 100\%}{As \times Vstd \times Wsam}$$

or

$$Oxymatrine\ (mg/unit) = \frac{Aa \times Wsand \times Vsam \times UW}{As \times Vstd \times Wsam}$$

Here
Aa = Peak area of oxymatrine in sample solution
As = Peak area of oxymatrine in standard solution
Wsand = Weight of oxymatrine standard (mg)
Wsam = Weight of sample (mg)
Vstd = Total volume of standard solution (ml)
Vsam = Total volume of sample solution (ml)
UW = Unit weight (mg/unit)

4.74 Aucubin Test Method

Aucubin is extracted from *Eucommiaceae*. Its main functions are as an anti-inflammatory agent and for pain relief.

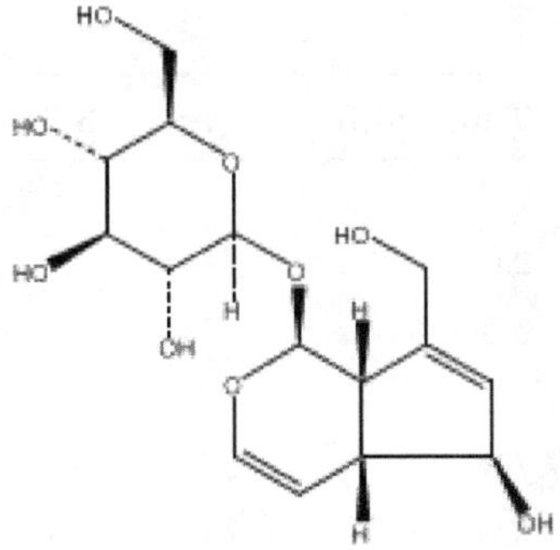

Aucubin

(i) *Test procedure*

Solvent 1 preparation — To 250 ml of methanol add 750 ml of water, shake well, and sonicate for 10 min.

Preparation of standard solution — Accurately weigh about 20 mg of aucubin standard, and transfer to a 100 ml volumetric flask. Add 60 ml of solvent 1, and shake to dissolve the standard completely. Add solvent 1 to mark, and shake well, the standard solution is ready for injection.

Preparation of sample solution — Accurately weigh a certain amount of ground sample containing about 20 mg of aucubin, and transfer it to a 100 ml volumetric flask. Add 10 ml of water, and sonicate for 5 min. Then add 60 ml solvent 1, and sonicate for 10 min when testing extract materials or 40 min for *eucommiaceae* powder. Cool to room temperature, and then add solvent 1 to mark. Shake well, centrifuge (10,000 rpm) for 5 min, the clear solution can be injected.

(ii) *UPLC conditions*

Column: Acquity HSS T3 C18, 1.8 μm, 2.1 × 150 mm
Flow rate: 0.4 ml/min
Injection volume: 2 μL
UV wavelength: 210 nm
Mobile phase A: 0.1% phosphoric acid in water
Mobile phase B: Acetonitrile
Colum temperature: 45°C

Gradient:

Time (min)	A%	B%
0	97	3
2.0	97	3
6.0	92	8
6.8	50	50
7.8	50	50
8.0	97	3
10.0	97	3

(iii) *Results and calculation*

$$Aucubin\ (\%) = \frac{Aa \times Wstand \times Vsam \times 100\%}{As \times Vstd \times Wsam}$$

or

$$Aucubin\ (mg/unit) = \frac{Aa \times Wsand \times Vsam \times UW}{As \times Vstd \times Wsam}$$

Here
Aa = Peak area of aucubin in sample solution
As = Peak area of aucubin in standard solution

Wsand = Weight of aucubin standard (mg)
Wsam = Weight of sample (mg)
Vstd = Total volume of standard solution (ml)
Vsam = Total volume of sample solution (ml)
UW = Unit weight (mg/unit)

4.75 Mogroside V Test Method

Mogroside V is extracted from *s. grsvenorii*. It is 200 times sweeter than sucrose.

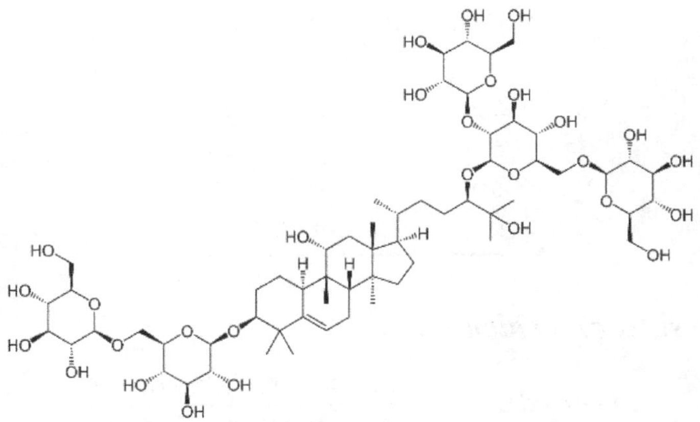

Mogroside V

(i) *Test procedure*

Preparation of standard solution — Accurately weigh about 10 mg of mogroside V standard, and transfer it to a 50 ml volumetric flask. Add 30 ml methanol, and shake to dissolve all of the standard. Then add methanol to 50 ml volume, and shake well. The standard is ready for injection.

Preparation of sample solution — Accurately weigh a certain amount of ground sample containing about 10 mg of Mogroside V, and transfer it to a 50 ml volumetric flask. Add 5 ml of water, and sonicate for 5 min. Then add 30 ml methanol, sonicate 40 min for *s. grsvenorii* powders; or 10 min when testing extract materials. Cool to room temperature, and then add methanol to the mark. Shake well, and centrifuge (10,000 rpm) for 5 min. Take the clear solution for injection.

(ii) *UPLC conditions*

Column: Acquity UPLC® HSS Ts, C18, 1.8 μm, 2.1 × 150 mm
Flow rate: 0.4 ml/min
Injection volume: 2.0 μL
UV wavelength: 210 nm
Mobile phase A: 0.1% phosphoric acid in water
Mobile phase B: Acetonitrile
Column temperature: 45°C

Gradient:

Time (min)	A%	B%
0	90	10
5.0	50	50
5.6	50	50
6.0	90	10
8.0	90	10

(iii) *Results and calculation*

$$Mogroside\,V\ (\%) = \frac{Aa \times Wstand \times Vsam \times 100\%}{As \times Vstd \times Wsam}$$

or

$$Mogroside\,V\ (mg/unit) = \frac{Aa \times Wsand \times Vsam \times UW}{As \times Vstd \times Wsam}$$

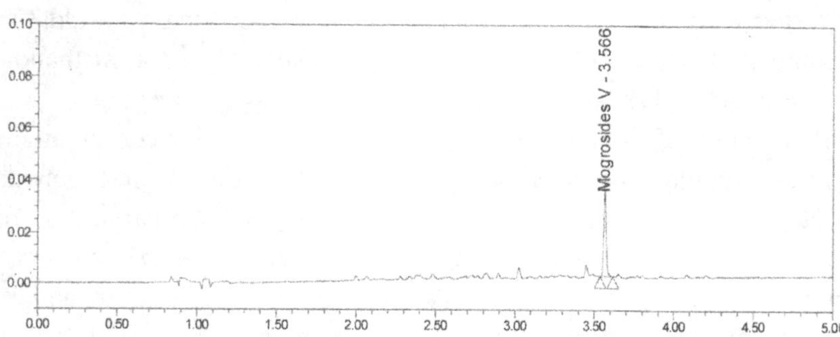

Figure 4.47: Chromatogram of mogroside V.

Here
Aa = Peak area of mogroside V in sample solution
As = Peak area of mogroside V in standard solution
Wsand = Weight of mogroside V standard (mg)
Wsam = Weight of sample (mg)
Vstd = Total volume of standard solution (ml)
Vsam = Total volume of sample solution (ml)
UW = Unit weight (mg/unit)

4.76 6-Paradol Test Method

6-paradol is a chemical compound contained in the roots of ginger plants. Experiments have shown that 6-paradol has antioxidant and anti-tumor effect in mice.

With the chemical structure shown as below, 6-paradol is a non-polar compound. It can be separated and identified by reversed phase UPLC C18 column.

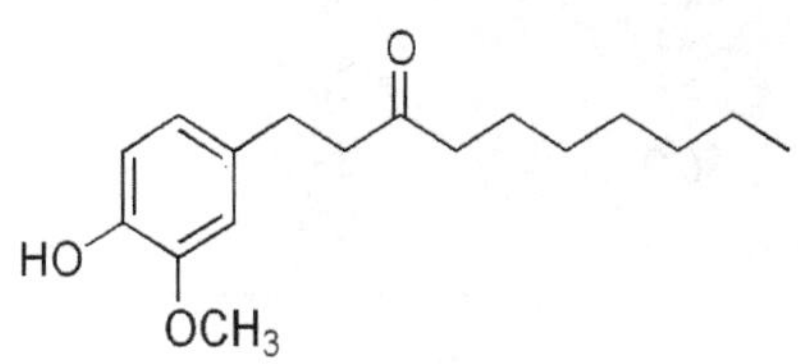

6-Paradol

(i) *Test procedure*

Preparation of standard solution — Accurately weigh 10 mg of 6-paradol standard, and transfer it to a 100 ml volumetric flask. Add 60 ml of methanol, and shake until all the standards are dissolved completely. Then add methanol to the 100 ml volume, shake well, and the standard solution is ready to inject.

Preparation of sample solution — Accurately weigh a certain amount of ground sample containing about 10 mg of 6-paradol, and transfer it to 100 ml volumetric flask. Add 10 ml of water, and sonicate for 10 min. Then add 60 ml of ethanol, and sonicate for 40 min for ginger root powder or 10 min if extract powders are being tested. Cool to room temperature, and then add methanol to the mark. Shake well, centrifuge (10,000 rpm) for 5 min, and draw the top clear solution to an injection vail. It is ready for injection.

(ii) *UPLC conditions*

Column: Acquity UPLC® HSS Ts, C18, 1.8 μm, 2.1 × 150 mm
Flow rate: 0.4 ml/min
Injection volume: 1.0 μL
UV wavelength: 280 nm
Mobile phase A: 0.1% phosphoric acid in water
Mobile phase B: Acetonitrile
Column temperature: 45°C

Gradient:

Time (min)	A%	B%
0	45	55
5.0	20	80
5.6	20	80
6.0	45	55
8.0	45	55

(iii) *Results and calculation*

$$Paradol\ (\%) = \frac{Aa \times Wstand \times Vsam \times 100\%}{As \times Vstd \times Wsam}$$

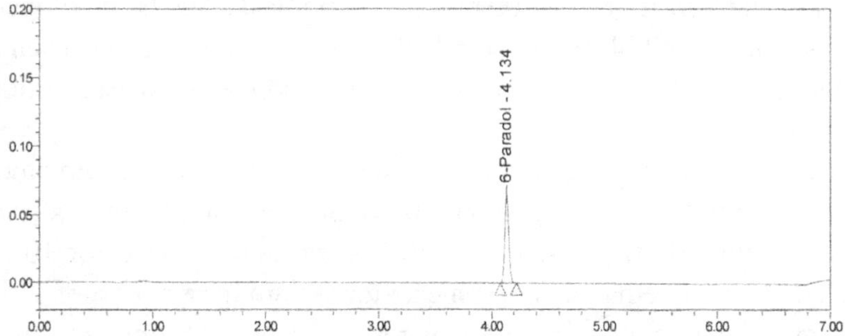

Figure 4.48: Chromatogram of 6-paradol.

or

$$Paradol\ (mg/unit) = \frac{Aa \times Wsand \times Vsam \times UW}{As \times Vstd \times Wsam}$$

Here
Aa = Peak area of paradol in sample solution
As = Peak area of paradol in standard solution
Wsand = Weight of paradol standard (mg)
Wsam = Weight of sample (mg)
Vstd = Total volume of standard solution (ml)
Vsam = Total volume of sample solution (ml)
UW = Unit weight (mg/unit)

4.77 Stevia Glycosides Test Method

Natural stevia contains a variety of stevia glycosides which are 200 times sweeter than sugar. They can be used as a sweetener. This method tests stevia glycosides contained in natural stevia, steviaside, rebaudioside A, rebaudioside C, dulcoside and steviolbioside.

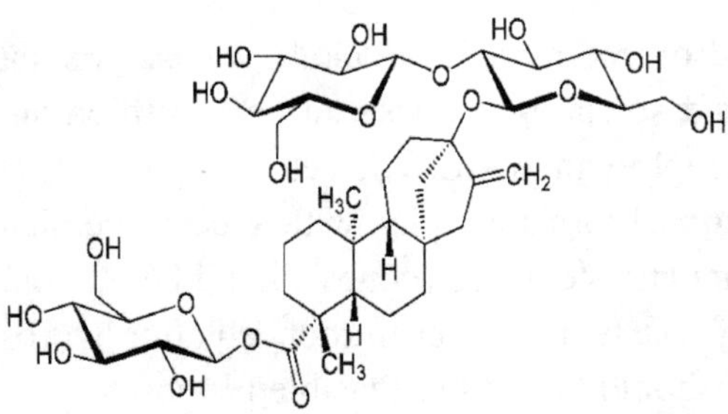

Steviaside

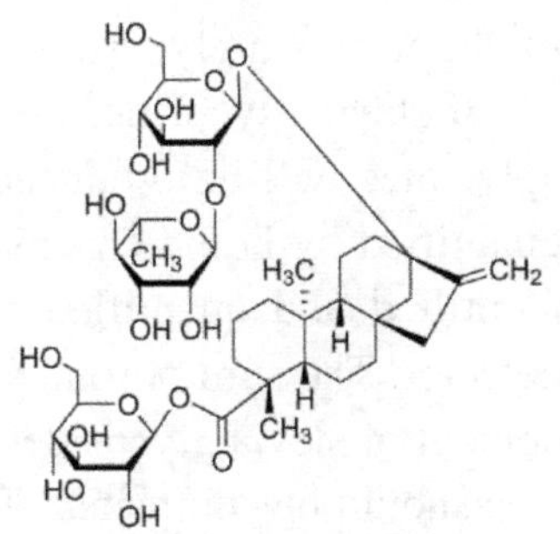

Dulcoside

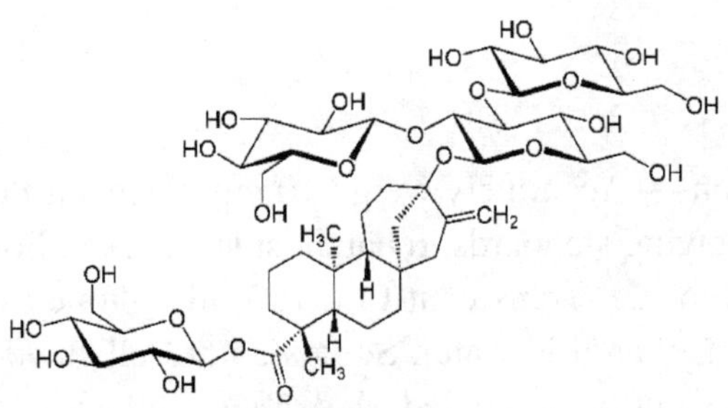

Rebaudioside A

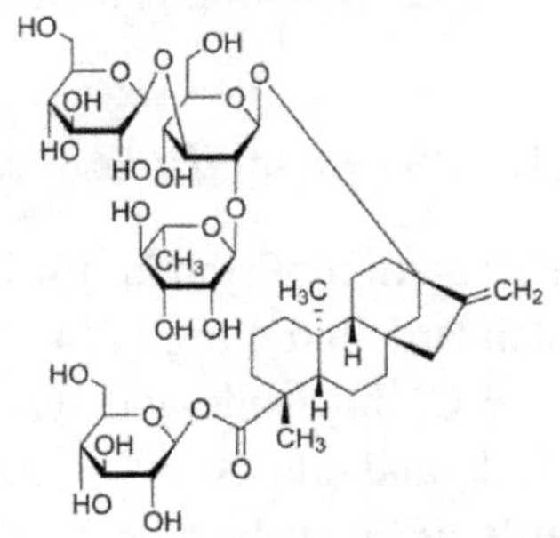

Rebaudioside C

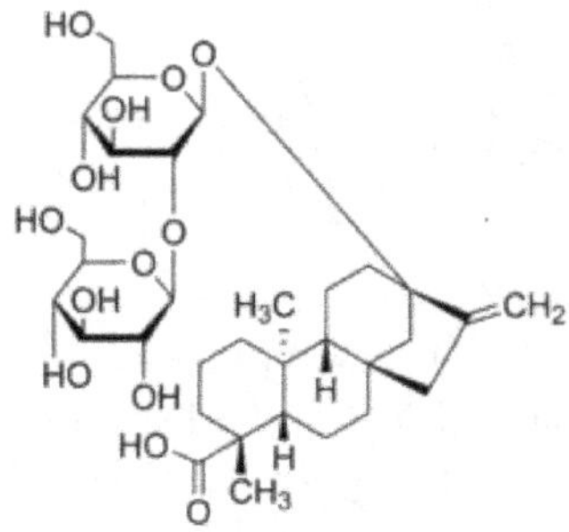

Steviolbioside

At present, there are also enzyme-modified stevia glycosides. Depending on the activity of enzymes, additional sugars are bonded to different carbon positions of stevia aglycones, and can form more than 20 stevia glycosides. This can greatly improve the yield.

However, it is difficult to identify and quantify each individual glycoside after enzyme modification. Some companies currently use LC-MS/MS to identify each stevia glycoside. Due to the availability of reference standards of each glycoside, and the requirements for the instruments, it is difficult for general laboratories to identify and quantify each enzyme-modified stevia glycoside.

If stevia glycosides are hydrolyzed by acid or alkali, free sugars and aglycones will be produced, and stevia aglycones can be identified and quantified by liquid chromatography tandem UV detector. Sugars can be identified and quantified by ion chromatography with electrochemical detector. The sum of total sugars and stevia aglycones should be the total content of stevia glycosides. Of course, the water introduced after hydrolysis should be subtracted. This should be a more feasible proposal.

The following is a chromatographic test method for natural stevia.

(i) *Test procedure*

Preparation of standard solution — Accurately weigh 10 mg of steviaside standard, and 5 mg of the following standards, rebaudioside A, rebaudioside C, dulcoside and steviolbioside. Transfer it to a 100 ml volumetric flask, and add 60 ml of 50% methanol in water. Sonicate until all standards are dissolved. After the solution is cooled, add 50% methanol in water to 100 ml mark, and shake well. This standard solution is ready for injection.

Preparation of sample solution (stevia extract materials) — Accurately weigh a certain amount of ground sample which contains about 20 mg of total stevia glycosides, and transfer it to a 100 ml volumetric flask. Add 60 ml 50% of methanol aqueous solution, and sonicate for 10 min. After the solution is cooled, add 50% methanol aqueous solution to the mark, and shake and mix well. Centrifuge (10,000 rpm) for 5 min, and take the clear solution to make injections.

Preparation of sample solution (stevia leaf powder) — Accurately weigh about 1 g of stevia leaf powder, and transfer it to a 250 ml round bottom flask. Add exactly 100 ml 50% of methanol water solution, and reflux for 1 h. After cooling take out 10 ml of the reflux solution, centrifuge (10,000 rpm) for 5 min, and take the clear solution for injection.

(ii) *HPLC conditions*

Column: Supelco Discovery LC-NH2, 5 μm, 4.6 × 250 mm
Flow rate: 1.8 ml/min
Column temperature: Room temperature
Injection volume: 20.0 μL
UV wavelength: 210 nm
Mobile phase A: 10 mM KH_2PO_4, pH 5.0
Mobile phase B: Acetonitrile
Mobile phase A 90%, mobile phase B 10% isocratic
Run time: 30 min

(iii) *Results and calculation*

$$Individual\ glycoside\ (\%) = \frac{Aa \times Wstand \times Vsam \times 100\%}{As \times Vstd \times Wsam}$$

or

$$Individual\ glycoside\ (mg/unit) = \frac{Aa \times Wsand \times Vsam \times UW}{As \times Vstd \times Wsam}$$

Here
Aa = Peak area of corresponding stevia glycoside in sample solution
As = Peak area of corresponding stevia glycoside in standard solution
Wsand = Weight of corresponding stevia glycoside standard (mg)
Wsam = Weight of sample (mg)
Vstd = Total volume of standard solution (ml)
Vsam = Total volume of sample solution (ml)
UW = Unit weight (mg/unit)

Total stevia glycosides = Sum of individual stevia glycoside detected.

4.78 Ephedrine Test Method

Ephedrine can be extracted from ephedra sinica, ephedra equisetina and ephedra intermedia. Along with ephedrine pseudoephedrine, methyl ephedrine, methyl pseudoephedrine, other active ingredients including demethylephen and amethyst pseudoephedrine active ingredients will be extracted. As a result of its curative effects on coughing, dilating trachea and relieving nasal mucosa congestion, it is often used to treat common diseases such as colds, coughs and asthma. Ephedrine remains a controlled substance.

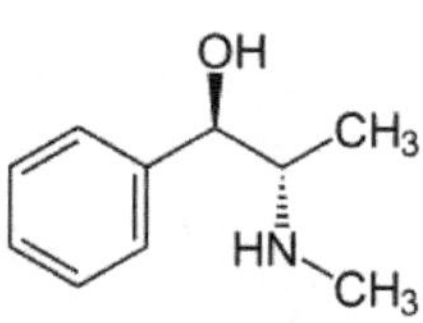

Ephedrine

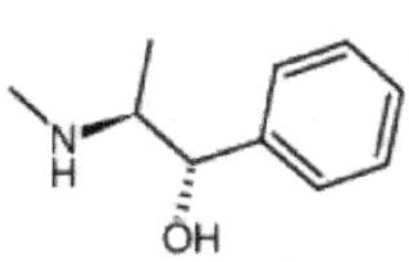

Pseudoephedrine

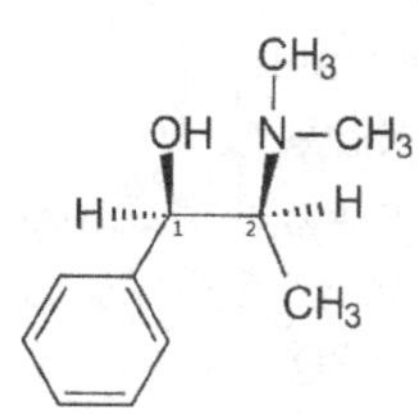

Methylephedrine

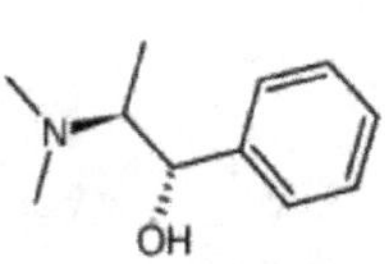

Methylpseudoephedrine

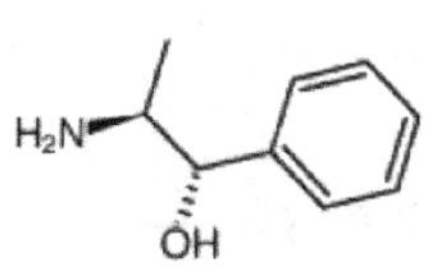

Norephedrine

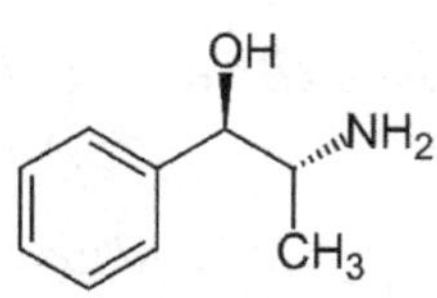

Norpseudoephedrine

From the molecular structures it can be seen that ephedrines and the corresponding pseudoephedrines are enantiomers. Due to the stereoscopic structures being different, this will cause the alkaline strength (pKa) to change between enantiomers, so it can be separated using ion exchange column chromatography.

(i) *Test procedure*

0.01 N hydrochloric acid solution preparation — In a 1,000 ml volumetric flask add about 600 ml of deionized water, add 1 ml of concentrated hydrochloric acid slowly into the volumetric flask, and shake a few times. Then add deionized water to the mark, and shake well.

Preparation of pH 6.3 buffer solution — Weigh 2.8 g of KH_2PO_4 and 0.8 g of K_2HPO_4, and dissolve it in 1,000 ml of deionized water. Filter with a filter film of 0.25 um.

Preparation of standard solution — Ephedrines are controlled items, so some standards are not easy to obtain. It is best to have four basic standards, ephedrine, pseudoephedrine, methyl ephedrine and norephydrine. Accurately weigh about 25 mg of ephedrine, 15 mg of pseudoephedrine, 5 mg of methyl ephedrine and norephydrine, and transfer it to a 50 ml volumetric flask. Add 30 ml 0.01 N hydrochloric acid solution, and shake until all standards are dissolved. Then fill with 0.01 N hydrochloric acid solution to mark, shake well, and label "Standard stock solution". Transfer 10 ml of the stock standard solution to a 50 ml volumetric flask, add 0.01N hydrochloric acid solution to the mark. Shake well, and label as "Standard solution". This standard solution can be injected.

Preparation of sample solution (herb powder) — Accurately weigh a certain amount of ground sample containing about 10 mg of ephedrines, and transfer it to a 200 ml round bottom flask. Add 95 ml pH 6.3 buffer solution and 5 ml of methanol, then reflux for 1 h. After the solution is cooled, filter the reflux solution through a 0.45 μm filter paper, and the filtrate can be injected.

Preparation of sample solution (for extract powder) — Accurately weigh a certain amount of ground sample which contains about 5 mg of ephedrines, and transfer it to a 50 ml volumetric flask. Add 30 ml of 0.01 N hydrochloric acid solution, and shake for 15 min with a wrist action shaker. Then sonicate for 5 min. After cooling, fill with 0.01 N hydrochloric acid to the mark, and filter through a 0.45 μm filter paper. The filtrate is ready for injection.

(ii) *HPLC conditions*

Column: Suplcosil LC-SCX, 5 um, 4.6 × 250 mm
Flow rate: 1.2 ml/min
Injection volume: 20 μL
UV wavelength: 254 nm
Mobile phase A: pH 6.3 buffer solution
Mobile phase B: Acetonitrile
Mobile phase A/ Mobile phase B = 90/10 isocratic
Column temperature: Room temperature

(iii) *Results and calculation*

$$Individual\,ephedrine\ (\%) = \frac{Aa \times Wstand \times Vsam \times 100\%}{As \times Vstd \times Wsam}$$

or

$$Individual\,ephedrine\,(mg/unit) = \frac{Aa \times Wsand \times Vsam \times UW}{As \times Vstd \times Wsam}$$

Here

Aa = Peak area of corresponding individual ephedrine in sample solution
As = Peak area of corresponding individual ephedrine in standard solution
Wsand = Weight of corresponding individual ephedrine standard (mg)
Wsam = Weight of sample (mg)
Vstd = Total volume of standard solution (ml)
Vsam = Total volume of sample solution (ml)
UW = Unit weight (mg/unit)

Calculation of methyl pseudoephedrine and norpseudoephedrine content: Since methylephedrine/methyl pseudoephedrine and norephedrine/norpseudoephedrine are enantiomers, their UV spectrum and molecular weight are the same, so methyl ephedrine standard can be used to calculate methyl pseudoephedrine content. The same will be true of norephedrine and norpseudoephedrine.

Total ephedrines = Sum of individual ephedrine detected

4.79 Spirulina Test Method

Spirulina contains many nutrients such as protein, vitamins, minerals and carotenoids. Protein is the main nutrient constituent of spirulina. Spirulina contains phycobiliproteins which have antioxidant properties and may enhance immunity. Phycobiliproteins are divided into two main classes: c-phycocyanin (cPC; max. UV abs, 610–620 nm) and andallophycocyanin (aPC, max. UV abs, 650–655 nm). Both cPC and aPC are macromolecules, and are difficult to isolate and quantify with chromatography. This method was developed in accordance with the method published by Yoshikawa and Belay in *Journal of AOAC International*, 91(3), 2008.

(i) *Test procedure*

Chemicals:

Disodium hydrogen phosphate dodecahydrate: Reagent grade
Sodium dihydrogen phosphate dihydrate: Reagent grade
Sodium azide: Reagent grade

Preparation of standard and sample solutions — Grind the sample into a powder, and accurately weigh about 300 mg of the spirulina standard, or the equivalent of 300 mg of spirulina standard samples. Transfer into different 50 ml centrifuge tubes, respectively, and add 25 ml of 100 mM disodium hydrogen phosphate buffer solution pH adjusted to 6.0 with dilute phosphoric acid. Stir with a stirring stick, and culture at a temperature of 30°C, for 16 h. Then stir well with a stir stick, centrifuge for 10 min, and transfer 1 ml of clear solution to 50 ml volumetric flask. Add 100 mM disodium hydrogen phosphate, pH 6.0 buffer to the mark, and shake well. If necessary, further dilutions can be made with the pH 6.0 buffer solution.

Remove 1 ml of standard or sample solution and place into 1 cm spectral tubes. Run UV/visible scanning 300–700 nm. The maximum absorption of standard or sample solution should be within the range of 0.3–0.9, and further dilution or correction should be made if the range is exceeded.

The proportion of cPC and aPC should be about 70:30.

Results and calculation:

Extinction coefficients for cPC and aPC

Extinction coefficients (mg/ml × cm)	**620 nm**	**650 nm**
cPC	7.20	1.67
aPC	3.91	6.45

Calculation:

$$OD_{620nm} = C_C \times 7.20 + C_A \times 3.91$$

$$OD_{650nm} = C_C \times 1.67 + C_A \times 6.45$$

Here

620 nm is the maximum absorption wavelength of cPC
650 nm is the maximum absorption wavelength of aPC
C_C = Concentration of cPC (mg/ml)
C_A = Concentration of aPC (mg/ml)
7.20 = Absorption of 1 mg/ml cPC solution at 620 nm
3.91 = Absorption of 1 mg/ml aPC solution at 620nm
1.67 = Absorption of 1 mg/ml cPC solution at 650nm
6.45 = Absorption of 1 mg/ml aPC solution at 650nm
OD = Optical density (UV absorption)

Set up,
$C_C = X$
$C_A = Y$
A_{620nm} = Absorption of sample solution at 620 nm
B_{650nm} = Absorption of sample solution at 650 nm

Yield

$$A_{620nm} = X \times 7.20 + Y \times 3.91$$

$$B_{650nm} = X \times 1.67 + Y \times 6.45$$

Solve the above linear equation with two unknows, get

$$X = 0.162\text{A} - 0.098\text{B}$$

$$Y = 0.18\text{B} - 0.042\text{A}$$

Final

$$cPC\ \% = \frac{X \times sample\,volume(ml) \times 100\%}{weight\ of\ sample(mg)}$$

$$aPC\ \% = \frac{Y \times sample\,volume(ml)}{weight\ of\ sample(mg)}$$

Total phycobiliproteins (%) = cPC(%) + cPA(%)

Comparing total phycobiliproteins (%) in the test sample with the level in the spirulina standard can give you an idea of the sample quality.

4.80 Garlic Test Method

Garlic has two active or marker compounds, alliin and allicin. Fresh garlic contains 1%–2% alliin. Garlic releases allinase when the cloves are pressed or crushed. The allinase reacts with alliin to produce allicin. Therefore, the fresh and whole garlic cloves mainly contain alliin, and the processed garlic such as garlic powder, should mainly contain allicin. For testing alliin, the fresh and whole cloves of garlic should be treated under high temperature to deactivate the allinase. This prevents the conversion to allicin during the sample processing and extraction.

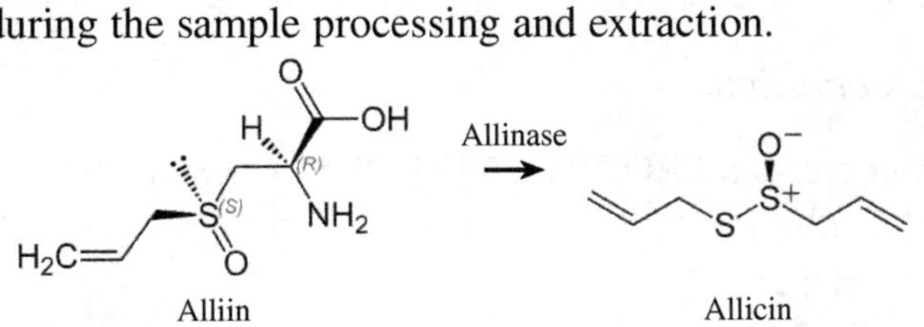

Alliin and allicin are polar compounds. When using reverse phase chromatography column, the retention time is short, and it is easy to have interferences. By adding an ion pair reagent (tetrabutyl ammonia salt) in the mobile phase, the retention time can be extended and help facilitate the separation of impurities. See Chapter 1, Section 1.1.2 "Mobile phase application".

4.80.1 *Allicin testing method*

(i) *Test procedure*

Preparation of pH 5.5 buffer — Weigh 1 g of potassium dihydrogen phosphate and 0.2 g of dipotassium hydrogen phosphate. Dissolve in 1,000 ml of deionized water, with 0.1 N hydrochloric acid and 0.01 N sodium hydroxide to adjust pH to 5.5.

Preparation of standard solution — Accurately weigh about 5 mg of allicin standard, transfer it to a refrigerator cooled 50 ml volumetric flask, add 30 ml cooled pH 5.5 buffer. Vortex until all standard is dissolved, and then add pH 5.5 buffer to the mark. Shake this solution well, avoid light, and store in the refrigerator, until injection.

Preparation of sample solution — Take 500 mg of fresh garlic, or dried garlic powder, or other samples equivalent to 5 mg of allicin. Transfer it to a proper utensil or instrument to grind. After grinding, rinse the utensil with 10 ml of cold pH 5.5 buffer, and transfer the slurry to a 50 ml volumetric flask. Rinse the utensil two more times, and combine the rinse solutions together in the 50 ml volumetric flask. Shake for 2 min, then add pH 5.5 buffer to mark. Shake well, then remove 5 ml of sample solution and place in a 10 ml centrifuge tube. Place a cap on the tube, centrifuge it for 10 min, and take the clear solution for injection.

(ii) *HPLC conditions*

Column: Phenomenex PRODIGY ODS (2) 5 μm 4.6 × 150 mm 100A
Flow rate: 1.0 ml/mi
Injection volume: 20 μL
UV wavelength: 240 nm

Mobile phase A: 5 mM tetra butyl ammonium chloride, pH 5.5
Mobile phase B: Acetonitrile

Gradient:

Time (min)	A%	B%
0	75	25
15.0	30	70
18.0	30	70
18.5	75	25
25.0	75	25

(iii) *Results and calculation*

$$Allicin\ (\%) = \frac{Aa \times Wstand \times Vsam \times 100\%}{As \times Vstd \times Wsam}$$

or

$$Allicin\ (mg/unit) = \frac{Aa \times Wsand \times Vsam \times UW}{As \times Vstd \times Wsam}$$

Here
Aa = Peak area of allicin in sample solution
As = Peak area of allicin in standard solution
Wsand = Weight of allicin standard (mg)
Wsam = Weight of sample (mg)
Vstd = Total volume of standard solution (ml)
Vsam = Total volume of sample solution (ml)
UW = Unit weight (mg/unit)

4.80.2 *Test method for alliin*

(i) *Test procedure*

Preparation of standard solution — Accurately weigh about 5 mg of alliin standard, and transfer it to a 50 ml of volumetric flask. Add 30 ml of 20%

methanol/water solution, and vortex until the standard completely dissolved. Then add 20% of methanol/water solution to the mark, and shake well. The standard solution is ready for injection.

Preparation of sample solution — Take about 20 g of fresh and completely peeled whole garlic clove sample, transfer to a vessel with cover, and add about 200 ml of water. Cover, and place in a 90°C water bath for 30 min to deactivate the enzyme. Mash the sample, then put in 100°C water bath for 30 min, after cooling take about 500 mg of sample, and transfer to 50 ml volumetric flask. Add 30 ml of 20% methanol/water solution, and vortex for 5 min. Shake with a wrist action shaker for another 10 min, then add 20% methanol/water solution to the mark. Shake well, and after centrifuging, take the clear solution for injection.

(ii) *HPLC conditions*

Same as the aforementioned allicin test method.

(iii) *Results and calculation*

$$Alliin\ (\%) = \frac{Aa \times Wstand \times Vsam \times 100\%}{As \times Vstd \times Wsam}$$

or

$$Alliin\ (mg/unit) = \frac{Aa \times Wsand \times Vsam \times UW}{As \times Vstd \times Wsam}$$

Here
Aa = Peak area of alliin in sample solution
As = Peak area of alliin in standard solution
Wsand = Weight of alliin standard (mg)
Wsam = Weight of sample (mg)
Vstd = Total volume of standard solution (ml)
Vsam = Total volume of sample solution (ml)
UW = Unit weight (mg/unit)

4.81 Ferulic Acid Test Method

Ferulic acid is found in rice, bamboo shoots, popcorn and some vegetables. It has shown antioxidant and anti-inflammatory functions.

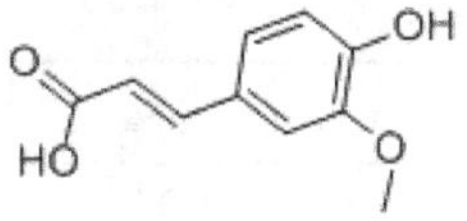

Ferulic acid

Ferulic acid is an acidic compound that is soluble in water and is negatively charged when the pH is greater than 5. In order to increase its chromatographic retention time, this method uses tetrahexyl ammonium chloride in the mobile phase, which can be paired with negative ferulic acid, to achieve this purpose. It helps extend the retention time and facilitate the separation of impurities. See Chapter 1, Section 1.1.2 "Mobile phase application".

(i) *Test procedure*

Preparation of standard solution — Accurately weigh about 10 mg ferulic acid standard, and transfer it to 100 ml volumetric flask. Add 60 ml of water, and sonicate until the standard gets completely dissolved. Then add water to 100 ml volume, and shake well. The standard solution is ready for injection.

Preparation of sample solution — Accurately weigh a certain amount of ground sample that contains about 10 mg of ferulic acid, and transfer it to a 100 ml volumetric flask. Add 60 ml of water, and sonicate for 10 min. After the solution is cooled add water to the mark, and shake well. Then centrifuge (10,000 rpm) for 5 min, and draw the clear solution into a 2 ml injection vail. It is ready for injection.

(ii) *HPLC conditions*

Column: Supelco Discovery C18, 5 um, 4.6 × 150 mm
Flow rate: 1.0 ml/min
Injection volume: 10 μL
UV wavelength: 300 nm

Mobile phase A: 2 mM tetrahexylammonium chloride, pH 6.0
Mobile phase B: Acetonitrile
Column temperature: 45°C

Gradient:

Time (min)	A%	B%
0	95	5
10	75	25
14.0	75	25
14.5	95	5
18.0	95	5

(iii) ***Results and calculation***

$$Ferulic\ acid\ (\%) = \frac{Aa \times Wstand \times Vsam \times 100\%}{As \times Vstd \times Wsam}$$

or

$$Ferulic\ acid\ \ (mg/unit) = \frac{Aa \times Wsand \times Vsam \times UW}{As \times Vstd \times Wsam}$$

Here
Aa = Peak area of ferulic acid in sample solution
As = Peak area of ferulic acid in standard solution
Wsand = Weight of ferulic acid standard (mg)
Wsam = Weight of sample (mg)
Vstd = Total volume of standard solution (ml)
Vsam = Total volume of sample solution (ml)
UW = Unit weight (mg/unit)

4.82 Testing Methods for Phytosterols

The richest natural occurring phytosterol sources are vegetable oils. Phytosterols can reduce blood cholesterol levels. The main compounds include B-sitosterol, stigmasterol, campesterol and brassicasterol.

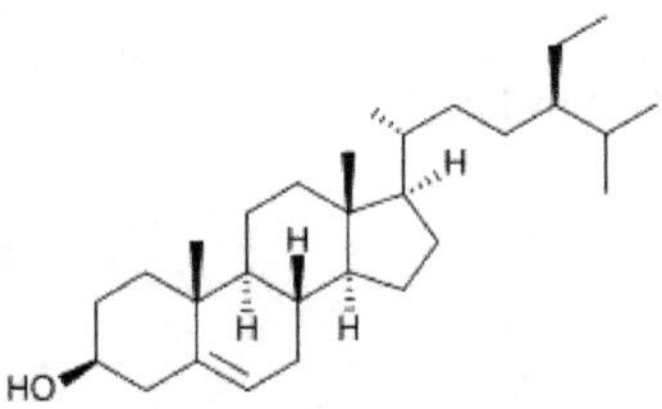

B-sitosterol

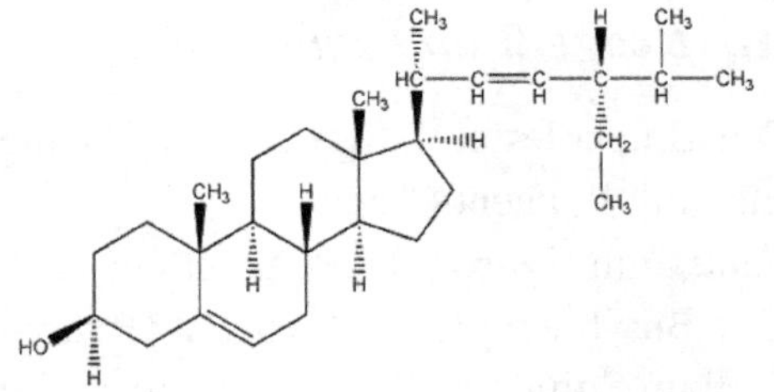

stigmasterol

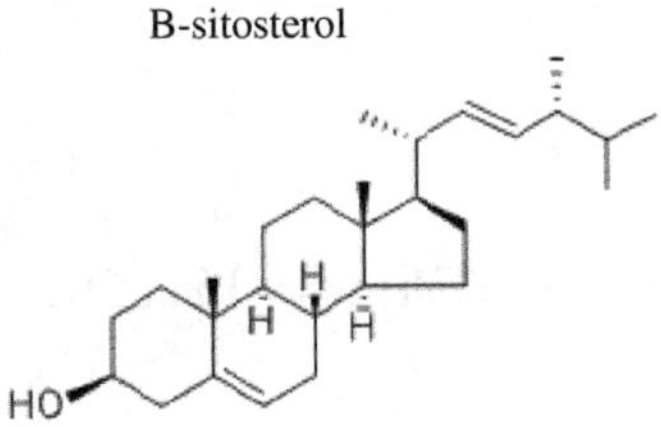

Brassicasterol

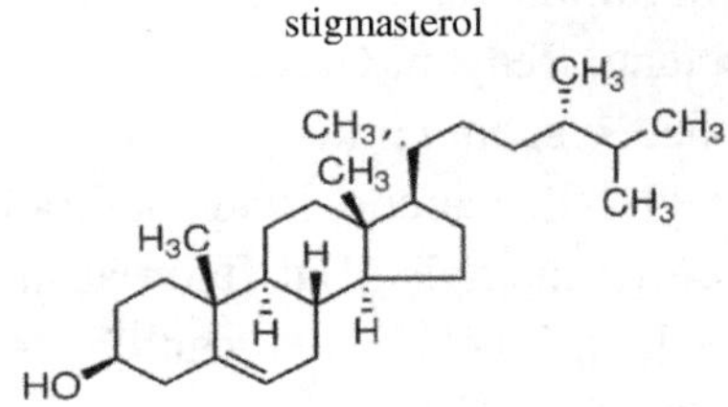

Campesterol

Sterols in plants are present in the form of various fatty acid esters. Due to the many types of fatty acids, the test method uses hydrolysis to convert the sterol esters into free sterols and fatty acids. Then gas chromatography (GC) is used to separate and measure them. Because sterol molecules contain hydroxyls, the boiling point is higher under the force of hydrogen bonds, if the temperature of the GC is raised, the sterol molecule may be decomposed. Thus, the free sterols must undergo silanization to reduce the boiling point before being injected into the GC.

(i) *Apparatus and equipment*

GC: Hewlett-Packard 5890 with FID detection
GC Column: Restek Rtx®-5, 5% diphenyl — 95% dimethyl polysiloxane, 60m × 0.25mm, 0.25 μm film thickness
10mL glass tubes with screw caps
Vortex
Centrifuge
Ultrasonic water bath
Analytical balance
2 mL glass vial with screw cap (PTFE/SIL)
Weighing paper
Disposable pipettes
Volumetric pipettes

(ii) *Reagent and standard*

Dihydrocholesterol, Sigma, D6128 (Internal Standard)
Ethanol, Reagent Grade
Potassium Hydroxide, Reagent Grade
Tert-Butylmethylether, Reagent Grade
Sodium Sulfate, anhydrous, Reagent Grade
N-Heptane, Reagent Grade
Pyridine, Reagent Grade
4-Methyl-2-Pantanone, Reagent Grade
N, O-bis (trimethylsilil) trifluoroacatamide (BSTFA) with 1% of trimethyl chlorosilane (TMCS), Reagent Grade
Nanopure Water

(iii) *Preparation of sample solution*

Extraction and hydrolysis:

(1) Accurately weigh about 2 g of oil samples, or 10 g of blended raw plants into a 200 ml round bottem reflux flask. Add 15 mg of internal standard (dihydrocholesterol). Then add 50 ml of 7.5% KOH in methanol and a stirring bar, and reflux for 60 min.
(2) Cool to room temperature, then add 5 ml water. Use 50 mL *n*-hexane: petroleum ether (50:50, v/v) to extract the saponified sterols three times. The upper layer (organic phase, about 150 mL) is collected into a separatory funnel and the lower layer is discarded. Wash the organic extract with 40 mL of water by gently rotating the separatory funnel. After allowing the layers to separate the lower aqueous phase can be discarded.
(3) Desiccate the organic extract by pouring through a glass funnel containing 20 g sodium sulfate in a filter paper, into a clean 250-mL Erlenmeyer flask.
(4) Evaporate the organic extract to dryness on a rotary evaporator at 40 ± 1°C.
(5) Add 1 ml of pyridine and 4 ml of 4-methyl-2-pantanone, sonicate for 10 min to dissolve the residue, centrifuge 10 min and take the top clear solution to derivatization procedure.

Note: The volume of solvents can be modified as long as the ratio of pyridine to 4methyl-2-pantanone is 1 to 4.

(iv) *Preparation of standard solution*

(1) Accurately weigh about 10 mg of each B-sitosterol, stigmasterol, campesterol, brassicasterol standards and internal standard (dihydrocholesterol) into a 10 mL glass tube with a screw cap.
(2) Add 1 mL of pyridine and sonicate the tube for 15 min.
(3) Add 4 mL of 4-methyl-2-pantanone and sonicate the tube for another 10 min.
(4) After filtration the filatant is ready for derivatization procedure.
Note: The volume of solvents can be modified as long as the ratio of pyridine to 4methyl-2-pantanone is 1 to 4.

(v) *Derivatization procedure*

(1) Take 500 μL standard, or sample solution, or blank (pyridine: 4-methyl-2-pantanone, 1:4) solutions to individual 2 ml injection vials.
(2) In each injection vial, add 100 μL of N, O-bis (trimethylsilil) trifluoroacatamide (BSTFA) with 1% of trimethyl chlorosilane (TMCS) and mix well.
(3) The vial is capped and put in a hot water bath at 100°C for 10–15 min. The water level is just as high as the solution level in the injection vial.
(4) Cool the vial to room temperature and it is ready for GC injection.

(vi) *GC condition*

Instrument: Hewlett-Packard GC 5890 with FID
Column: Restek Rtx®-5, 5% diphenyl — 95% dimethyl polysiloxane, 60m × 0.25mm, 0.25 μm film thickness
Condition: Initial Oven Temperature: 200°C hold for 1 min, then increase to 340°C at 15°C/min, hold for 10 min
Detector: 355°C
Injector: 345°C

Injection Volume: 2 μL
Carry gase(nitrogen)flow rate: 1 ml/min

(vii) *Result and calculation*

$$Individual\ phytosterol\ (\%) = \frac{Cs \times PARu \times Vu \times C'u \times 100\%}{PARs \times Wu \times C's}$$

Here

Cs = Concentration of corresponding phytosterol in standard solution (mg/ml)

C'u = Concentration of internal standard in sample solution

C's = Concentration of internal standard in standard solution

PARu = The peak area ratio of corresponding phytosterol/internal standard in sample solution

PARs = The peak area ratio of corresponding phytosterol/internal standard in standard solution

Vu = Total volume of sample solution (ml)

Wu = Sample weight (mg)

Total phytosterol = Sum of individual phytosterol detected

Chapter 5
Other Nutritional Ingredients Test Methods

5.1 Iodine Test Method

This method is modified from one of the AOAC methods, and can be used to test the total iodine content in dietary supplements and food products. All forms of iodine are reduced by sodium thiosulfate to the iodide anion, and then the iodide ions are determined by ion chromatography. A reversed phase chromatography method with ion pairing is introduced as well.

(i) *Test procedure*

Preparation of standard solution — Accurately weigh about 10 mg of potassium iodide, and transfer it to a 50 ml volumetric flask. Dissolve in a 0.2 N sodium thiosulfate solution and fill to volume mark. Shake well, and label as "Stock standard solution". Transfer 1 ml of the stock standard solution to a 50 ml volumetric flask and dilute to mark with 0.2 N sodium thiosulfate solution. Shake this well, and it is ready for injection. (Concentration of iodide ions is approximately 3 ppm.)

Preparation of sample solutions

(1) If the iodine in the sample comes entirely from potassium iodide, or other iodide salt: Accurately weigh a certain amount of the ground sample which contains about 200 micrograms of iodide, and transfer

it to a 50 ml of volumetric flask. Add about 30 ml of 0.2 N sodium thiosulfate solution, and sonicate for 30 min. After cooling, fill to the volume mark with sodium thiosulfate solution, and shake well. Centrifuge (10,000 rpm) for 5 min, and the above mentioned clear solution can be injected.

(2) If the iodine in the sample comes from natural plants or other form of iodine: Accurately weigh a certain amount of ground sample containing about 200 micrograms of iodine, and transfer it to 50 ml of metal crucible. Add 1.5 g of potassium hydroxide, and 15 ml of ethanol. Heat the crucible on an electric heating plate until all the ethanol is evaporated. Increase the temperature of the electric plate and continue to heat until the sample is completely dried and there is no more white smoke. Place the crucible in a 510°C muffle furnace and bake for 4 h. After cooling, add about 25 ml of 0.2 N sodium thiosulfate solution to rinse and dissolve the residue in the crucible. Sonicate for 20 min to ensure that the iodide ions have been all dissolved. Then transfer the solution to a 50 ml volumetric flask. Continue to rinse the crucible several times with a small amount of sodium thiosulfate solution, and combine all the rinse solutions into the 50 ml volumetric flask. Fill to volume with 0.2 N sodium thiosulfate solution, and shake well. Centrifuge (10,000 rpm) for 5 min, and take the clear solution to an injection vail. It is ready for injection.

(ii) *Ion chromatography (IC) conditions*

Column: Dionex IonPac®AS11-HC, 4 × 250 mm
Detector: Conductivity
Suppressor: Dionex ASRS_4 mm
Suppressor current: 120 mA
Flow rate: 1.0 ml/min
Injection volume: 25 μl
Elute: 50 mM NaOH
Run time: 30 min

Same sample and standard solution can be run with reversed phase chromatography/Ion pair method.

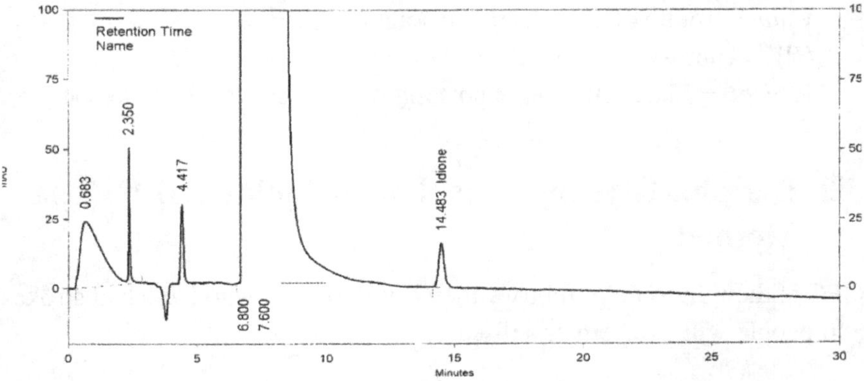

Figure 5.1: IC chromatogram of iodide.

(iii) *UPLC conditions*

Column: Acquity UPLC® BEH C18, 1.7 μm, 2.1 × 150 mm
Flow rate: 0.4 ml/min
Injection volume: 2 μL
UV wavelength: 225 nm
Mobile phase A: 7.5 mM tetrabutylammonium salt, pH 5.5
Mobile phase B: Acetonitrile
A:B = 92:8
Run time: 12 min

(iv) *Results and calculation (applicable for both methods)*

$$Total\,iodine\,(ug)\,per\,unite = \frac{Aa \times Cstd \times Vsam \times 126 \times UW}{As \times Wsam \times 166}$$

or

$$Total\,iodine\;(ug/g) = \frac{Aa \times Cstd \times Vsam \times 126}{As \times Wsam \times 166}$$

Aa = Peak area of iodide in sample solution
$Cstd$ = Concentration of iodide in standard solution (ug/ml)
As = Peak area of iodide in standard solution
$Wsam$ = Weight of sample (g)

Vsam = Total volume of sample solution (ml)
UW = Unit weight (g)
126/166 = The coefficient of potassium iodide conversion to iodide ions.

5.2 L-alpha-GlycerylphosphorylCholine (GPC) Test Method

GPC is thought to help improve memory in people who have had strokes and people with Alzheimer's disease.

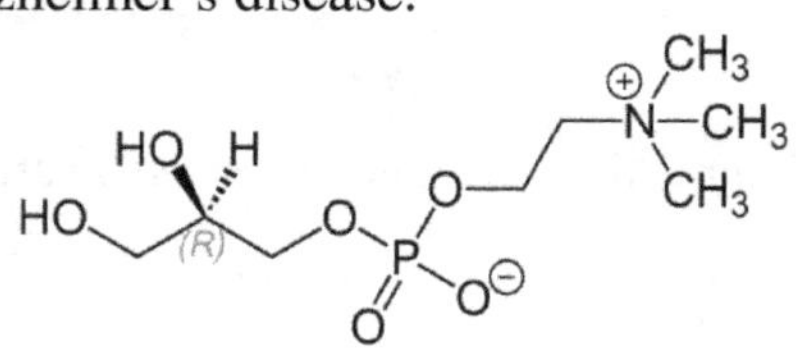

α-GPC

The molecular structure shows that GPC is a strong polar compound, and reversed phase column chromatography will not work. The molecule also has poor UV absorption and cannot be detected by UV detector.

The method presented here uses a normal phase LC column coupled with MS/MS detector to test the GPC. Of course, if the laboratory has ELSD this may be attempted for use. The ELSD detector is not as selective, and it is easy to be disrupted.

(i) *Test procedure*

Because GPC is a polar compound, the MS/MS (ESI) detector is extremely sensitive. To get good linearity and to reduce the concentration of impurities, the overall concentration of the standard and sample solutions can be set at ppb level. The sensitivity of different instruments is different, each laboratory can adjust the solution concentrations according to their actual situation.

Preparation of standard solutions — Accurately weigh about 20 mg of L-alpha-GPC, and transfer to a 100 ml volumetric flask. Add water to dissolve, and dilute up to 100 ml. Make further dilutions to obtain three different standard solutions: 100 ppb, 20 ppb and 5 ppb.

Preparation of sample solution — Accurately weigh a certain amount of sample containing 20 mg GPC, and transfer it to a 100 ml volumetric flask. Add about 60 ml of water and shake with a wrist action shaker for 15 min. Then sonicate for 5 min, and fill to the mark with water. Shake well, centrifuge (10,000 rpm) for 5 min, and transfer 25 μl of the clear solution into 100 ml volumetric flask. Add water, dilute to the mark, and shake well. This solution can be injected.

Spike solution preparation — Transfer 995 μl of the aforementioned sample solution to another injection vail, add 5 μl of 10 ppm stock solution, and mix well. This is ready for injection.

(ii) *UPLC conditions*

Column: Acquity UPLC® BEH Amide, 1.7 μm, 2.1 × 100 mm
Flow rate: 0.40 mL/min
Column temperature: 45°C
Injection volume: 1 μL
Mobile phase A: 0.01% formic acid in nano pure water
Mobile phase B: 0.01% formic acid in acetonitrile

Gradient:

Time (min)	A%	B%
0	10	90
0–1.5	20	80
1.5–2.0	20	80
2.0–2.3	10	90
5.0	10	90

MS/MS parameter

Model	MRM
Ion	ES+
Inter Channel Delay (sec)	–1.000
InterScan Time (sec)	–1.000
Span (Da)	0.0
Start Time (min)	0.0
End Time (min)	5.0

α-GPC

Ch	Prnt (Da)	Dau (Da)	Dwell (s)	Cone (V)	Coll (eV)	Delay (s)	Compound	Formula
1	258.13	86.11	0.080	30.00	24.00	−1.000	GPC	257.1
2	258.13	104.14	0.080	30.00	14.00	−1.000	GPC	257.1
3	258.13	125.03	0.080	30.00	24.00	−1.000	GPC	257.1

(iii) *Results and calculation*

First, calculate the spike recovery (see Chapter 1, Section 1.1.5 "Qualitative and quantitative testing of LC-MS/MS"). If the recovery is good, you can use the TIC to calculate the results. The calculated result should be corrected by the spike recovery. If the recovery is not good, follow the steps in Chapter 1, Section 1.1.5 "Qualitative and quantitative testing of LC-MS/MS".

$$GPC\ (\%) = \frac{Csam \times Vsam \times DF \times 100\%}{Wsam \times 1000000 \times R}$$

Csam = Concentration of the sample solution (ppb, ng/ml)
Vsam = Volume of sample solution (100 ml)
DF = Dilution factor (4,000)
Wsam = Weight of sample (mg)
1000000 = mg/ng
R = spike recovery

5.3 Test Method for Free Amino Acids (Direct HPLC Method)

According to different health care needs, dietary supplements could contain a single or multiple free form of amino acids. Amino acids are polar compounds that are difficult to stay on reversed phase columns. Ion pairing is used in this method for the purpose of effectively increasing the retention times and helping to quantify the free amino acids in dietary supplements. To make the ion pairs work efficiently, the amino acids under analysis must be charged, either positively or negatively.

Amino acid	Isoelectric point
Glycine	5.97
Alanine	6.00
Valine	5.96
Leucine	5.98
Isoleucine	6.02
Phenylalanine	5.48
Serine	5.68
Threonine	6.16
Tyrosine	5.66
Cysteine	5.05
Methionine	5.74
Proline	6.30
Tryptophan	5.89
Lysine	9.74
Arginine	10.76
Histidine	7.59
Aspartic acid	2.77
Glutamate	3.22
Asparagine	5.41
Glutamine	5.65

From this list it can be seen that all amino acids isoelectric points are higher than 5, except aspartic acid and glutamate. As long as the pH of the mobile phase is less than 3, the amino acids are positively charged except aspartic acid and glutamate. By adding negative ions (such as hexane sulfonic acid salt) to the mobile phase, neutral ion pairs will be formed with amino acids under test. This will help interactions with the reversed phase column, and extend the retention time. This facilitates the separation of impurities.

For testing of aspartic acid and glutamate, the pH of the mobile phase can be adjusted to 6, so aspartic acid and glutamate will be negatively charged. Adding cations to the mobile phase can form ion pairs with aspartic acid and glutamate. Commonly used cations are tetrabutylammonium salt, or others. See Chapter 1, Section 1.1.2 "Mobile phase application".

The following is a reversed phase separation with ion pairing test method for amino acids.

(i) *Test procedure*

Preparation of standard solution — Accurately weigh 20 mg of each amino acid standards needed, and transfer it to a 50 ml volumetric flask. Add 30 ml of water, and vortex until all standards get dissolved. Then add water to 50 ml mark and shake well. The standard solution is ready for injection.

Preparation of sample solution — Weigh a certain amount of ground sample containing about 20 mg of amino acids under test, and transfer it to a 50 ml volumetric flask. Add 30 ml of water, and shake for 15 min with a wrist action shaker. Then sonicate for 5 min. After cooling, fill with water to the mark, shake well, and centrifuge (10,000 rpm) for 5 min. The clear solution can be injected.

(ii) *UPLC conditions (except aspartic acid and glutamate testing)*

Column: Acquity Hss T3 C18, 1.8 um, 2.1 × 150 mm
Mobile phase A: 10 mM hexane sulfonic acid sodium salt, pH 2.0
Mobile phase B: Acetonitrile
Flow rate: 0.4 ml/min
Column temperature: 45°C
UV wavelength: 210 nm

Gradient:

Time (min)	A%	B%
0	97	3
0–8.0	75	30
8.0–9.0	75	30
9.0–9.3	97	3
12.0	97	3

(iii) *Results and calculation*

$$Individual\,amino\,acid\,(mg/unit) = \frac{Aa \times Wstd \times Vsam \times UW}{As \times Wsam \times Vstd}$$

or

$$Individual\,amino\,acid\,(\%) = \frac{Aa \times Wstd \times Vsam \times 100\%}{As \times Wsam \times Vstd}$$

Aa = Peak area of corresponding amino acid in sample solution
As = Peak area of corresponding amino acid in standard solution
Wstd = Weight of standard (mg)
Wsam = Weight of sample (mg)
Vsam = Total volume of sample solution (ml)
Vstd = Total volume of standard solution (ml)
UW = Unit weight (mg)

This method is not suitable for testing carnitine, because carnitine and its degradant crotonoylbetaine cannot be separated using this method. In addition, crotonoylbetaine contains a conjugated double bond, the UV absorption is much more intense than carnitine. The signal strength of 0.5% crotonoylbetaine is equivalent to 100% carnitine signal strength. Even a trace amount of crotonoylbetaine can cause a large error if it cannot be separated from the carnitine peak. The Carnitine test should follow Section 5.53 "Betaine, carnitine and acetyl-carnitine test method".

If the ion pair method experiences problems, the ion exchange method can be attempted. Under low pH conditions, most amino acids are positively charged, and the cations can be separated using a cation exchange column. Because the electrostatic force is relatively strong, some amino acids under analysis could not be eluded, or may be retained too long, and cause peak widening. To control the interaction forces between the amino acids and the stationary phase, competitive cations (e.g., NH4+, etc.) can be added to the mobile phase. The amino acid ions can be "squeezed out" by NH4+ ion (see Chapter 1, Section 1.1.2 "Mobile phase application"). The following section describes how to determine amino acids with ion exchange method.

IC test procedure

Standard and sample solution preparation are same as above "Ion Pair" method.

IC condition

Column: Supelcosil LC-SCX, 5 μm, 4.6 mm × 250 mm
Flow rate: 1.5 ml/min
UV wavelength: 210 nm
Injection volume: 20.0 μL
Mobile phase A: 10 mM potassium dihydro phosphate, 20 mM ammonia chloride, pH 2.0
Mobile phase B: Acetonitrile
Mobile phase A: mobile phase B = 25:75

The concentration of ammonia chloride in the mobile phase can be adjusted. The greater the concentration of ammonia chloride, the faster the amino acids will be eluted; the lower the concentration of ammonia chloride, the slower amino acids will be eluted.

Results and calculation

Same as above "Ion pair" method.

5.4 Test Method for Amino Acids (Pre-Column Derivatization)

Protein or peptides can be hydrolyzed which results in a variety of amino acids with different proportions. There are many hydrolysis methods. Acid hydrolysis method is the most commonly used. The hydrolysis steps used for proteins or peptides are not included in this method.

There are various amino acids obtained after protein or peptide hydrolysis, with large differences in content and complexity. The direct HPLC method cannot test the amino acids produced through hydrolysis.

In order to extend the retention time of amino acids and improve specificity and sensitivity of the measurement, it is suggested to use a pre column derivatization method.

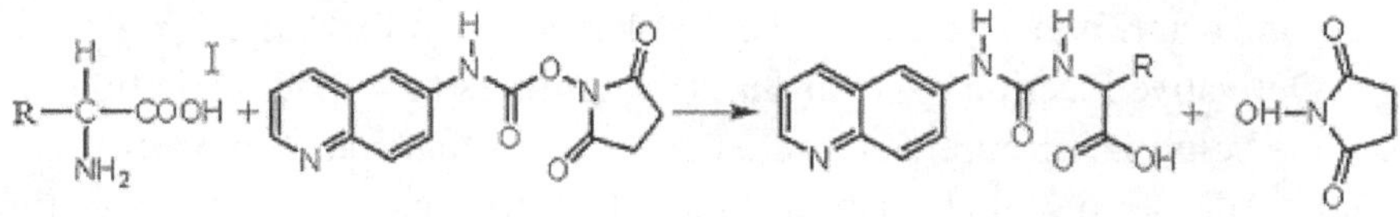

Several derivative reagents can be used to derivatize amino acids. This method uses 6-amino-quinoly-N-hydroxysuccinimidyl carbamate (AQC) as the derivative reagent.

After derivatization, the resulting molecule (AQC-amino acids) becomes larger, with less polarity and a higher UV sensitivity. It is easier to separate and quantify by reversed phase liquid chromatography. In addition, the resulting molecules increase the alkalinity, so in the low pH mobile phase conditions, all AQC-amino acids become cations. The ion pair method will work more efficiently and facilitate separation and quantification of each AQC-amino acid. See Chapter 1, Section 1.1.2 "Mobile phase application".

(i) *Test procedure*

(i) *Derivatization procedure*

Boric acid buffer solution preparation — Weigh 12.4 g of boric acid, and dissolve in 400 ml of water, with 40% sodium hydroxide solution to adjust pH to 8.8. Then add water to 500 ml.

Preparation of QAC solution — Weigh 10 mg of AQC powder, dissolve it in 10 ml of acetonitrile and shake well.

Preparation of standard solution — Accurately weigh 5 mg of each amino acid standard, and transfer it to a 100 ml volumetric flask. Add 60 ml of 0.15 N hydrochloric acid, and vortex until all standards dissolve. Fill to the volume mark with 0.15 N hydrochloric acid, and shake well. The solution is ready for derivatization. The concentrations of amino acid can be adjusted base on the sample.

Preparation of sample solution — Accurately weigh a certain amount of ground sample that contains about 0.1–10 mg of the aforementioned amino acids, and transfer it to a 100 ml volumetric flask. Add 60 ml 0.15 N hydrochloric acid and shake for 15 min with a wrist action shaker. Then sonicate for 10 min. After cooling, fill to the volume mark with 0.15 N hydrochloric acid, and centrifuge for 5 min. Take the clear solution for derivatization.

Derivative reaction — Transfer 20 microliters of standard solution, or sample solution, or pure water to each 200microliter injection vails separately. Add 80 microliter of boric acid buffer to each vail, and vortex for 10 sec. Then add 20 microliters of QAC solution to each vail, and vortex for 10 sec. Put the vials in 50°C water bath for 10 min. After cooing, centrifuge for 5 min, and the clear solution can be injected.

(ii) *UPLC conditions*

Column: Acquity UPLC® BEH, Phenyl, 1.7 μm, 2.1 × 150 mm
Flow rate: 0.4 ml/min
Injection volume: 1.0 μL
UV wavelength: 248 nm
Mobile phase A: 10 mM hexane sulfonic acid sodium salt, pH 2.5
Mobile phase B: Methanol
Column temperature: 50°C

Gradient:

Time (min)	A%	B%
0	95	5
1	95	5
4	80	20
7.0	60	40
7.6	60	40
8.0	95	5
10.0	95	5

(iii) *Results and calculation*

$$Individual\,amino\,acid\ (mg/unit) = \frac{Aa \times Wstd \times Vsam \times UW}{As \times Wsam \times Vstd}$$

or

$$Individual\ amino\ acid\ (\%) = \frac{Aa \times Wstd \times Vsam \times 100\%}{As \times Wsam \times Vstd}$$

Aa = Peak area of corresponding amino acid in sample solution
As = Peak area of corresponding amino acid in standard solution
$Wstd$ = Weight of standard (mg)
$Wsam$ = Weight of sample (mg)
$Vsam$ = Total volume of sample solution (ml)
$Vstd$ = Total volume of standard solution (ml)
UW = Unit weight (mg)

5.5 Identification and Quantification of Amino Acid Enantiomers by UPLC-UV/CD

CD is an abbreviation for Circular Dichroism. The absorption intensity of left and right-handed light is not equal for the optically active molecules in a solution. The resulting differential can be used to determine the D or L forms of molecules. Nearly all natural amino acids from protein are L-type, and synthetic amino acids are the D-type. In order to determine whether the form of amino acid contained in a dietary supplement is natural or synthetic, CD detection system is utilized.

See Figures 5.2–5.4. Figure 5.2 is a UV chromatogram of 6 amino acids. The peak area is proportional to the sum of D/L molecules. Figure 5.3 is a CD chromatogram of the L-type molecules. The peak area is proportional to the concentration of L-type molecule. Figure 5.4 is the CD chromatogram of the D-type molecule. The peak area is proportional to the concentration of D-type molecule, even though the peaks are inverted. But if 50% of the amino acids in the sample are in L form, and the other 50% is D form, then the CD signal is offset. It becomes a racemate, so the CD chromatogram is a straight line, without any peaks. However, the UV chromatogram does not change, and the peak area is dependent on the total of D and L molecules.

If 95% of the amino acids in the sample are the L-type, and 5% are the D-type, the UV signal is not affected, but the peak area of the CD

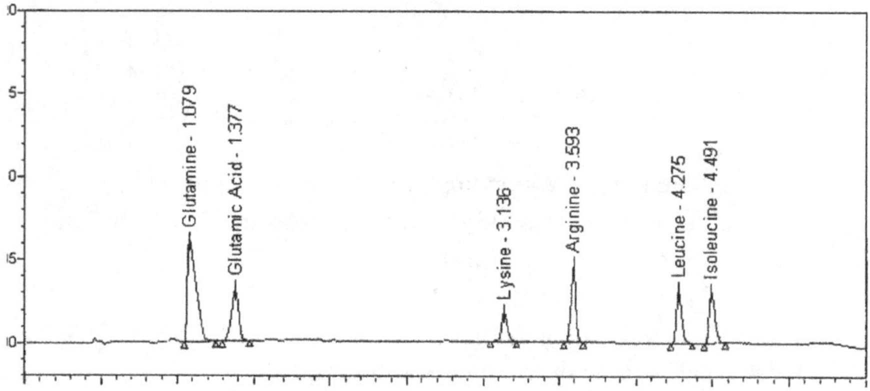

Figure 5.2: UV chromatogram of 6 amino acids, in 50 mg/50 ml water solution.

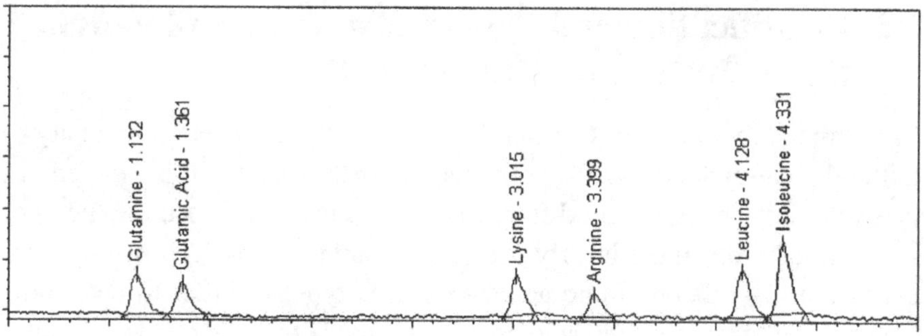

Figure 5.3: CD Chromatogram of 6 L form of amino acids.

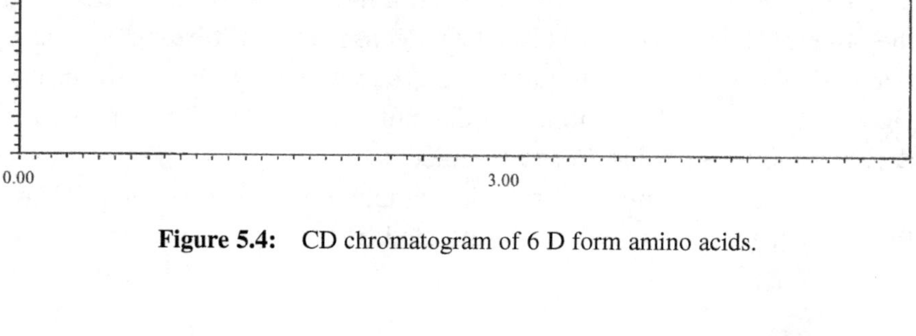

Figure 5.4: CD chromatogram of 6 D form amino acids.

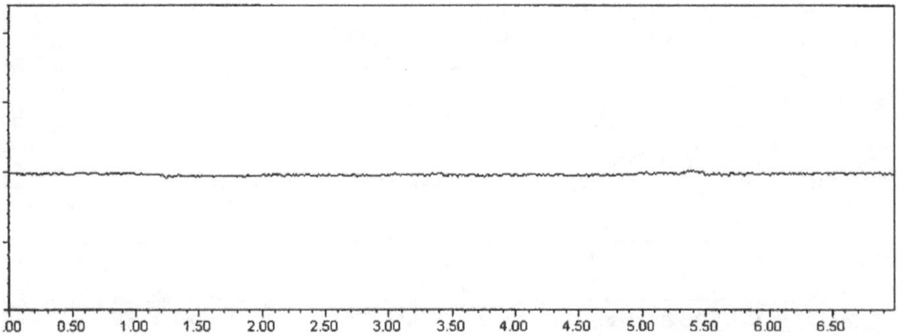

Figure 5.5: CD chromatogram of 6 amino acids, 50% L, 50% D.

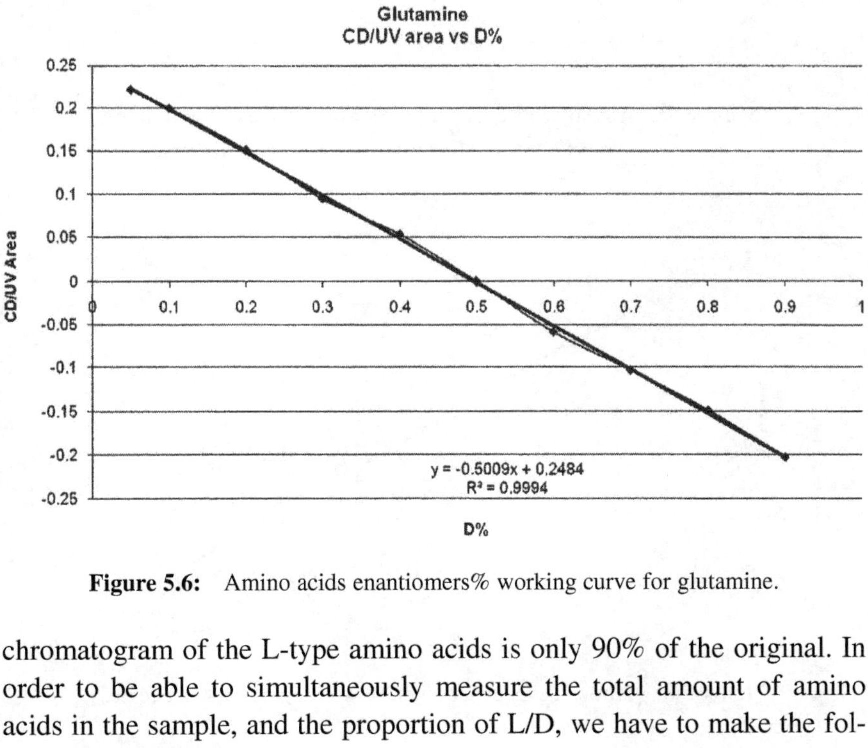

Figure 5.6: Amino acids enantiomers% working curve for glutamine.

chromatogram of the L-type amino acids is only 90% of the original. In order to be able to simultaneously measure the total amount of amino acids in the sample, and the proportion of L/D, we have to make the following working curve.

As in Figure 5.6 the CD peak area/UV peak area is the vertical coordinate, with D% as the horizontal coordinate. A working curve can be made by the difference in D%. With the working curve (temporarily referred to amino acid enantiomers% working curve), you can measure

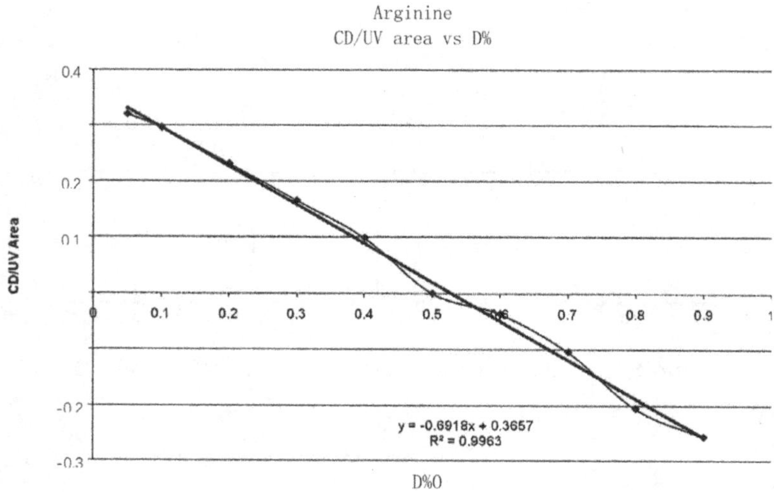

Figure 5.7: Amino acids enantiomers% working curve for arginine.

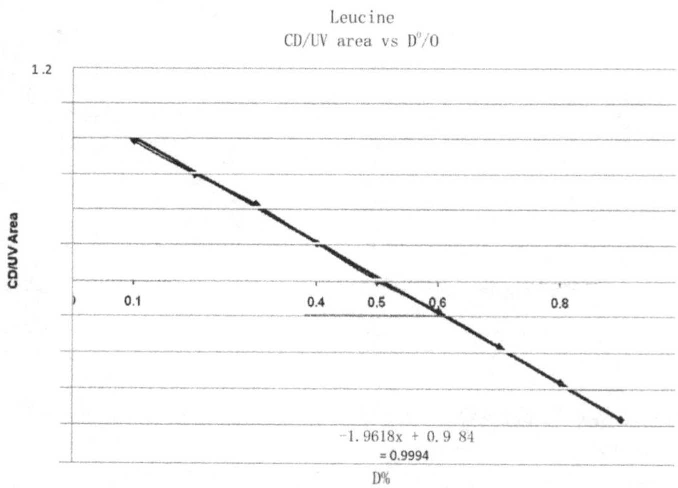

Figure 5.8: Amino acids enantiomers% working curve for leucine.

the percentage of L-type amino acid in the sample, based on the CD area/UV area ratio.

Figures 5.6–5.11 are 6 amino acids, glutamine, glutamate, lysine, arginine, leucine, and isoleucine, "Amino acids enantiomers % working curve". These are essentially linear.

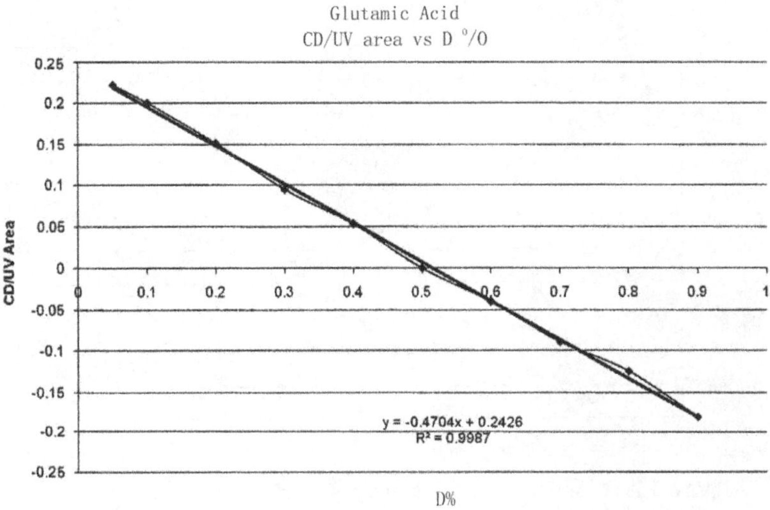

Figure 5.9: Amino acids enantiomers% working curve for glutamic acid.

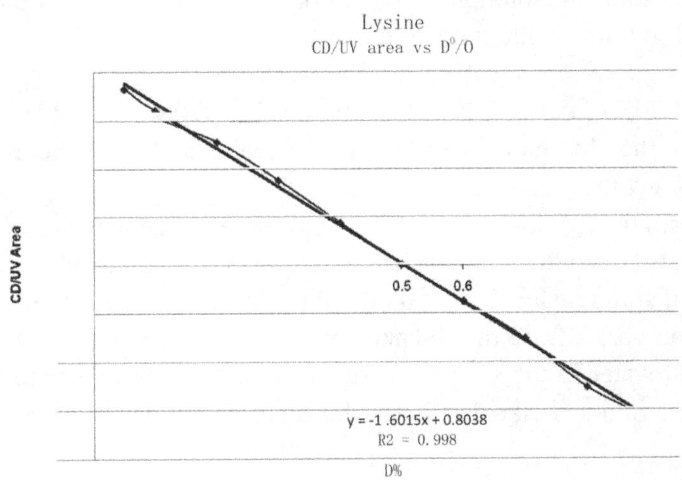

Figure 5.10: Amino acids enantiomers% working curve for lysine.

(i) *Test procedure*

Preparation of standard solution — Accurately weigh 50 mg of pure L-type amino acids (anyone to be tested), and transfer it to a 50 ml volumetric flask. Add water to dissolve, dilute to 50 ml, and shake well. The

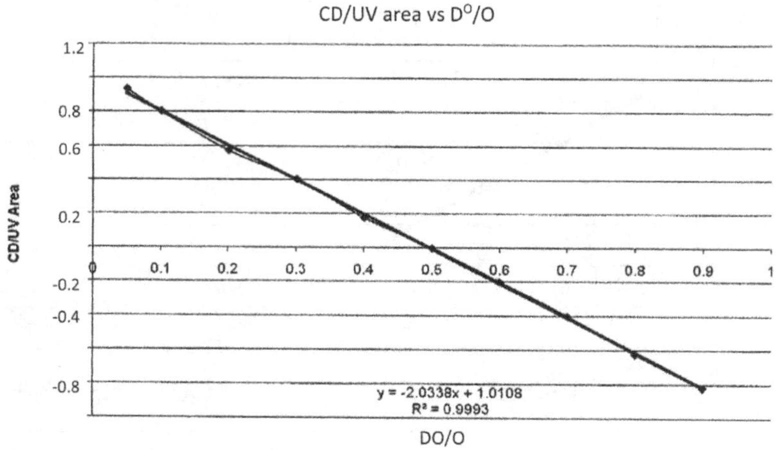

Figure 5.11: Amino acids enantiomers% working curve for Isoleucine.

first point standard solution is ready. Follow the same procedure to make standard solutions with: total amino acid 50 mg, L95%, D5%; total amino acid 50 mg, L90%, D10%; then L80%, D20%; L70%, D30%; L60%, D40%; L50%, D50%; L40%, D60%; L30%, D70% and L20%, D80%. Based on the aforementioned nine points make an "Amino acids enantiomers % working curve".

Preparation of sample solution — Accurately weigh a certain amount of ground sample that contains about 50 mg of any of the amino acids to be tested, and transfer it to a 50 ml volumetric flask. Add about 30 ml of water, and vortex for 2 min. Shake with a wrist action shaker for 15 min. Then add water to the volume mark and shake well. Centrifuge (10,000 rpm) for 5 min and take the clear solution for injection.

(ii) *UPLC-CD conditions*

Column: Acquity Hss T3 C18, 1.8 um, 2.1 × 150 mm
Mobile phase A: 10 mM hexane sulfonic acid sodium salt, pH 2.0
Mobile phase B: Acetonitrile
Flow rate: 0.40 ml/min
Column temperature: 45°C

UV wavelength: 210
CD wavelength: 220
CD temperature: 35°C
Injection volume: 2 ul

Gradient:

Time (min)	A%	B%
0	97	3
0–8.0	75	30
8.0–9.0	75	30
9.0–9.3	97	3
12.0	97	3 End

(iii) *Results and calculation*

Calculate peak area ratio of CD/UV of sample solution, from the "Amino acids enantiomers% working curve" fine D%, 100-D% = L%.

Calculate total D and L form amino acid

$$Total\ D/L\ amino\ acid\ (mg/unit) = \frac{Aa \times Wstd \times Vsam \times UW}{As \times Wsam \times Vstd}$$

or

$$Total\ D/L\ amino\ acid\ (\%) = \frac{Aa \times Wstd \times Vsam \times 100\%}{As \times Wsam \times Vstd}$$

Aa = UV peak area of corresponding amino acid in sample solution
As = UV peak area of corresponding amino acid in standard solution
Wstd = Weight of standard (mg)
Wsam = Weight of sample (mg)
Vsam = Total volume of sample solution (ml)
Vstd = Total volume of standard solution (ml)
UW = Unit weight (mg)

Total amino acid (%) × *D%* = *content of D-type amino acid*
Total amino acid (%) × *(100%-D%)* = *content of L-type amino acids*

5.6 Test Method for 10-Hydroxydecanoic Acid and 10-Hydroxydecenoic Acid in Royal Jelly

10-Hydroxydecanoic acid and 10-Hydroxydecenoic acid are considered as active and marker compounds in royal jelly.

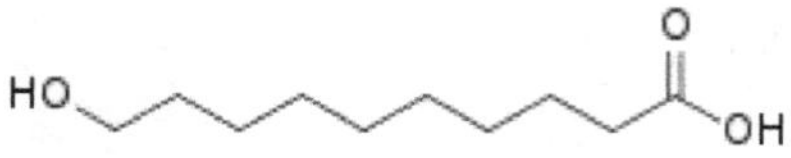

10-hydroxydecanoic acid

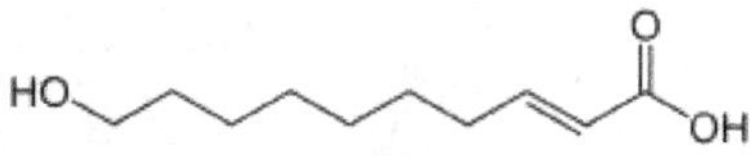

10-hydroxydecenoic acid

As the above molecular structures show, both compounds are non-polar, contain one hydroxyl group and 10 carbon fatty acids. The only difference is 10-hydroxydecenoic acid contains a conjugated double bond. This may create an additional π–π interaction with a phenyl column, and make it easier to be separated (see Chapter 1, Section 1.1.1 "Types of stationary phases").

(i) *Test procedure*

Preparation of standard solution — Accurately weigh about 10 mg of 10-Hydroxydecanoic acid and 10 mg of 10-Hydroxydecenoic acid standards, and transfer to a 100 ml volumetric flask. Add 60 ml of ethanol, and vortex until all standards dissolve. Then add ethanol to the mark, and shake well. It is ready for injection.

Preparation of sample solution — Accurately weigh a certain amount of evenly mixed sample that contains 10 mg of 10-Hydroxydecanoic acid and/or 10-Hydroxydecenoic acid, and transfer it to a 100 ml volumetric flask.

If the sample is a solid powder, add about 10 ml of water, and sonicate for 5 min. Then add about 60 ml of isopropyl alcohol, and shake for 5 min. Sonicate for 10 min. After the solution is cooled, add ethanol to 100 ml mark, and shake well. Centrifuge (10,000 rpm) for 5 min, and take the clear solution for injection.

If the sample is liquid, just add 60 ml of ethanol, and sonicate for 10 min. After cooling, fill to volume with ethanol, and shake well. Centrifuge for 5 min, and take the clear solution to inject.

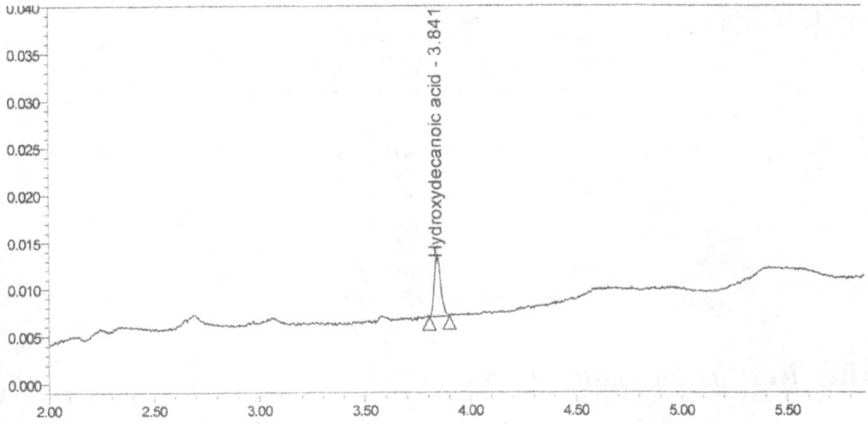

Figure 5.12: UPLC chromatogram of 10-hydroxydecanoic acid.

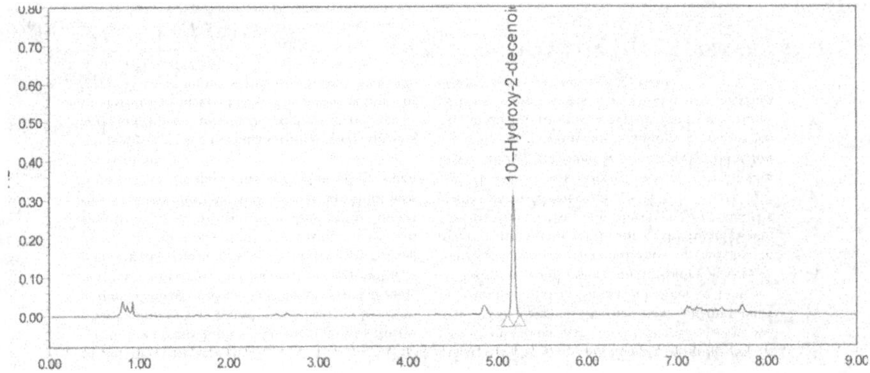

Figure 5.13: UPLC chromatogram of 10-hydroxydecenoic acid.

(ii) *UPLC conditions*

Column: Acquity UPLC® BEH Phenyl 1.7 μm, 2.1 × 150 mm
Flow rate: 0.4 ml/min
Injection volume: 2 μL
UV wavelength: 210 nm
Mobile phase A: 0.1% phosphoric acid in water
Mobile phase B: Acetonitrile
Column temperature: 45°C

Gradient:

Time (min)	A%	B%
0	80	20
7.0	30	70
8.0	30	70
8.5	80	20
12.0	80	20

(iii) ***Results and calculation***

$$Hydroxydecanoic/Hydroxydecenoic\,acid\ (mg/unit) = \frac{Aa \times Wstd \times Vsam \times UW}{As \times Wsam \times Vstd}$$

or

$$Hydroxydecanoic/Hydroxydecenoic\,acid\ (\%) = \frac{Aa \times Wstd \times Vsam \times 100\%}{As \times Wsam \times Vstd}$$

Aa = Peak area of hydroxydecanoic/hydroxydecenoic acid in sample solution
As = Peak area of hydroxydecanoic/hydroxydecenoic acid in standard solution
Wstd = Weight of standard (mg)
Wsam = Weight of sample (mg)
Vsam = Total volume of sample solution (ml)
Vstd = Total volume of standard solution (ml)
UW = Unit weight (mg)

5.7 Test Method of α-Ketoglutaric Acid

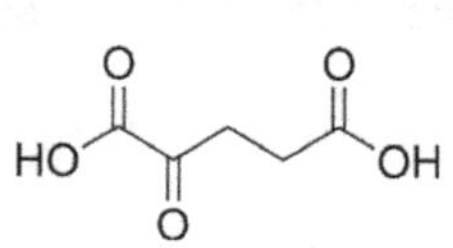

α-Ketoglutaric Acid

α-ketoglutaric acid (AKG) is a precursor to glutamic acid, and in combination with L-glutamate it can reduce body ammonia levels, and prevent nitrogen excesses in body tissues and fluids. In addition, AKG is often used in sport supplements, to help athletes reach their peak performance.

AKG is a polar compound containing two carboxy acid groups. In order to extend the retention time with a reversed phase column, the pH of the mobile phase can be reduced, or an ion pairing reagent (such as tetrabutylammonium hydrochloride) can be added to the mobile phase. This will form ion pairs with AKG, reducing the polarity and increasing retention time.

(i) *Test procedure*

Preparation of standard solution — Accurately weigh about 30 mg of AKG standard, and transfer it to a 100 ml volumetric flask. Add 60 ml of water, and vortex until the standard is completely dissolved. Fill to the volume mark with water, shake well, and the standard is ready to inject.

Preparation of sample solution — Accurately weigh a certain amount of ground sample that contains about 30 mg of AKG, and transfer it to a 100 ml volumetric flask. Add 60 ml of water, and shake for 5 min. Then sonicate for 10 min. After the solution is cooled, fill to volume with water, and shake well. Centrifuge (10,000 rpm) for 5 min, and take the clear solution for injection.

(ii) *UPLC conditions*

Column: Acquity Hss T3 C18, 1.8 um, 2.1 × 150 mm
Flow rate: 0.4 ml/min
Injection volume: 2 μL
UV wavelength: 210 nm
Mobile phase A: 0.5% phosphoric acid in water
Mobile phase B: Acetonitrile
A:B = 97:3
Run time: 10 min

In case the aforementioned method fails to separate interferences, try the following method.

Column: Acquity Hss T3 (C18), 1.7 um, 2.1 × 150 mm
Flow rate: 0.4 ml/min

Injection volume: 2 ul
UV wavelength: 210 nm
Column temperature: 45°C
mobile phase A: 5 mM tetrabutylammonium hydrochloride, pH 5.5
Mobile phase B: Acetonitrile

Gradient:

Time (min)	A%	B%
0	95	5
7	60	40
8	60	40
8.5	95	5
12.0	95	5 End

(iii) *Results and calculation*

$$AKR\ (mg/unit) = \frac{Aa \times Wstd \times Vsam \times UW}{As \times Wsam \times Vstd}$$

or

$$AKG\ (\%) = \frac{Aa \times Wstd \times Vsam \times 100\%}{As \times Wsam \times Vstd}$$

Aa = Peak area of AKG in sample solution
As = Peak area of AKG in standard solution
Wstd = Weight of standard (mg)
Wsam = Weight of sample (mg)
Vsam = Total volume of sample solution (ml)
Vstd = Total volume of standard solution (ml)
UW = Unit weight (mg)

5.8 Aminobutyric Acid (GABA) Test Method

Since the 1990s, GABA has been used in dietary supplements to improve the quality of sleep.

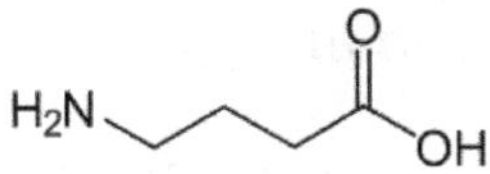

Aminobutyric Acid

GABA is a polar compound that does not work with reverse phase columns, because the retention time is too short. The isoelectric point of GABA is pH 7.3. This means that while the pH < 7.3 the molecule is positively charged; when the pH > 7.3 the molecule is negatively charged. In order to effectively separate GABA and other interfering compounds, this method adds hexane sulfonic acid sodium salt to the mobile phase to form an ion pair with GABA. This extends the retention time. The mobile phase pH is adjusted to around 2.0 to ensure that the GABA is in a positive ion state (see Chapter 1, Section 1.1.2 "Mobile phase application").

(i) *Test procedure*

Preparation of standard solution — Accurately weigh about 100 mg of GABA standard, and transfer it to a 100 ml volumetric flask. Add 60 ml of water, and shake until all of the standard is dissolved. Then add water to 100 ml volume, and shake well. The standard solution can be injected.

Preparation of sample solution — Accurately weigh a certain amount of ground sample which contains about 100 mg GABA, and transfer it to a 100 ml volumetric flask. Add 60 ml of water, and shake with wrist action shaker for 15 min. Then sonicate for 5 min. After cooling, fill with water to the mark, and shake well. Centrifuge (10,000 rpm) for 5 min, and take the clear solution for injection.

(ii) *UPLC conditions*

Column: Acquity UPLC® BEH C18 1.7 μm, 2.1 × 150 mm
Flow rate: 0.4 ml/min
Injection volume: 2 μL
UV wavelength: 210 nm
Mobile phase A: 10 mM hexane sulfonic acid sodium salt, pH 2.0
Mobile phase B: Acetonitrile
Mobile phase A/mobile phase B = 90/10
Run time: 6 min

(iii) *Results and calculation*

$$GABA\ (mg/unit) = \frac{Aa \times Wstd \times Vsam \times UW}{As \times Wsam \times Vstd}$$

or

$$GABA\ (\%) = \frac{Aa \times Wstd \times Vsam \times 100\%}{As \times Wsam \times Vstd}$$

Aa = Peak area of GABA in sample solution
As = Peak area of GABA in standard solution
Wstd = Weight of standard (mg)
Wsam = Weight of sample (mg)
Vsam = Total volume of sample solution (ml)
Vstd = Total volume of standard solution (ml)
UW = Unit weight (mg)

5.9 Test Method for Nicotinamide Adenine Dinucleotide (NADH)

According to recent research, NADH may have anti-aging effects.

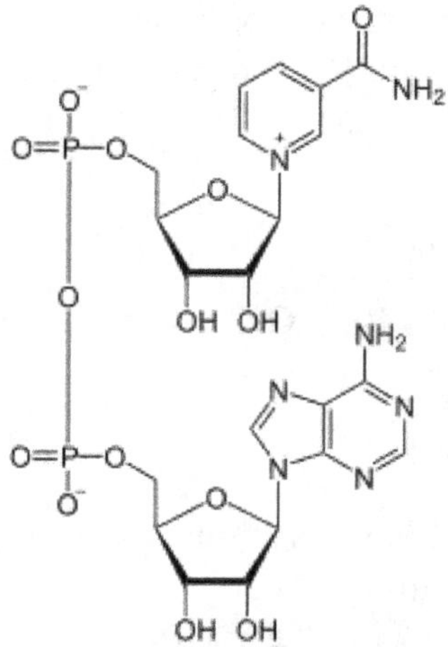

NADH

NADH is a polar compound, if you are using a reverse phase column to separate and quantify it, the proportion of organic solvent in mobile phase should be low.

(i) *Test procedure*

Preparation of standard solution — Accurately weigh about 10 mg of NADH standard, and transfer it to a 100 ml volumetric flask. Add 60 ml of water, and shake until the standard is completely dissolved. Then add water to the volume mark, shake well, and the standard solution is ready for injection.

Preparation of sample solution — Accurately weigh certain amount of ground sample which contains about 10 mg of NADH, and transfer it to a 100 ml volumetric flask. Add 60 ml of water, and shake with wrist action shaker for 15 min. Then sonicate for 5 min. After the solution is cooled add water to the mark, and shake well. Centrifuge for 5 min, and then take the solution for injection.

(ii) *UPLC conditions*

Column: Acquity UPLC® HSS T3 1.8 μm, 2.1 × 150 mm
Flow rate: 0.4 ml/min
Injection volume: 1 μL
UV wavelength: 258 nm
Mobile phase A: 1 mM potassium hydro phosphate in water, pH 5
Mobile phase B: Acetonitrile
Column temperature: 45°C

Gradient:

Time (min)	A%	B%
0	97	3
1	97	3
5	75	25
6.0	75	25
6.5	97	3
8.5	97	3

(iii) *Results and calculation*

$$NADH\ (mg/unit) = \frac{Aa \times Wstd \times Vsam \times UW}{As \times Wsam \times Vstd}$$

or

$$NADH\ (\%) = \frac{Aa \times Wstd \times Vsam \times 100\%}{As \times Wsam \times Vstd}$$

Aa = Peak area of NADH in sample solution
As = Peak area of NADH in standard solution
Wstd = Weight of standard (mg)
Wsam = Weight of sample (mg)
Vsam = Total volume of sample solution (ml)
Vstd = Total volume of standard solution (ml)
UW = Unit weight (mg)

5.10 Test Method for Phytic Acid (IP6)

Phytic acid has a wide range of uses. The food industry uses phytic acid in oil products to help block the oxidation chain, and extend the oil shelf life. Phytic acid in dietary supplements is used as post-operative health care for cancer patients.

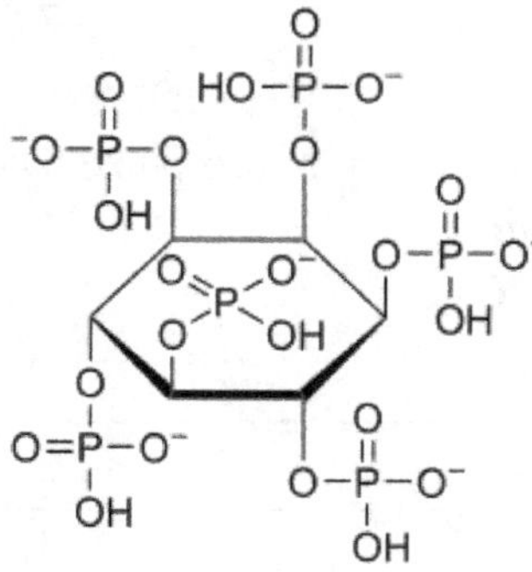

Phytic acid

Phytic acid is a polyatomic acid. In chromatography it is difficult to obtain a symmetrical peak. Peak shape tends to have severe tailing, and cannot even be completely eluded. This makes it difficult to quantify. At the same time, the phytic acid molecule has poor UV absorption, so a UV detector cannot be used to measure phytic acid.

Introduced here is a "Counter ion exchange" chromatography tandem MS/MS method. Phytic acid is anion at normal pH range, so if it is injected on a cation exchange column (the active sites are negative charged), the phytic acid molecule will be repelled by the active sites of the column, and eluted even faster than neutral solvents. Therefore, you get a negative retention time. However, a nice symmetric peak is obtained, with no tailing, and no broadening (see Figure 5.14).

Using "Counter ion exchange" chromatography, phytic acid can be separated from cations and neutral compounds, but the separation from other anions is questionable. Though the repel forces intensity in the column could be different for different anions, we cannot expect them to completely separate all of the anions during a negative retention period. Fortunately, the MS/MS can distinguish and quantify phytic acid, even with co-eluted anions.

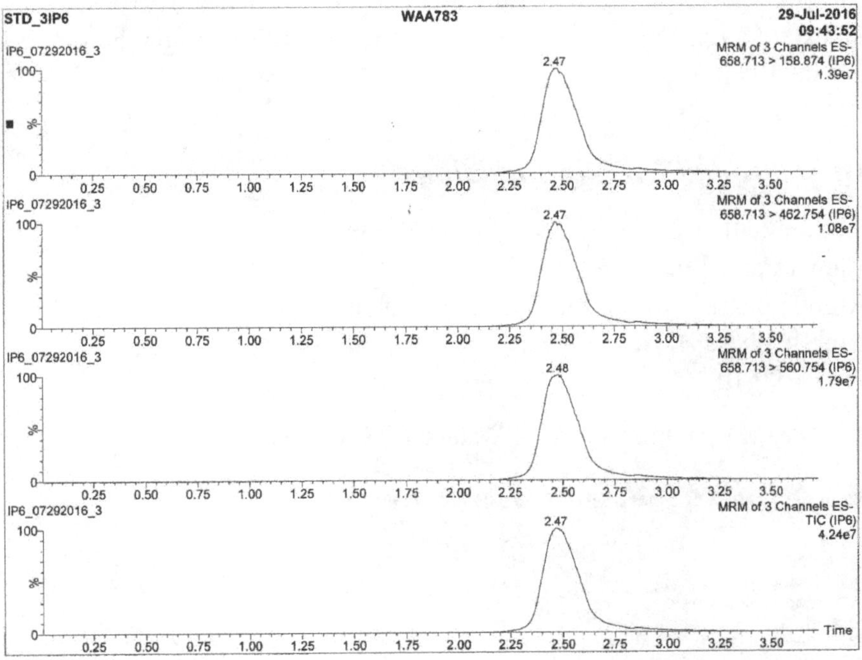

Figure 5.14: Chromatogram of phytic acid, three ion pairs and TIC from MS/MS detector.

(i) *Test procedure*

Preparation of standard solution — Accurately weigh about 25 mg of phytic acid standard, and transfer it to a 100 ml volumetric flask. Add about 60 ml of water, then add 1 ml of 1:5 hydrochloric acid. Sonicate for 2–5 min until all standards dissolve. Then add water to the mark, and shake well. Label the solution as "Phytic acid stock solution". Make further dilutions with water to obtain three different concentrations of standard solutions: 1 ppm, 5 ppm and 25 ppm.

Preparation of sample solution — Accurately weigh certain amount of sample equivalent to 25 mg of phytic acid, and transfer it to a 100 ml volumetric flask. Add 60 ml of water and 1 ml of 1:5 hydrochloric acid, then sonicate for 10 min. After cooling, add water to volume, and shake well. Centrifuge for 5 min, and take the clear solution to dilute to about 5 ppm for injection.

Preparation of spike sample solution — Pipette 980 μl of the aforementioned sample solution into 2 ml injection vail, and add 20 μl standard stock solution. Vortex and mix the solution well. It can now be directly injected.

(ii) *Chromatography conditions*

Column: Dionex IonPac CS14, 4 × 250 mm
Flow rate: 0.6 mL/min
Mobile phase A: 0.1% formic acid in water
Mobile phase B: Acetonitrile
A:B = 90:10

MS/MS parameters (from Waters TQS MS/MS)

Function 1 : MRM of 3 mass pairs, Time 0.00 to 3.00, ES- (IP6)

Type	MRM
Ion Mode	ES-
Inter Channel Delay (sec)	-1.000
InterScan Time (sec)	-1.000
Span (Da)	0.0
Start Time (min)	0.0
End Time (min)	3.0

Ch	Prnt(Da)	Dau(Da)	Dwell(s)	Cone(V)	Coll(eV)	Delay(s)	Compound	Formula	Comments
1	658.71	158.87	0.100	74.00	58.00	-1.000	IP6	660	IntelliStart Generated
2	658.71	462.75	0.100	74.00	32.00	-1.000	IP6	660	IntelliStart Generated
3	658.71	560.75	0.100	74.00	24.00	-1.000	IP6	660	IntelliStart Generated

(iii) *Results and calculation*

Inject three different concentration standard solutions to create a standard working curve. Inject sample and spiked sample solution, calculate the spike recovery, if the recovery rate is within control range (see Chapter 1, Section 1.1.5 "*Qualitative and quantitative testing of LC-MS/MS*"), then calculate the result as follows.

$$Phytic\,acid\ (mg/unit) = \frac{Aa \times Wstd \times Vsam \times UW}{As \times Wsam \times Vstd \times R}$$

or

$$Phytic\,acid\ (\%) = \frac{Aa \times Wstd \times Vsam \times 100\%}{As \times Wsam \times Vstd \times R}$$

Aa = Peak area of sample solution
As = Peak area of standard solution
$Wstd$ = Weight of standard (mg)
$Wsam$ = Weight of sample (mg)
$Vsam$ = Total volume of sample solution (ml)
$Vstd$ = Total volume of standard solution (ml)
UW = Unit weight (mg)
R = Spike recovery (see Chapter 1, Section 1.1.5 "*Qualitative and quantitative testing of LC-MS/MS*").

If spike recovery is not within the control range, then follow see Chapter 1, Section 1.1.5 "*Qualitative and quantitative testing of LC-MS/MS*" steps.

5.11 Diosmin Test Method

Diosmin is a prescription drug in some European countries but is classified as a dietary supplement in the United States and some other countries. The main function of diosmin is to prevent hypertension and arterial hardening.

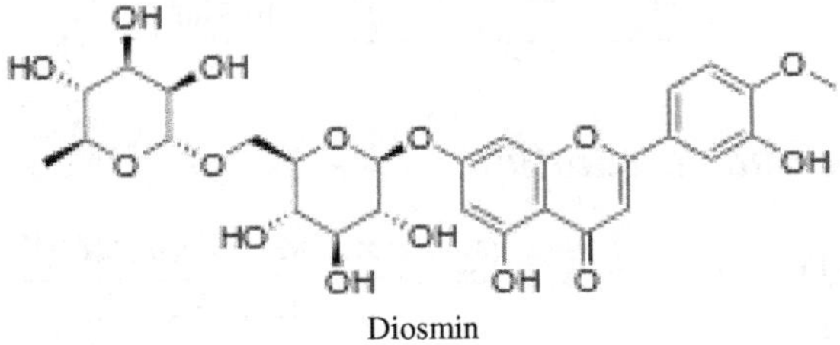

Diosmin

(i) *Test procedure*

Preparation of standard solution — Accurately weigh about 10 mg of diosmin standard, and transfer it to a 100 ml volumetric flask. Add 20 ml of DMSO/methanol (50/50), and sonicate until the standard completely dissolves. Then add methanol to the volume mark, shake well, and the standard is ready to inject.

Preparation of sample solution — Accurately weigh a certain amount of ground sample which contains about 10 mg of the diosmin, and transfer it to a 100 ml volumetric flask. Add 30 ml of DMSO / methanol (50%/50%), and sonicate for 20 min. After the solution has cooled add methanol to the mark, and shake well. Centrifuge (10,000 rpm) for 5 min, and take the clear solution for injection.

(ii) *UPLC conditions*

Column: Acquity UPLC® BEH C18 1.7 μm, 2.1 × 150 mm
Flow rate: 0.4 ml/min
Injection volume: 1 μL
UV wavelength: 345 nm
Mobile phase A: 0.1% phosphoric acid in water
Mobile phase B: Acetonitrile
Column temperature: 45°C

Gradient:

Time (min)	A%	B%
0	90	10
3.0	80	20
4.0	50	50
4.8	50	50
5.0	90	10
7.0	90	10 End

(iii) *Results and calculation*

$$Diosmin\ (mg/unit) = \frac{Aa \times Wstd \times Vsam \times UW}{As \times Wsam \times Vstd}$$

or

$$Diosmin\ (\%) = \frac{Aa \times Wstd \times Vsam \times 100\%}{As \times Wsam \times Vstd}$$

Aa = Peak area of diosmin in sample solution
As = Peak area of diosmin in standard solution
Wstd = Weight of standard (mg)
Wsam = Weight of sample (mg)
Vsam = Total volume of sample solution (ml)
Vstd = Total volume of standard solution (ml)
UW = Unit weight (mg)

5.12 Dehydroepiandrosterone (DHEA) Test Method

The main function of DHEA is to improve memory and slow aging. DHEA is a non-polar compound, and can be tested using reverses phase chromatography.

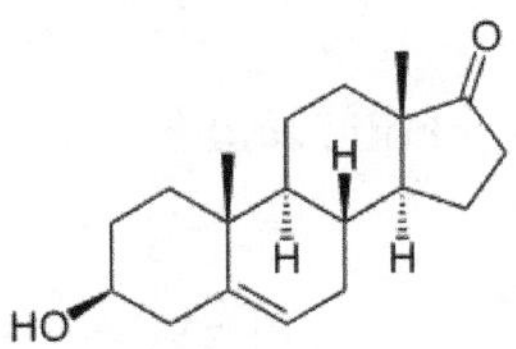

DHEA

(i) *Test procedure*

Preparation of standard solution — Accurately weigh approximately 25 mg of DHEA standard and transfer it to a 100 ml volumetric flask. Add 60 ml of methanol, and sonicate until the standard completely dissolves. Then add methanol to the mark, shake well, and the standards is ready to be injected.

Preparation of sample solution — Accurately weigh certain amount of ground sample that contains about 25 mg of DHEA, and transfer it to a 100 ml volumetric flask. Add 10 ml of water, and sonicate for 10 min. Then add 60 ml of ethanol and sonicate for 15 min. After cooling, fill with methanol up to the volume mark, and shake well. Centrifuge (10,000 rpm) for 5 min, and the clear solution can be injected.

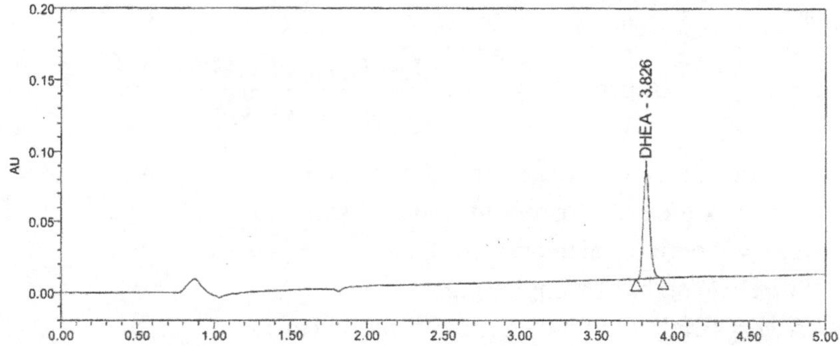

Figure 5.15: UPLC chromatogram of DHEA.

(ii) *UPLC conditions*

Column: Acquity UPLC® HSS Ts C18 1.8 μm, 2.1 × 150 mm
Flow rate: 0.4 ml/min
Injection volume: 1 μL
UV wavelength: 210 nm
Mobile phase A: 0.1% phosphoric acid in water.
Mobile phase B: Acetonitrile
Column temperature: 45°C

Gradient:

Time (min)	A%	B%
0	65	35
5.0	20	80
5.8	20	80
6.0	65	35
8.0	65	35 End

(iii) *Results and calculation*

$$DHEA\ (mg/unit) = \frac{Aa \times Wstd \times Vsam \times UW}{As \times Wsam \times Vstd}$$

or

$$DHEA\ (\%) = \frac{Aa \times Wstd \times Vsam \times 100\%}{As \times Wsam \times Vstd}$$

Aa = Peak area of DHEA in sample solution
As = Peak area of DHEA in standard solution
Wstd = Weight of standard (mg)
Wsam = Weight of sample (mg)
Vsam = Total volume of sample solution (ml)
Vstd = Total volume of standard solution (ml)
UW = Unit weight (mg)

5.13 3,3-Diindolymethane Test Method

3,3-Diindolymethane is thought to have anti-cancer properties. It is mainly found in vegetables, especially broccoli.

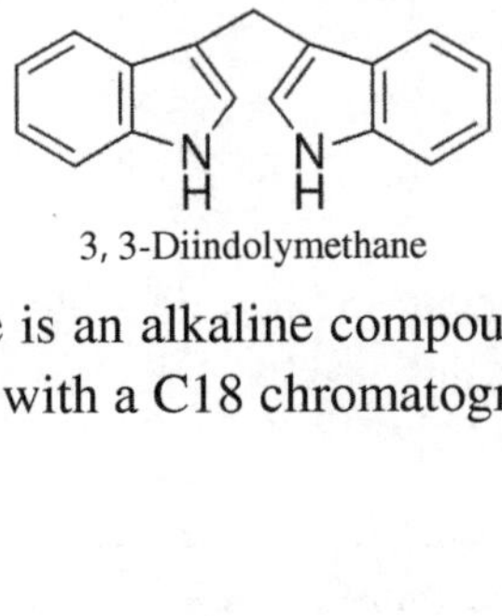

3, 3-Diindolymethane

3,3-Diindolymethane is an alkaline compound, and is relatively non-polar. It can be analyzed with a C18 chromatography column.

(i) *Test procedure*

Preparation of standard solution — Accurately weigh approximately 10 mg of 3,3-Diindolymethane standard, and transfer it to a 100 ml volumetric flask. Add 60 ml of methanol, and vortex until the standard completely dissolves. Then add methanol to the volume mark, and shake well. The standard solution is ready for injection.

Preparation of sample solution — Accurately weigh a certain amount of ground sample contains about 10 mg of 3,3-Diindolymethane, and transfer it to a 100 ml volumetric flask. Add 20 ml of DMSO, and sonicate for 5 min. Add 50 ml of ethanol, sonicate for another 10 min. After the solution is cooled, add methanol to the volume mark, and shake well. Centrifuge for 5 min, and take the clear solution for injection.

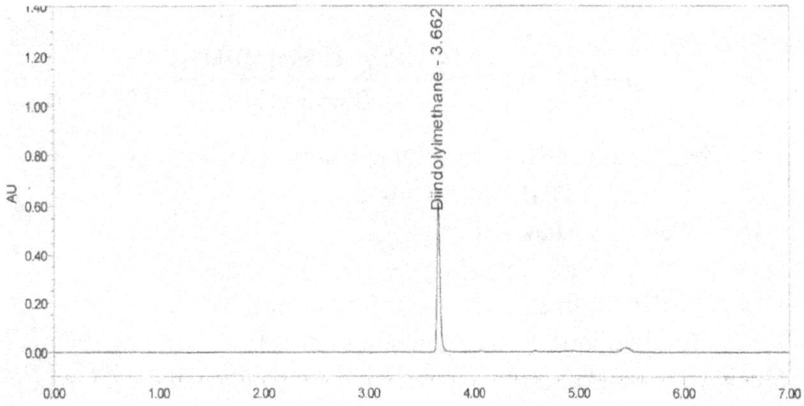

Figure 5.16: UPLC chromatogram of 3,3-Diindolymethane.

(ii) *UPLC conditions*

Column: Acquity UPLC® HSS T3 C18, 1.8 μm, 2.1 × 100 mm
Column temperature: 45°C
Flow rate: 0.4 ml/min
Injection volume: 1 μL
UV wavelength: 282 nm
Mobile phase A: 0.1% phosphoric acid in water
Mobile phase B: Acetonitrile

Gradient:

Time (min)	A%	B%
0	70	30
4	20	80
4.8	20	80
5.0	70	30
7.0	70	30 End

(iii) *Results and calculation*

$$Diindolymethane\ (mg/unit) = \frac{Aa \times Wstd \times Vsam \times UW}{As \times Wsam \times Vstd}$$

or

$$Diindolymethane\ (\%) = \frac{Aa \times Wstd \times Vsam \times 100\%}{As \times Wsam \times Vstd}$$

Aa = Peak area of diindolylmethane in sample solution
As = Peak area of diindolylmethane in standard solution
Wstd = Weight of standard (mg)
Wsam = Weight of sample (mg)
Vsam = Total volume of sample solution (ml)
Vstd = Total volume of standard solution (ml)
UW = Unit weight (mg)

5.14 Choline Test Method

Choline is a strong alkaline organic compound with no double bonds. Therefore, a reversed phase chromatography system with UV detection is unable to test choline.

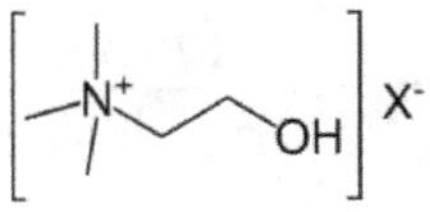

Choline

Choline in a water solution is a cation, so a cation exchange column can be used to separate it from other compounds. Since ions have conductivity, a conductivity detector can be used to measure the choline ion.

(i) *Test procedure*

Preparation of standard solution — Accurately weigh about 10 mg of choline standard, and transfer it to a 100 ml volumetric flask. Add water to dissolve the standard, then fill the flask with water to the mark, and shake well. Pipette 2 ml of the solution to a 10 ml volumetric flask, add water to 10 ml mark, and shake well. The standard solution can be injected.

Preparation of sample solution — Accurately weigh a certain amount of ground sample which contains about 10 mg choline, and transfer it to a 100 ml volumetric flask. Add 60 ml of water, and shake for 15 min. Then sonicate for 5 min. After cooling add water to the volume mark, and shake well. Centrifuge for 10 min, and transfer 2 ml of the upper-level clear solution to a 10 ml volumetric flask. Add water to volume mark, shake well, and the solution is ready for injection.

(ii) *Ion chromatography conditions*

Column: Thermo/Dionex IonPac®CS 14, 4 × 250 mm
Suppressor: Dionex CSRS 4 mm
Suppressor current: 100 mA
Elute: 40 mM methylsulfonic aid
Flow rate: 1 ml/min
Injection volume: 25 μl
Run time: 10 min

(iii) *Results and calculation*

$$Choline\ (mg/unit) = \frac{Aa \times Wstd \times Vsam \times UW}{As \times Wsam \times Vstd}$$

or

$$Choline\ (\%) = \frac{Aa \times Wstd \times Vsam \times 100\%}{As \times Wsam \times Vstd}$$

Aa = Peak area of choline in sample solution
As = Peak area of choline in standard solution
Wstd = Weight of standard (mg)
Wsam = Weight of sample (mg)
Vsam = Total volume of sample solution (ml)
Vstd = Total volume of standard solution (ml)
UW = Unit weight (mg)

5.15 Vinpocetine Test Method

Vinpocetine functions as a cerebral vascular dilator, which can improve brain circulation and help patients with memory impairment and dyskinesia. The US Food and Drug Administration (FDA) did not approve vinpocetine as a drug, so it only can be sold as a dietary supplement.

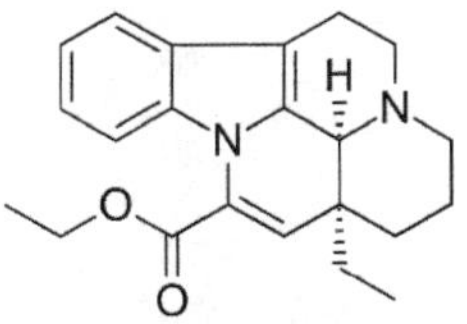

Vinpocetine

Vinpocetine is an alkaline compound with little polarity and contains low energy π electrons. A phenyl UPLC column can be used to attract vinpocetine by both dispersion and π–π interaction forces. See Chapter 1, Section 1.1.1 "Types of stationary phases".

(i) *Test procedure*

Preparation of standard solution — Accurately weigh about 10 mg of vinpocetine standard, and transfer it to a 100 ml volumetric flask. Add 60 ml methanol, and shake until all standard dissolve. Fill to volume with methanol, shake well, and the standard solution is ready for injection.

Preparation of sample solution — Accurately weigh a certain amount of ground sample that contains about 10 mg of vinpocetine, and transfer it to a 100 ml volumetric flask. Add 10 ml of water, and sonicate for 5 min. Add 60 ml methanol and sonicate for another 15 min. After cooling fill to the volume mark with methanol, and shake well. Centrifuge for 10 min, and take the upper clear solution for injection.

(ii) *UPLC conditions*

Column: Acquity UPLC® Phenyl, 1.7 μm, 2.1 × 150 mm
Flow rate: 0.4 mL/min
Injection volume: 1 μL
UV wavelength: 270 nm
Mobile phase A: 0.1% phosphoric acid in water
Mobile phase B: Acetonitrile
Column temperature: 45°C

Gradient:

Time (min)	A%	B%
0	80	20
5.0	50	50
5.8	50	50
6.0	80	20
8.0	80	20 End

(iii) *Results and calculation*

$$Vinpocetine\ (mg/unit) = \frac{Aa \times Wstd \times Vsam \times UW}{As \times Wsam \times Vstd}$$

or

$$Vinpocetine\ (\%) = \frac{Aa \times Wstd \times Vsam \times 100\%}{As \times Wsam \times Vstd}$$

Aa = Peak area of vinpocetine in sample solution
As = Peak area of vinpocetine in standard solution
Wstd = Weight of standard (mg)
Wsam = Weight of sample (mg)
Vsam = Total volume of sample solution (ml)
Vstd = Total volume of standard solution (ml)
UW = Unit weight (mg)

5.16 Test Method for Bile Acids

Bile acids are hydroxylated steroids, synthesized in the liver from cholesterol. Bile acids facilitate digestion of dietary fats and oils. There are two groups of bile acids: the first group is conjugated bile acids and include taurocholic acid, taurochenodeoxycholic acid, taurodeoxycholic acid, glycholic acid and glycochenodeoxycholic acid. The second group is unconjugated bile acids, which includes cholic acid and deoxycholic aid.

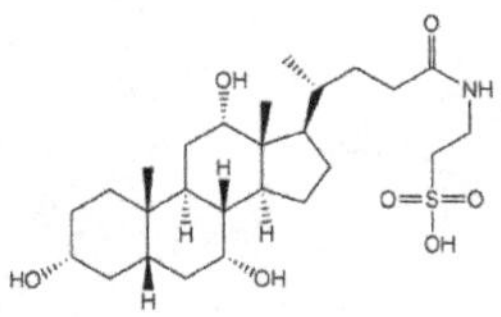

Taurocholic acid

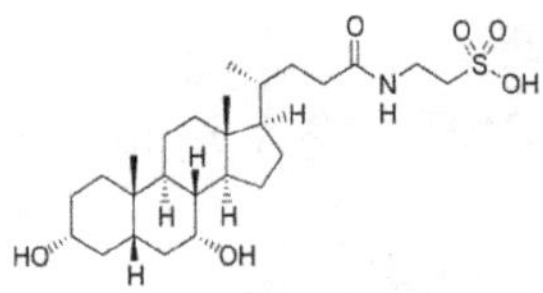

Taurochenodeoxycholic acid

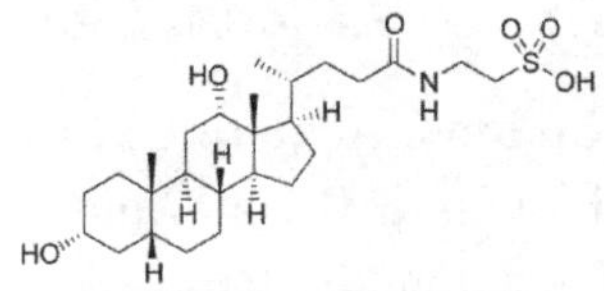

Taurodeoxycholic acid

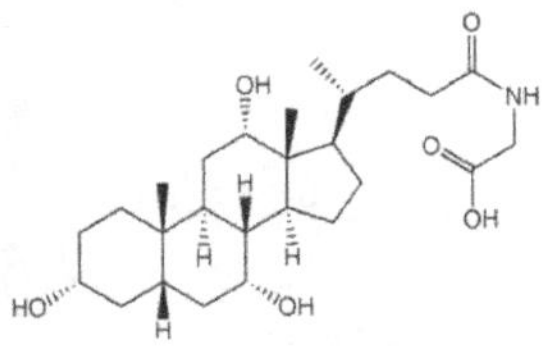

glycholic acid

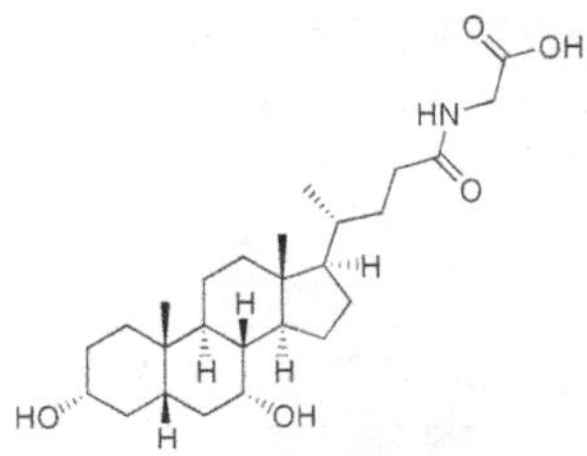

glycochenodeoxycholic acid

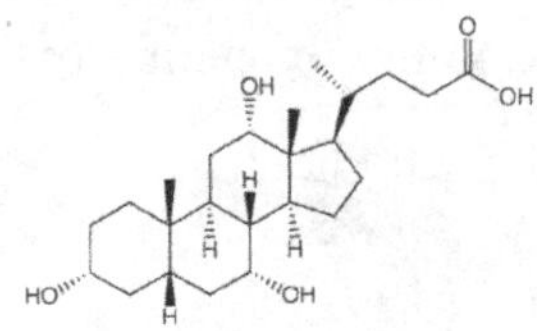

cholic acid

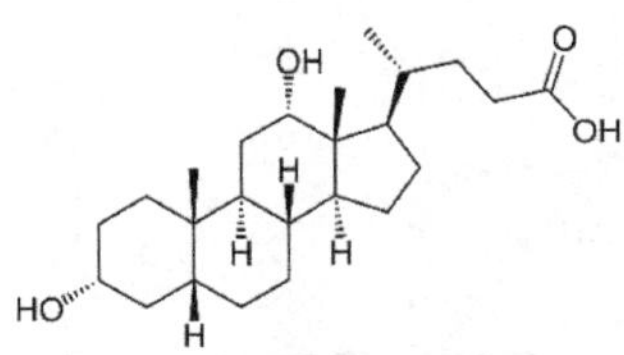

Deoxycholic acid

According to the molecular structures, bile acids are non-polar compounds which can be separated and quantified by a C18 UPLC column.

(i) *Test procedure*

Preparation of standard solution — Accurately weight about 10 mg of each bile acid standard, and transfer it to a 50 ml volumetric flask. Add about 30 ml of methanol, and sonicate until all standards dissolve. After cooling, fill to volume with methanol, shake well, and the standard solution is ready for injection.

Preparation of sample solution — Accurately weigh a certain amount of ground sample equivalent to 10 mg of bile acids, and transfer it to 50 ml volumetric flask. Add 10 ml of DMSO, and sonicate for 5 min. Then add 25 ml methanol, and sonicate for 10 min. After cooling, add methanol to the volume mark, and shake well. Centrifuge for 5 min, and take the upper clear solution for injection.

(ii) *UPLC conditions*

Column: Acquity UPLC®, BEH C18, 1.7 μm, 2.1 × 150 mm
Flow rate: 0.4 mL/min
Injection volume: 2 μL
UV wavelength: 210 nm
Mobile phase A: 0.1% phosphoric acid in water
Mobile phase B: Acetonitrile
Column temperature: 45°C

Gradient:

Time (min)	A%	B%
0	85	15
10.0	45	55
10.2	30	70
10.8	30	70
11.0	85	15
13.0	85	15 End

(iii) *Results and calculation*

$$Individual\,bile\,acid\;(mg/unit) = \frac{Aa \times Wstd \times Vsam \times UW}{As \times Wsam \times Vstd}$$

or

$$Individual\,bile\,acid\;(\%) = \frac{Aa \times Wstd \times Vsam \times 100\%}{As \times Wsam \times Vstd}$$

Aa = UV peak area of corresponding bile acid in sample solution
As = UV peak area of corresponding bile acid in standard solution
Wstd = Weight of standard (mg)
Wsam = Weight of sample (mg)
Vsam = Total volume of sample solution (ml)
Vstd = Total volume of standard solution (ml)
UW = Unit weight (mg)

Total bile acids = sum of each individual bile acid determined.

5.17 4-Methylimidazole Test Method

Caramel is used in food, beverages and dietary supplements. It may contain 4-methylimidazole, which is thought to be carcinogenic. Because the caramel content in food and beverages is relatively low, the possible 4-methylimidazole content would be at trace levels. To improve the detection limit, this method uses the UPLC-MS/MS.

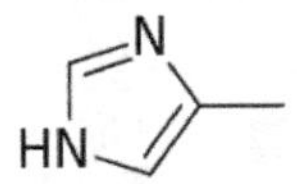

4-methylimidazole

(i) *Test procedure*

Preparation of standard solution — Accurately weigh about 10 mg of 4-methylimidazole standard, and transfer it to a 100 ml volumetric flask. Add about 60 ml of water, and sonicate until the standard completely dissolves. After cooling add 0.1% of formic acid water solution to the volume mark, and shake well. Label this solution as "4-methylmine stock standard solution". Further dilutions are made with water to get 5, 10, 20, 40 ppb standard solutions. Use the four solutions to make a working standard curve.

Preparation of sample solution — Accurately weigh a certain amount of ground sample, designed to meet the required detection limit, and transfer to a suitable flask. Accurately transfer 100 ml of water to the flask, and sonicate for 10 min. Shake well, and transfer 5 ml of the solution to a 10 ml centrifuge tube. Centrifuge for 10 min, and then pipette 1000 μl of upper-level clear solution to a 2 ml injection vail. Cover the vial, and label as "Sample solution". In addition, pipet 997 μl of the clear solution to another 2 ml injection vail and add 3 μl of 5 ppm standard stock solution. Shake this well, and label it as "spiked sample solution".

(ii) *UPLC conditions*

Column: Acquity UPLC®, HSS T3 C18, 1.7 μm, 2.1 × 150 mm
Flow rate: 0.4 mL/min
Injection volume: 2 μL

Mobile phase A: 20 mM ammonia acetate water solution, pH 4.0
Mobile phase B: Acetonitrile
Column temperature: 45°C

Gradient:

Time (min)	A%	B%
0	95	5
1	95	5
5	70	30
6.5	60	40
7.2	60	40
7.5	95	5
10.0	95	5 End

MS/MS parameter (from Waters TQS MS/MS)

Function 1 : MRM of 3 mass pairs, Time 0.00 to 3.00, ES+ (Methylimidazol)

```
Type                              MRM
Ion Mode                          ES+
Inter Channel Delay (sec)         -1.000
InterScan Time (sec)              -1.000
Span (Da)                         0.0
Start Time (min)                  0.0
End Time (min)                    3.0
  Ch Prnt(Da) Dau(Da) Dwell(s) Cone(V) Coll(eV) Delay(s) Compound          Formula


   1   82.97    28.15    0.050    56.00    14.00    -1.000 Methylimidazol 82

ted
   2   82.97    42.14    0.050    50.00    14.00    -1.000 Methylimidazol 82

ted
   3   82.97    56.06    0.050    38.00    12.00    -1.000 Methylimidazol 82

ted
```

(iii) *Results and calculation*

Check the spike recovery, if the recovery rate is within control range (see Chapter 1, Section 1.1.5 “Qualitative and quantitative testing of LC-MS/MS”), then calculate the result as follows.

$$4\text{-}methylimidazole\,(ppb) = \frac{Ca \times Vsam}{Wsam \times R}$$

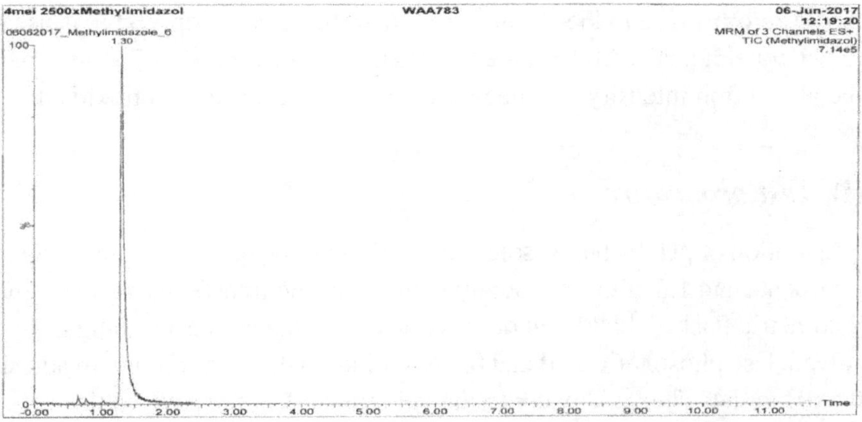

Figure 5.17: LC-MS/MS TIC chromatogram of 4-methylimidazole.

Ca = concentration of sample solution (ppb, or ng/ml)
Vsam = Weight of sample (g)
Wsam = Total volume of sample solution (ml)
R = spike recovery

$$4\text{-}methylimidazole\left(ppb\right)=\frac{Aa\times Cstd\times Vsam}{As\times Wsam\times R}$$

Aa = Peak area of 4-methylimidazole in sample solution
As = Peak area of 4-methylimidazole in standard solution
Cstd = concentration of standard solution (ppb, or ng/ml)
Wsam = Weight of sample (g)
Vsam = Total volume of sample solution (ml)
R = spike recovery

If the recovery out of the control range, follow Chapter 1, Section 1.1.5 "Qualitative and quantitative testing of LC-MS/MS" procedures.

5.18 Oxygen Radical Absorbance Capacity (ORAC) Test Method

The antioxidant capacity of any substance can be measured by comparing its antioxidant capacity with the antioxidant capacity of Trolox. In this method, the quantitation unit is established as "the antioxidant capacity of one micromole trolox in one gram of sample". The reporting unit as abbreviated as TEμmole/g.

2, 2-Azino-bis (3-ethylbenzothiazoline-6-sulfonic acid), or ABTS, is used to generate radicals. ABTS has a maximum UV absorption at 734 nm, and the absorption intensity will decrease with the presence of antioxidants.

(i) *Test procedure*

Preparation of pH 7.4 buffer solution — Weigh 6.8 g potassium dihydrogen phosphate and 1.6 grams of sodium hydroxide, and transfer it to a 1,000 ml volumetric flask. Add 800 ml of water, and sonicate until everything is dissolved. Use phosphoric acid and 0.1 N sodium hydroxide solution to adjust the pH to 7.4. Then add water to the volume mark, and shake well.

Preparation of ABTS solution — Accurately weigh 384 mg of ABTS, and 66.5 mg of peroxydisulfuric acid, and transfer it to a 100 ml volumetric flask. Add water to dissolve and then fill to volume. Shake this solution well. The solution can be kept for 24 h. Take 2 ml of the solution to 100 ml volumetric flask, add pH 7.4 buffer solution to 100 ml, and shake well.

Standard solution — Accurately weigh about 74 mg of water-soluble vitamin E (Trolox), and transfer it to a 100 ml volumetric flask. Add 20 ml of water and 20 ml of ethanol, then sonicate for 5 min. Next, add ethanol to the volume mark, and shake well. Dilute 25 times with ethanol.

Preparation of sample solution — Accurately weigh a certain amount of sample equivalent to 3 mg of trolox, and transfer it to a 100 ml volumetric flask. Add 20 ml of water and 20 ml of ethanol, then sonicate for 10 min. After cooling, add ethanol to 100 ml volume mark, and shake well. Centrifuge for 5 min, and take the clear solution to process the test. If necessary, further dilutions can be made with ethanol.

(ii) *Operation procedure*

Mix the solutions as below in a 10 ml test tube with cap.

	Solution 1 (0.5ml)	**Solution 2 (5ml)**
Blank	Ethanol	ABTS solution
Standard	Standard solution	ABTS solution
Sample	Sample solution	ABTS solution

Cap the test tube and shake well. Then put the tube in 30°C water bath 10 min. After it is cooled, measure the UV absorption at 734 nm.

(iii) *Results and calculation*

$$TE\ \mu mole/g = \frac{(Ab - A) \times Ws \times V \times 10^6}{(Ab - As) \times Vs \times W \times 250.29}$$

A = UV absorption of sample solution
As = UV absorption of standard solution
Ab = UV absorption of blank solution
V = Total volume of sample solution (ml)
Vs = Total volume of standard solution (ml)
Ws = Weight of standard (g)
W = Weight of sample (g)
250.29 = Trolox molecule weight
10^6 = Mole/μMole
TE = Trolox Equivalent

5.19 Ibuprofen Test Method

Ibuprofen is a Western medicine used as an anti-inflammatory and pain relief product. It has certain side effects, especially for people with heart disease. If ibuprofen is spiked in natural products, either unintentionally or as an adulterant, long-term use in this type of dietary supplement may have adverse consequences. This method is designed to detect ibuprofen contained in natural products. It uses LC-UV-MS/MS method to improve sensitivity and accuracy.

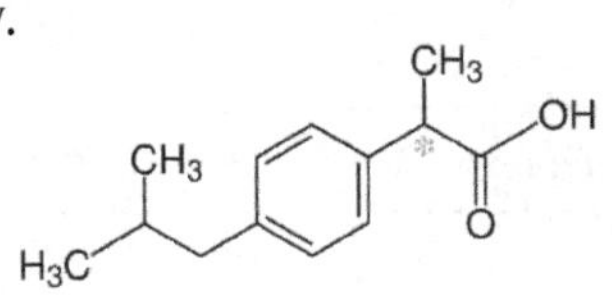

Ibuprofen

(i) *Test procedure*

Preparation of standard solution — Accurately weigh about 10 mg of ibuprofen standard, and transfer it to a 50 ml volumetric flask. Add about

30 ml of methanol, and sonicate until the standard is dissolved. After the standard is cooled, add methanol to the volume mark, and shake well. Label as "Ibuprofen stock standard solution". Make further dilutions to 1, 5, and 25 ppm with methanol. Use the three standard solutions to establish a working curve for both UV and MS/MS detectors.

Preparation of sample solution — Accurately weigh a certain amount of ground sample to meet the required minimum ibuprofen content allowed. Transfer it to a 100 ml volumetric flask, and accurately add 15 ml of water. Sonicate 10 min, then add 60 ml ethanol, and sonicate for another 15 min. Cool the solution to room temperature, then add methanol to volume mark. Shake well, then centrifuge 10 min, and take the clear solution for injection. Further dilutions can be made with methanol if required.

In addition, transfer 990 μl of sample solution into a 2 ml injection vail, and add 10 μl of stock standard solution. Vortex and mix this solution well. This is the spiked sample solution, and it is used to check the recovery of MS/MS detector.

(ii) *UPLC conditions*

Column: Acquity UPLC® BEH Phenyl, 1.7 μm, 2.1 × 150 mm
Flow rate: 0.4 mL/min
Injection volume: 2 μL
Mobile phase A: 10 mM ammonia acetate in water, pH4.0
Mobile phase B: 10 mM ammonia acetate, in acetonitrile
UV wavelength: 254 nm
Column temperature: 45°C

Gradient:

Time (min)	A%	B%
0	65	35
6	35	65
6.5	35	65
6.8	65	35
9.0	65	35

MS/MS parameter

Type	MRM
Ion model	ESI^-
Ion pair	204.94 → 94 (single pair)
Dwell	0.200 second
Cone (V)	16.00
Collision (eV)	10.00

(iii) *Results and calculation*

Calculation by UV detector

$$Ibuprofen\ (mg/unite) = \frac{Aa \times Wstd \times Vsam \times UW}{As \times Wsam \times Vstd}$$

or

$$Ibuprofen\ (\%) = \frac{Aa \times Wstd \times Vsam \times 100\%}{As \times Wsam \times Vstd}$$

Aa = Peak area of ibuprofen in sample solution
As = Peak area of ibuprofen in standard solution
Wstd = Weight of standard (mg)
Wsam = Weight of sample (mg)
Vsam = Total volume of sample solution (ml)
Vstd = Total volume of standard solution (ml)
UW = Unit weight (mg)

Calculation by MS/MS detector (for lower detection limit required)

Check the spike recovery, if the recovery rate is within control range (see Chapter 1, Section 1.1.5 "Qualitative and quantitative testing of LC-MS/MS"), then calculate the result as follows.

$$Ibuprofen\ (\%) = \frac{Csam \times Vsam \times 100\%}{Wsam \times R}$$

Csam = concentration of sample solution (mg/ml), obtained from the MS/MS working curve

Wsam = weight of sample (mg)
Vsam = Total volume of sample solution (ml)
R = Spike recovery

If spike recovery is out the control range, follow Chapter 1, Section 1.1.5 "Qualitative and quantitative testing of LC-MS/MS" procedures.

5.20 Test Method for Thymol

Thymol is an isomer of carvacrol, which is derived from thyme. It is often used in dietary supplements and in food as a preservative.

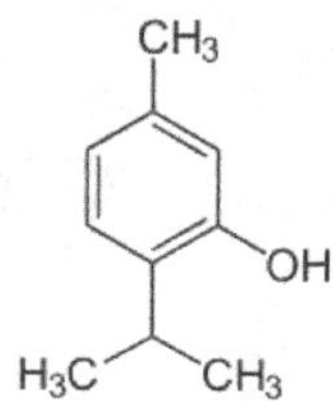

Thymol

(i) *Test procedure*

Preparation of standard solution — Accurately weigh about 5 mg of a thymol standard, and transfer it to a 50 ml volumetric flask. Add 30 ml of methanol, and sonicate for 5 min. Then add methanol to the volume mark and shake well. Dilute with methanol 10-fold, and this standard solution can be injected.

Preparation of sample solution — Accurately weigh a certain amount of ground sample containing about 0.5 mg of thymol, and transfer it to 50 ml volumetric flask. Add 10 ml of DMSO and sonicate for 5 min. Then add 30 ml of ethanol and sonicate for another 10 min. After the solution is cooled, add methanol to the volume mark, and shake well. Centrifuge this for 5 min, and take the clear solution, to inject directly.

(ii) *UPLC conditions*

Column: Acquity UPLC® HSS T3 1.8 μm, 2.1 × 150 mm
Flow rate: 0.4 ml/min

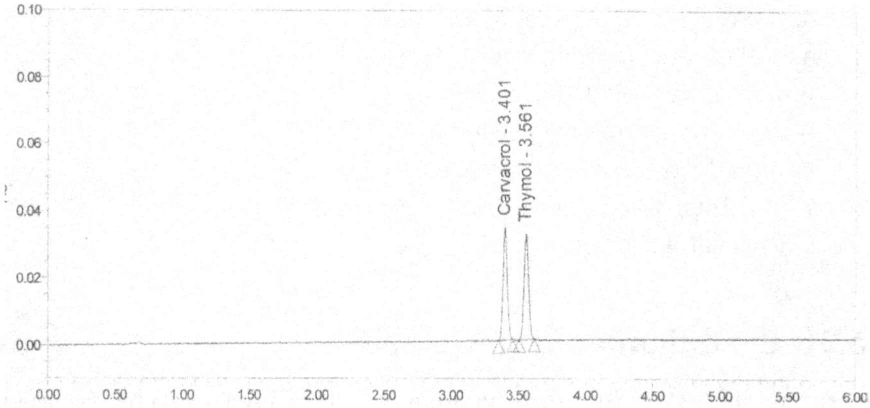

Figure 5.18: UPLC chromatogram of thymol and carvacrol.

Injection volume: 1.0 μL
UV wavelength: 275 nm
Mobile phase A: 0.1% phosphoric acid in water
Mobile phase B: Acetonitrile
Column temperature: 45°C

Gradient:

Time (min)	A%	B%
0	60	40
4	35	65
4.8	35	65
5.0	60	40
7.0	60	40

(iii) *Results and calculation*

$$Thymol\ (mg/unite) = \frac{Aa \times Wstd \times Vsam \times UW}{As \times Wsam \times Vstd}$$

or

$$Thymol\ (\%) = \frac{Aa \times Wstd \times Vsam \times 100\%}{As \times Wsam \times Vstd}$$

Aa = Peak area of thymol in sample solution
As = Peak area of thymol in standard solution
Wstd = Weight of standard (mg)
Wsam = Weight of sample (mg)
Vsam = Total volume of sample solution (ml)
Vstd = Total volume of standard solution (ml)
UW = Unit weight (mg)

5.21 Benfotiamine Test Method

Benfotiamine is a derivative of vitamin B_1, which is easier to be absorbed than vitamin B_1. It has antioxidant, and anti-aging properties and is thought to be helpful in the treatment of diabetes.

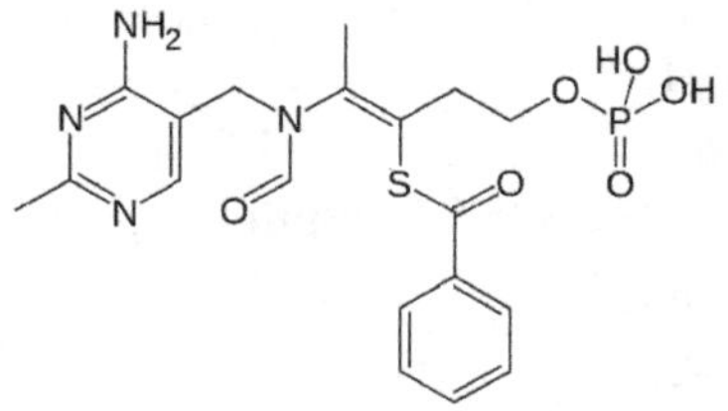

Benfotiamine

(i) *Test procedure*

Preparation of standard solution — Accurately weigh about 10 mg of benfotiamine standard, into 100 ml volumetric flask, add 60 ml 0.05 N sodium hydroxide solution. Shake for 15 min, to ensure that the standard is all dissolved. Then add 0.05 N sodium hydroxide solution to the volume mark, and shake well. This standard is ready for injection.

Preparation of sample solution — Accurately weigh a certain amount ground sample which contains about 10 mg of benfotiamine, and transfer it to a 100 ml volumetric flask. Add 60 ml 0.05 N sodium hydroxide solution, and shake 10 min. Then sonicate for 5 min, and cool to room temperature. Next, add 0.05 N sodium hydroxide solution to volume mark, and shake well. After centrifuging for 5 min, the upper clear solution can be injected.

(ii) *UPLC conditions*

Column: Acquity UPLC® BEH C18 1.7 μm, 2.1 × 150 mm
Flow rate: 0.4 ml/min
Injection volume: 1.0 μL
UV wavelength: 244 nm
Mobile phase A: 0.1% phosphoric acid in water
Mobile phase B: 0.1% phosphoric acid in acetonitrile
Column temperature: 45°C

Gradient:

Time (min)	A%	B%
0	90	10
4	80	20
4.8	80	20
5.0	90	10
7.0	90	10

(iii) *Results and calculation*

$$Benfotiamine\ (mg/unite) = \frac{Aa \times Wstd \times Vsam \times UW}{As \times Wsam \times Vstd}$$

or

$$Benfotiamine\ (\%) = \frac{Aa \times Wstd \times Vsam \times 100\%}{As \times Wsam \times Vstd}$$

Aa = Peak area of benfotiamine in sample solution
As = Peak area of benfotiamine in standard solution
Wstd = Weight of standard (mg)
Wsam = Weight of sample (mg)
Vsam = Total volume of sample solution (ml)
Vstd = Total volume of standard solution (ml)
UW = Unit weight (mg)

5.22 Ipriflavone Test Method

Ipriflavone is a synthetic isoflavone which may be used to inhibit bone calcium desorption. This may help maintain bone density and prevent osteoporosis in postmenopausal women.

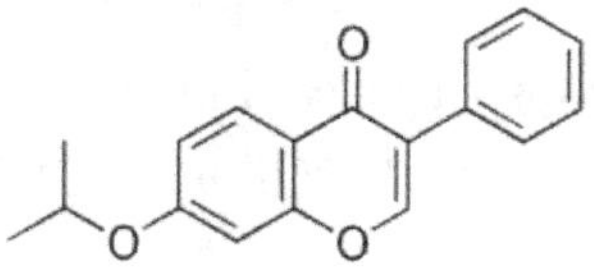

Ipriflavone

According to the molecular structure, ipriflavone is a non-polar compound, and a reversed phase C18 column can be used to measure ipriflavone in a sample matrix.

(i) *Test procedure*

Preparation of standard solution — Accurately weigh about 10 mg of an ipriflavone standard, and transfer it to a 100 ml volumetric flask. Add 60 ml methanol, and sonicate until the standard dissolved completely. After it is cooled, add methanol to the volume mark, and shake well. The standard solution can be injected.

Preparation of sample solution — Accurately weigh a certain amount of ground sample which contains about 10 mg of ipriflavone, and transfer it to a 100 ml volumetric flask. Add 10 ml of water, and sonicate for 5 min. Then add 60 ml of ethanol, and sonicate for another 15 min. After the solution is cooled, add methanol to the volume mark, and shake well. Centrifuge (10,000 rpm) for 5 min, and then take the clear solution for injection.

(ii) *UPLC conditions*

Column: Acquity UPLC® BEH C18, 1.7 μm, 2.1 × 150 mm
Flow rate: 0.4 ml/min
Injection volume: 1.0 μL
UV wavelength: 275 nm
Mobile phase A: 0.1% phosphoric acid in water
Mobile phase B: Acetonitrile
Column temperature: 45°C

Gradient:

Time (min)	A%	B%
0	70	30
5.0	10	90
5.8	10	90
6.0	70	30
8.0	70	30

(iii) *Results and calculation*

$$Ipriflavone\ (mg/unite) = \frac{Aa \times Wstd \times Vsam \times UW}{As \times Wsam \times Vstd}$$

or

$$Ipriflavone\ (\%) = \frac{Aa \times Wstd \times Vsam \times 100\%}{As \times Wsam \times Vstd}$$

Aa = Peak area of ipriflavone in sample solution
As = Peak area of ipriflavone in standard solution
Wstd = Weight of standard (mg)
Wsam = Weight of sample (mg)
Vsam = Total volume of sample solution (ml)
Vstd = Total volume of standard solution (ml)
UW = Unit weight (mg)

5.23 Chrysin Test Method

Chrysin is a flavone found in honey, propolis, the passion flowers, and other plants. Chrysin may have chemo-preventative activity in cancer treatments, but FDA has not approved it for that application. Chrysin is now used in dietary supplements only.

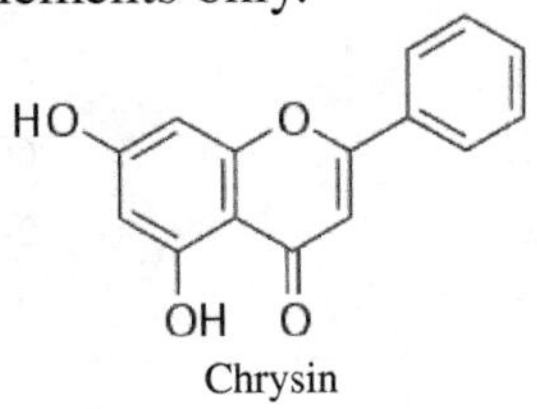

Chrysin

The molecular structure shows chrysin is a non-polar compound, and can be separated and quantified by C18 reversed phase column.

(i) *Test procedure*

Preparation of standard solution — Accurately weigh about 10 mg of a chrysin standard, and transfer it to a 100 ml volumetric flask. Add 60 ml of DMSO/methanol (50/50), and vortex until the standard is fully dissolved. Fill with DMSO/methanol (50/50) to the volume mark, and shake well. This standard can be injected.

Preparation of sample solution — Accurately weigh a certain amount of ground sample that contains about 10 mg of chrysin, and transfer it to a 100 ml volumetric flask. Add 60 ml of DMSO/methanol (50/50), and vortex for 2 min. Then sonicate for 15 min, and cool to room temperature. Next add DMSO/methanol (50/50) to the volume mark and shake well. Centrifuge (10,000 rpm) for 5 min, and the clear solution can be injected.

(ii) *UPLC conditions*

Column: Acquity UPLC® BEH C18, 1.7 μm, 2.1 × 150 mm
Flow rate: 0.4 ml/min
Injection volume: 1.0 μL
UV wavelength: 268 nm
Mobile phase A: 0.1% phosphoric acid in water
Mobile phase B: Acetonitrile
Column temperature: 45°C

Gradient:

Time (min)	A%	B%
0	80	20
5.0	40	60
5.8	40	60
6.0	80	20
8.0	80	20

(iii) *Results and calculation*

$$Chrysin\ (mg/unite) = \frac{Aa \times Wstd \times Vsam \times UW}{As \times Wsam \times Vstd}$$

or

$$Chrysin\ (\%) = \frac{Aa \times Wstd \times Vsam \times 100\%}{As \times Wsam \times Vstd}$$

Aa = Peak area of chrysin in sample solution
As = Peak area of chrysin in standard solution
Wstd = Weight of standard (mg)
Wsam = Weight of sample (mg)
Vsam = Total volume of sample solution (ml)
Vstd = Total volume of standard solution (ml)
UW = Unit weight (mg)

5.24 Pantethine Test Method

Pantethine can reduce low-density serum cholesterol and triglycerides at doses of 500–1200 mg/day. It is used as a dietary supplement.

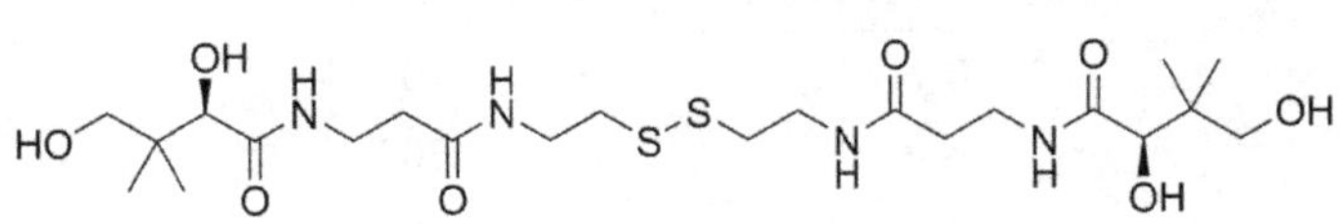

Pantethine

From the molecular structure it can be seen that pantethine is an alkaline molecule. If the testing method encounters interference, or if the following method does not work, an ion pairing mobile phase can be used to try extend the peak retention time (see Chapter 1, Section 1.1.2 "Mobile phase application"). Then the analysis can be performed using a reversed phase column and UV detector to quantify pantethine.

(i) *Test procedure*

Preparation of standard solution — Accurately weigh about 20 mg of a pantethine standard, and transfer it to a 100 ml volumetric flask. Add 60 ml of water, and vortex until the standard is fully dissolved. Then add water to the volume mark, and shake well. The standard solution can be injected.

Preparation of sample solution — Accurately weigh a certain amount of ground sample which contains about 20 mg of pantethine, and transfer it to a 100 ml volumetric flask. Add 60 ml of water, and shake for 15 min with a wrist action shaker. Then sonicate for 5 min, and after cooling, add water to the volume mark. Shake this solution well, and then centrifuge (10,000 rpm) for 5 min. Take the clear solution for injection.

(ii) *UPLC conditions*

Column: Acquity UPLC® HSS T3 C18 1.8 μm, 2.1 × 150 mm
Flow rate: 0.4 ml/min
Injection volume: 1.0 μL
UV wavelength: 211 nm
Mobile phase A: 0.1% phosphoric acid in water
Mobile phase B: Acetonitrile
Column temperature: 45°C

Gradient:

Time (min)	A%	B%
0	90	10
3	70	30
3.8	70	30
4.0	90	10
6.0	90	10

(iii) *Results and calculation*

$$Pantethine\ (mg/unite) = \frac{Aa \times Wstd \times Vsam \times UW}{As \times Wsam \times Vstd}$$

or

$$Pantethine\ (\%) = \frac{Aa \times Wstd \times Vsam \times 100\%}{As \times Wsam \times Vstd}$$

Aa = Peak area of pantethine in sample solution
As = Peak area of pantethine in standard solution
Wstd = Weight of standard (mg)
Wsam = Weight of sample (mg)
Vsam = Total volume of sample solution (ml)
Vstd = Total volume of standard solution (ml)
UW = Unit weight (mg)

5.25 Inositol Hexanicotinate Test Method

Inositol hexanicotinate has the function of lowering cholesterol and dilating the blood vessels. It can be used as an auxiliary treatment for high cholesterol and coronary heart disease. Inositol hexanicotinate can be dissolved in an acidic aqueous solution.

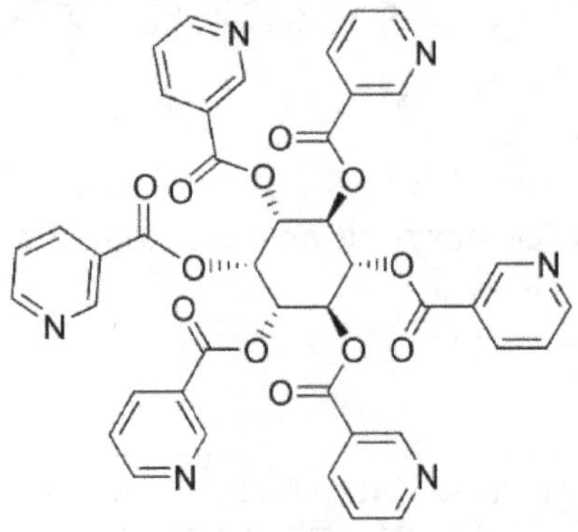

Inositol hexanicotinate

Based on the molecular structure, inositol hexanicotinate is an alkaline compound. In order to extend the retention time to improve the peak separation, this method uses an ion pairing mobile phase (see Chapter 1, Section 1.1.2 "Mobile phase application"). The analysis is conducted with a reversed phase column and PDF detector to perform the quantitative testing.

(i) *Test procedure*

Preparation of standard solution — Accurately weigh about 20 mg inositol hexanicotinate standard, and transfer it to a 100 ml volumetric flask.

Add 60 ml 0.1 N hydrochloric acid aqueous solution, and vortex until the standard completely dissolved. Then add 0.1 N hydrochloric acid aqueous solution to the volume mark, and shake well. The standard solution is ready for injection.

Preparation of sample solution — Accurately weigh a certain amount of ground sample which contains about 20 mg of inositol hexanicotinate, and transfer it to a 100 ml volumetric flask. Add 60 ml 0.1 N hydrochloric acid aqueous solution, and shake for 15 min. Then sonicate for 10 min, and after the solution is cooled add 0.1 N hydrochloric acid solution to the volume mark. Shake this solution well, and then centrifuge (10,000 rpm) for 5 min. Take the upper clear solution for injection.

(ii) *UPLC conditions*

Column: Acquity UPLC® HSS T3 C18 1.8 μm, 2.1 × 100 mm
Flow rate: 0.4 ml/min
Injection volume: 1.0 μL
UV wavelength: 264 nm
Mobile phase A: 10 mM hexansulfonate sodium, pH 3.30
Mobile phase B: Acetonitrile
Column temperature: 45°C

Gradient:

Time (min)	A%	B%
0	70	30
3	55	45
3.8	55	45
4.0	70	30
6.0	70	30

Note: The Inositol hexanicotinate peak in chromatogram is not symmetrical. It has "fronting", and is quite broad. It may be caused by sample overloading. To improve the chromatogram, it is suggested that the concentration of standard and sample solutions be reduced to 5 mg per 100 ml. See Figure 5.19.

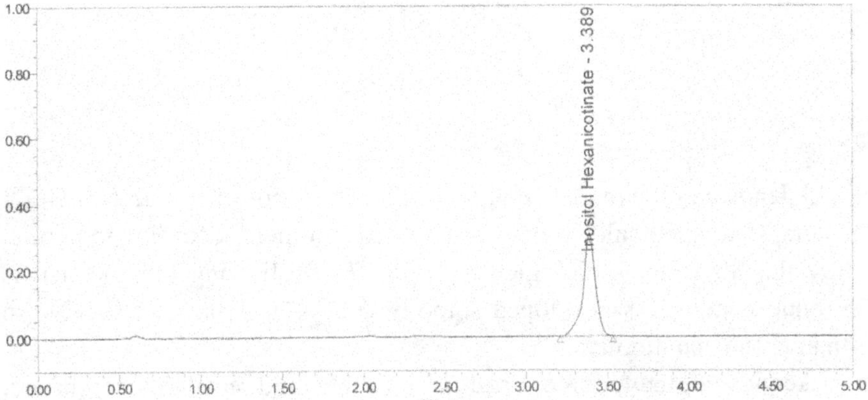

Figure 5.19: UPLC chromatogram of inositol hexanicotinate.

(iii) *Results and calculation*

$$Inositol\,hexanicotinate\ (mg/unite) = \frac{Aa \times Wstd \times Vsam \times UW}{As \times Wsam \times Vstd}$$

or

$$Inositol\,hexanicotinate\ (\%) = \frac{Aa \times Wstd \times Vsam \times 100\%}{As \times Wsam \times Vstd}$$

Aa = Peak area of inositol hexanicotinate in sample solution
As = Peak area of inositol hexanicotinate in standard solution
Wstd = Weight of standard (mg)
Wsam = Weight of sample (mg)
Vsam = Total volume of sample solution (ml)
Vstd = Total volume of standard solution (ml)
UW = Unit weight (mg)

5.26 S-Adenosyl-Methionine (SAMe) Test Method

Adenosylmethionine is classified as a dietary supplement in the United States, and is an auxiliary agent for the treatment of depression.

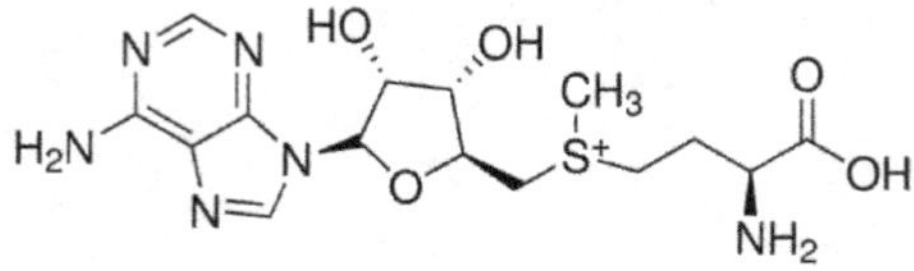

Adenosyl methionine

Adenosine methionine is an optically active molecule with two chiral centers, so there should be four different enantiomers according to 2^n rule. Only the SS form is biologically active. The following method that is introduced here was developed some time ago, and may not be able to separate the enantiomers.

Adenosine methionine itself is unstable and easily decomposed. When choosing a standard for testing, it is important to select a stable adenosine methionine salt. (S-(5'-Adenosyl)-L-methionine) P-toluene sulfonate salt (Sigma-Aldrich A2408) is stable and can be used as a standard.

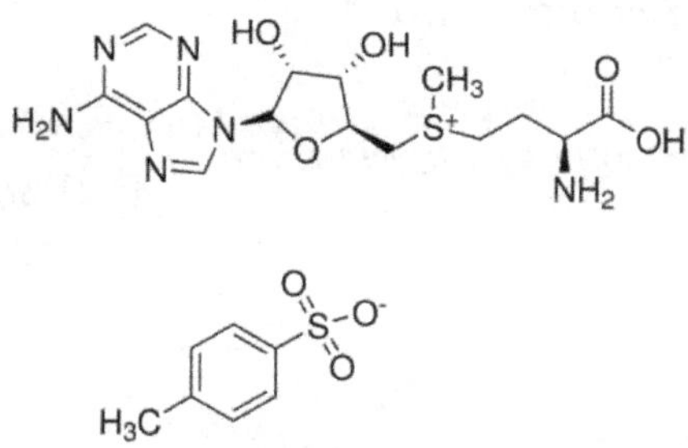

Adenosyl methionine p-toluene sulfonate

(i) *Test procedure*

Preparation of standard solution — Accurately weigh approximately 10 mg of adenosine methionine p-toluene sulfonate standard (contains about 36% SAMe, check the COA of the standard) into a 50 ml volumetric flask, add 30 ml of water, vortex until the standard is completely dissolved, then add water to the mark and shake well. The standard solution is ready for injection.

Preparation of sample solution — Accurately weigh a certain amount ground sample that contains about 10 mg of adenosine methionine p-toluene sulfonate equivalent, and transfer to 50 ml volumetric flask. Add 30 ml of water, and shake 15 min. Fill with water to the volume mark, and then shake well. Centrifuge (10,000 rpm) 5 min, and draw the upper clear solution for injection.

(ii) *UPLC conditions*

Column: Acquity UPLC® BEH C18 1.7 μm, 2.1 × 150 mm
Flow rate: 0.4 ml/min
Injection volume: 1 uL
UV wavelength: 260 nm
Mobile phase A: 10 mM hexane sulfonic acid sodium salt, pH 3.0
Mobile phase B: Acetonitrile
Column temperature: 45°C

Gradient:

Time (min)	A%	B%
0	95	5
3.0	80	20
3.5	80	20
4.0	50	50
4.8	505	50
5.5	95	5
8.0	95	5

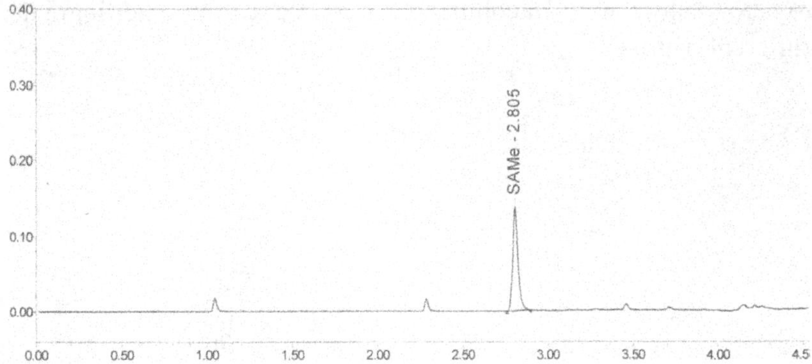

Figure 5.20: Chromatogram of SAMe.

(iii) *Results and calculation*

$$SAMe\ (mg/unite) = \frac{Aa \times Wstd \times Vsam \times UW}{As \times Wsam \times Vstd}$$

or

$$SAMe\ (\%) = \frac{Aa \times Wstd \times Vsam \times 100\%}{As \times Wsam \times Vstd}$$

Aa = Peak area of SAMe in sample solution
As = Peak area of SAMe in standard solution
Wstd = Weight of standard (mg)
Wsam = Weight of sample (mg)
Vsam = Total volume of sample solution (ml)
Vstd = Total volume of standard solution (ml)
UW = Unit weight (mg)

5.27 Co-Enzyme Q10 (Ubiquinone) Test Method

Coenzyme Q10 is an essential chemical that the body produces naturally. As a dietary supplement it may benefit patients with certain cardiac diseases including atherosclerosis, heart failure and other coronary artery diseases.

Co-enzyme Q10 (ubiquinone) is a strong non-polar compound, and can be dissolved in chloroform and other organic solvents. Reversed phase chromatography with C18 column can separate it from other ingredients in different matrices.

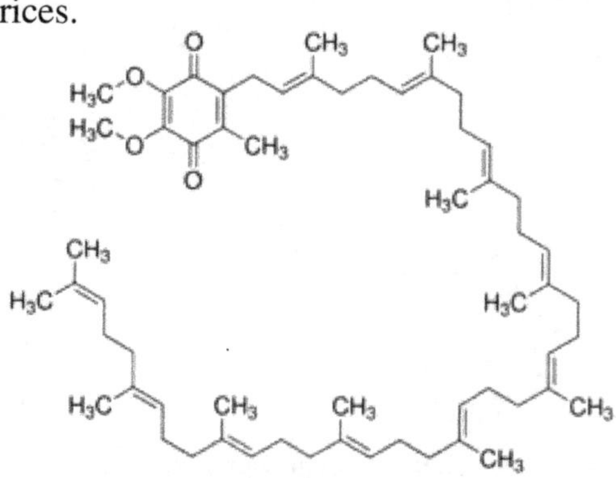

Co-enzyme Q10

(i) *Test procedure*

Preparation of standard solution — Accurately weigh about 5 mg of a coenzyme Q10 standard, and transfer it to a 100 ml volumetric flask. Add 20 ml of chloroform and sonicate until all of the standard is dissolved. After the solution is cooled, add isopropanol to the volume mark, and shake well. The standard solution is ready for injection.

Preparation of sample solution — Accurately weigh a certain amount of ground sample containing about 5 mg of coenzyme Q10, and transfer it to a 100 ml volumetric flask. Add 20 ml of chloroform, and sonicate for 10 min. Then add 40 ml of isopropyl alcohol, and sonicate for another 5 min. After cooling add isopropyl alcohol to the volume mark, and shake well. Centrifuge (10,000 rpm) for 5 min, and take the clear solution for injection.

(ii) *HPLC conditions*

Column: Phenomenex LUNA C18 (2) 5 μm, 4.6 × 250 mm 100 A
Flow rate: 1.0 ml/min
Injection volume: 10 μL
UV wavelength: 274 nm
Mobile phase: IPA/Acetonitrile (70/30)
Column temperature: Room temperature
Run time: 15 min

(iii) *Results and calculation*

$$CoQ10\ (mg/unite) = \frac{Aa \times Wstd \times Vsam \times UW}{As \times Wsam \times Vstd}$$

or

$$CoQ10\ (\%) = \frac{Aa \times Wstd \times Vsam \times 100\%}{As \times Wsam \times Vstd}$$

Aa = Peak area of CoQ10 in sample solution
As = Peak area of CoQ10 in standard solution
Wstd = Weight of standard (mg)

Wsam = Weight of sample (mg)
Vsam = Total volume of sample solution (ml)
Vstd = Total volume of standard solution (ml)
UW = Unit weight (mg)

5.28 Melatonin Test Method

Melatonin is a hormone primarily released by the human pineal gland at night. It has long been associated with helping control of the sleep–awake cycle. As a dietary supplement, melatonin is most commonly used for insomnia and improving sleep under different conditions.

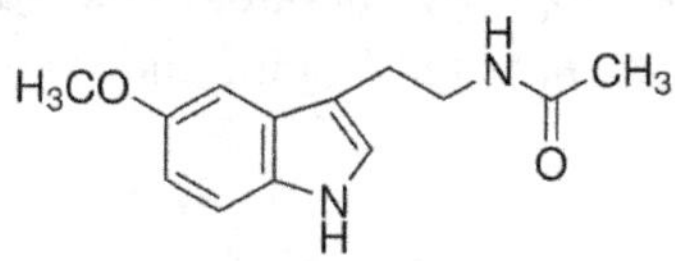

Melatonin

(i) *Test procedure*

Preparation of standard solution — Accurately weigh about 10 mg of a melatonin standard, and transfer it to a 100 ml volumetric flask. Add 60 ml methanol, and sonicate until the standard is dissolved completely. Then add methanol to the volume mark, shake well, and the standard solution can be injected.

Preparation of sample solution — Accurately weigh a certain amount of ground sample which contains about 10 mg of melatonin, and transfer it to a 100 ml volumetric flask. Add 10 ml of water, and sonicate for 5 min. Then add 60 ml of ethanol and sonicate for another 10 min. Cool to room temperature, then add methanol to the volume mark, and shake well. Centrifuge (10,000 rpm) 5 min, and draw the clear solution for injection.

(ii) *UPLC conditions*

Column: Acquity UPLC® HSS T3 C18 1.8 μm, 2.1 × 150 mm
Flow rate: 0.4 ml/min
Injection volume: 1 μL

UV wavelength: 280 nm
Mobile phase A: Water
Mobile phase B: Acetonitrile
Column temperature: 45°C

Gradient:

Time (min)	A%	B%
0	80	20
3.5	60	40
3.8	60	40
4.0	80	20
6.0	80	20

(iii) *Results and calculation*

$$Melatonin\ (mg/unite) = \frac{Aa \times Wstd \times Vsam \times UW}{As \times Wsam \times Vstd}$$

or

$$Melatonin\ (\%) = \frac{Aa \times Wstd \times Vsam \times 100\%}{As \times Wsam \times Vstd}$$

Aa = Peak area of melatonin in sample solution
As = Peak area of melatonin in standard solution
Wstd = Weight of standard (mg)
Wsam = Weight of sample (mg)
Vsam = Total volume of sample solution (ml)
Vstd = Total volume of standard solution (ml)
UW = Unit weight (mg)

5.29 Test Method of Isovitexin

Isovitexin is an isomer of vitexin; and both are active components of many traditional Chinese medicines. The pharmacological effects, include but are not limited to anti-oxidant, anti-cancer, anti-inflammatory, anti-hypoallergenic and neuroprotective effects. At present, isovitexin also can be used in dietary supplement for anti-hypoxia prevention, and treatment of oral ulcers health care products.

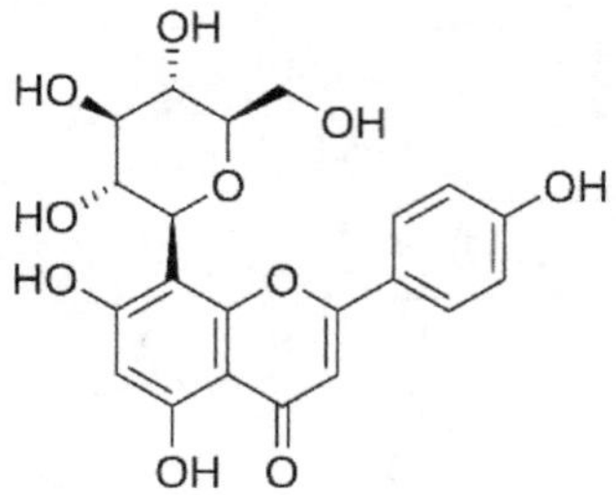

Vitexin

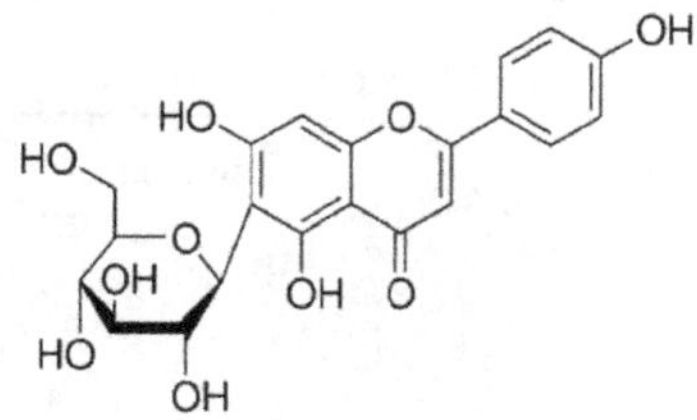

Isovitexin

(i) *Test procedure*

Preparation of standard solution — Accurately weigh about 10 mg of isovitexin standard, and transfer it to a 100 ml volumetric flask. Add 60 ml methanol and sonicate until all standards get dissolved. Then add methanol to the volume mark, and shake well. The standard solution is ready for injection.

Preparation of sample solution — Accurately weigh a certain amount of ground sample which contains about 10 mg of isovitexin, and transfer it to a 100 ml volumetric flask. Add 20 ml of water and sonicate for 5 min. Then add 60 ml of ethanol, and sonicate for another 10 min. After the solution is cooled, fill it with methanol to the volume mark, and shake well. Centrifuge (10,000 rpm) for 5 min, and draw the upper clear solution for injection.

(ii) *UPLC conditions*

Column: Acquity UPLC® BEH C18 1.7 μm, 2.1 × 150 mm
Flow rate: 0.4 ml/min
Injection volume: 1 μL
UV wavelength: 338 nm
Mobile phase A: 0.1% phosphoric acid in water
Mobile phase B: Acetonitrile
Column temperature: 45°C

Gradient:

Time (min)	A%	B%
0	90	10
4.0	70	30
4.8	40	60
5.8	40	60
6.0	90	10
8.0	90	10

(iii) *Results and calculation*

$$Isovitexin\ (mg/unite) = \frac{Aa \times Wstd \times Vsam \times UW}{As \times Wsam \times Vstd}$$

or

$$Isovitexin\ (\%) = \frac{Aa \times Wstd \times Vsam \times 100\%}{As \times Wsam \times Vstd}$$

Aa = Peak area of isovitexin in sample solution
As = Peak area of isovitexin in standard solution
$Wstd$ = Weight of standard (mg)
$Wsam$ = Weight of sample (mg)
$Vsam$ = Total volume of sample solution (ml)
$Vstd$ = Total volume of standard solution (ml)
UW = Unit weight (mg)

5.30 Determination of Omega-3 Fatty Acids in Fish Oil

Omega-3s are polyunsaturated fatty acids. In fish oil, the most abundant Omega-3s are eicosapentaenoic (EPA) and docosahexaenoic (DHA). Omega-3s work by lowering the body's production of triglycerides. High levels of triglycerides can lead to coronary artery disease, heart disease and stroke in humans.

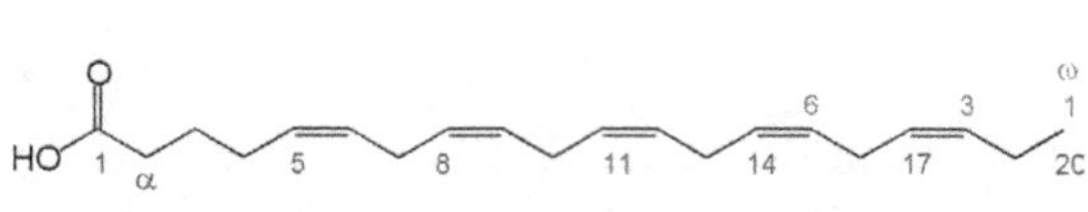

EPA

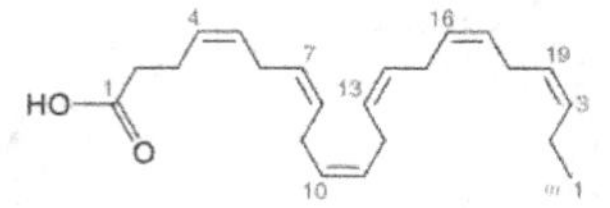

DHA

Omega-3s in fish oil are not free fatty acids but fatty acid esters. To determine omega-3 fatty acids, the sample should be hydrolyzed in alkaline ethanol. The free omega-3 fatty acids obtained after hydrolysis can be tested by gas chromatography with FID detection like other fatty acids. Here a UPLC-PDA method will be introduced. The advantage of this method is that it is faster than the gas chromatography method.

(i) *Test procedure*

Preparation of standard solution — Accurately weigh about 25 mg of EPA and 25 mg of DHA standards, in a 100 ml volumetric flask, and add 60 ml of ethanol. Sonicate until the standards are fully dissolved, and then add ethanol to the mark. Shake the solution well, and the standard solution is ready for injection.

Preparation of sample solution — Accurately weigh a certain amount of ground sample containing about 25 mg of EPA and/or 25 mg DHA, and transfer it to a 100 ml Erlenmeyer flask. Add 30 ml of ethanol and 800 mg of sodium hydroxide, and sonicate under a 60°C water bath for 40 min or until all sodium hydroxide is dissolved. After cooling transfer it to a 100 ml volumetric flask. Use a small amount of ethanol to wash the Erlenmeyer flask several times, and transfer all the wash solution into the 100 ml volumetric flask. Then add ethanol to the volume mark, and shake well. Centrifuge (10,000 rpm) for 5 min, and take the clear solution for injection.

(ii) *UPLC conditions*

Column: Acquity UPLC® BEH Phenyl 1.7 μm, 2.1 × 150 mm
Flow rate: 0.4 ml/min
Injection volume: 1.0 μL
UV wavelength: 211 nm

Mobile phase A: 0.1% phosphoric acid in water
Mobile phase B: Acetonitrile
Column temperature: 45°C

Gradient:

Time (min)	A%	B%
0	70	30
10	25	75
10.8	25	75
11.0	70	30
14.0	70	30

(iii) *Results and calculation*

$$EPA/DHA\ (mg/unite) = \frac{Aa \times Wstd \times Vsam \times UW}{As \times Wsam \times Vstd}$$

or

$$EPA/DHA\ (\%) = \frac{Aa \times Wstd \times Vsam \times 100\%}{As \times Wsam \times Vstd}$$

Aa = Peak area of EPA/DHA in sample solution
As = Peak area of EPA/DHA in standard solution

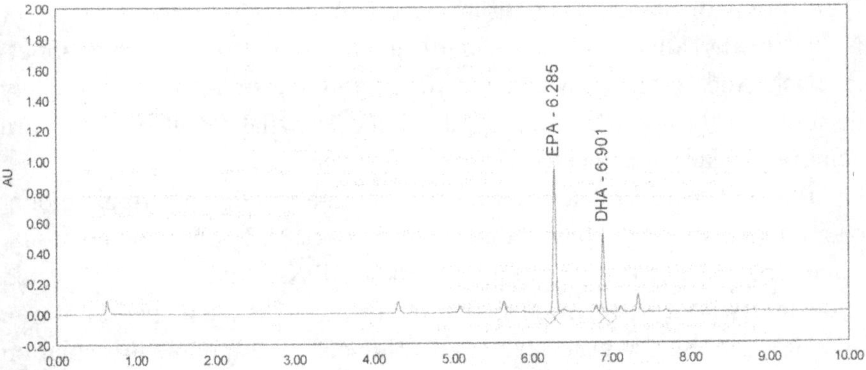

Figure 5.21: UPLC chromatogram of EPA and DHA.

Wstd = Weight of standard (mg)
Wsam = Weight of sample (mg)
Vsam = Total volume of sample solution (ml)
Vstd = Total volume of standard solution (ml)
UW = Unit weight (mg)

5.31 N, N-Dimethyl Ethanolamine (DMAE) Test Method

N, N-dimethyl ethanolamine is a compound that many people believe can positively affect mood, enhance memory and improve brain function. It is also thought to have benefits for aging skin. DMAE is a precursor to choline, and it complements choline in the body.

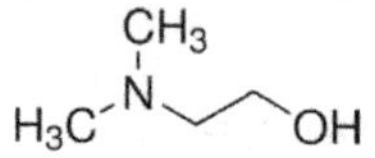

N, N-dimethyl ethanolamine

Bases on the molecular structure, N, N-dimethyl ethanolamine is a strong alkaline compound. Like choline it can be separated using a cation exchange column, and measured using a conductivity detector for quantitation.

(i) *Test procedure*

Preparation of standard solution — Accurately weigh about 5 mg of N, N-dimethyl ethanolamine standard, and transfer it to a 200 ml volumetric flask. Add 120 ml of water, and vortex until the standard is completely dissolved. Then add water to 200 ml volume, and shake well. The standard solution is ready for injection.

Preparation of sample solution — Accurately weigh a certain amount of ground sample which contains about 5 mg of N, N-dimethyl ethanolamine, and transfer it to a 200 ml volumetric flask. Add 120 ml of water, and shake with a wrist action shaker for 15 min. Then sonicate for 5 min, and after cooling add water to 200 ml volume. Shake and mix this solution well, then centrifuge (10,000 rpm) it for 5 min. Draw the clear solution for injection.

(ii) *IC conditions*

Column: IonPac® CS 14, 4 × 250 mm
Suppressor: Dionex CSRS Suppressor (4 mm)
Suppressor current: 120 mA
Flow rate: 1.0 ml/min
Elute: 40 mM methylsulfonic acid
Injection volume: 25 μL
Column temperature: 30°C

(iii) *Results and calculation*

$$DMAE\ (mg/unite) = \frac{Aa \times Wstd \times Vsam \times UW}{As \times Wsam \times Vstd}$$

or

$$DMAE\ (\%) = \frac{Aa \times Wstd \times Vsam \times 100\%}{As \times Wsam \times Vstd}$$

Aa = Peak area of DMAE in sample solution
As = Peak area of DMAE in standard solution
Wstd = Weight of standard (mg)
Wsam = Weight of sample (mg)
Vsam = Total volume of sample solution (ml)
Vstd = Total volume of standard solution (ml)
UW = Unit weight (mg)

5.32 Test Method of 5-Hydroxytrytophan (5-HTP)

5-hydroxytrytophan (5-HTP) is classified as drug in some countries, but in the United States and Canada it is classified as dietary supplements, which are complementary to the treatment of sleep improvement and depression.

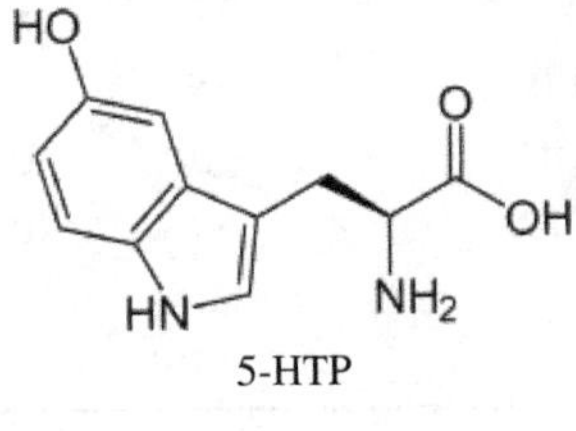

5-HTP

5-hydroxytryptophan is an amino acid, positively charged under acidic conditions. In order to extend the retention time, improve the peak shape, improve resolution and get a better separation effect, add hexansulfonate in the pH 2.0 mobile phase, to form an ion pair with 5-HTP (see Chapter 1, Section 1.1.2 "Mobile phase application").

(i) *Test procedure*

Preparation of standard solution — Accurately weigh about 5 mg of 5-hydroxytryptophan standard, and transfer it to a 100 ml volumetric flask. Add 60 ml methanol/water (80:20), and vortex until the standard is fully dissolved. Then add methanol/water (80:20) to the volume mark, and shake well. The standard solution can be injected.

Preparation of sample solution — Accurately weigh a certain amount of ground sample that contains about 5 mg 5-hydroxytryptophan, and transfer it to a 100 ml volumetric flask. Add 20 ml of water, and sonicate for 5 min. Then add 60 ml methanol, and sonicate for another 15 min. After the solution is cooled add methanol/water (80:20) to the volume mark, and shake well. Centrifuge for 5 min, and the upper clear solution can be injected.

(ii) *HPLC conditions*

Column: Supelcosil Discovery RP-Amide C16 column, 4.6 × 150 mm,
Flow rate: 1.0 ml/min
Injection volume: 10.0 μL
UV wavelength: 280 nm
Mobile phase A: 10 mM hexane sulfonic acid sodium salt, pH 2.0
Mobile phase B: Acetonitrile
Column temperature: Room temperature

Gradient:

Time (min)	A%	B%
0	95	5
1.0	95	5
10.0	60	40
11.0	60	40
11.5	95	5
15.0	95	5

(iii) *Results and calculation*

$$5\text{-}HTP\ (mg/unite) = \frac{Aa \times Wstd \times Vsam \times UW}{As \times Wsam \times Vstd}$$

or

$$5\text{-}HTP\ (\%) = \frac{Aa \times Wstd \times Vsam \times 100\%}{As \times Wsam \times Vstd}$$

Aa = Peak area of 5-HTP in sample solution
As = Peak area of 5-HTP in standard solution
Wstd = Weight of standard (mg)
Wsam = Weight of sample (mg)
Vsam = Total volume of sample solution (ml)
Vstd = Total volume of standard solution (ml)
UW = Unit weight (mg)

5.33 Ebselen Test Method

Ebselen is a synthetic organoselenium compound with anti-inflammatory and antioxidant activity.

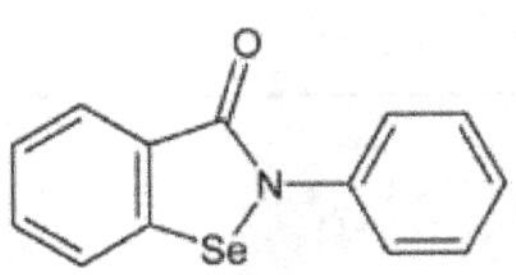

Ebselen

(i) *Test procedure*

Preparation of standard solution — Accurately weigh about 5 mg of an ebselen standard, and transfer it to a 100 ml volumetric flask. Add 60 ml methanol, and vortex until the standard completely dissolved. Then add methanol to 100 ml mark, shake well, and the standard can be injected.

Preparation of sample solution — Accurately weigh a certain amount of ground sample which contains about 5 mg ebselen, and transfer it to a 100 ml volumetric flask. Add 20 ml of DMSO and sonicate for 5 min. Then add 60 ml methanol, and sonicate for another 15 min. After the solution has cooled, add methanol to 100 ml mark, and shake well. Centrifuge

(10, 000 rpm) for 5 min, and draw the upper-level clear solution for injection.

(ii) *HPLC conditions*

Column: Supelcosil Discovery RP-Amide C16 column, 4.6 × 150 mm

Flow rate: 1.0 ml/min
Injection volume: 10.0 μL
UV wavelength: 325 nm
Mobile phase A: 0.1% phosphoric acid in water
Mobile phase B: Methanol
Column temperature: Room temperature

Gradient:

Time (min)	A%	B%
0	60	40
1.0	60	40
8	10	90
10.0	10	90
10.5	60	40
15.0	60	40

(iii) *Results and calculation*

$$Ebselen\ (mg/unite) = \frac{Aa \times Wstd \times Vsam \times UW}{As \times Wsam \times Vstd}$$

or

$$Ebselen\ (\%) = \frac{Aa \times Wstd \times Vsam \times 100\%}{As \times Wsam \times Vstd}$$

Aa = Peak area of ebselen in sample solution
As = Peak area of ebselen in standard solution
Wstd = Weight of standard (mg)
Wsam = Weight of sample (mg)
Vsam = Total volume of sample solution (ml)

Vstd = Total volume of standard solution (ml)
UW = Unit weight (mg)

5.34 Scopoletin Test Method

Scopoletin can be extracted from natural plants. It also can be synthesized. Biological activities include anti-inflammation and hypolipidemic activity. In traditional Chinese medicine it is used for rheumatoid arthritis therapy.

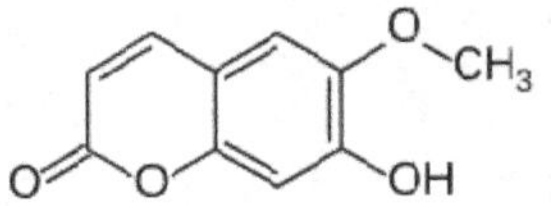

Scopoletin

Scopoletin is a non-polar compound, and it can be analyzed with reversed phase chromatography.

(i) *Test procedure*

Preparation of standard solution — Accurately weigh about 5 mg of a scopoletin standard, and transfer it to a 100 ml volumetric flask. Add 60 ml of methanol/water (50:50), and sonicate until the standard is completely dissolved. Then add methanol/water (50:50) to 100 ml volume, and shake well. This solution is ready to be injected.

Preparation of sample solution — Accurately weigh a certain amount of ground sample containing about 5 mg of scopoletin, and transfer it to a 100 ml volumetric flask. Add 30 ml of water, and sonicate for 5 min. Then add 30 ml methanol, and sonicate for another 10 min. Cool to room temperature, then add methanol/water (50:50) to the volume mark. Shake well, then centrifuge (10,000 rpm) for 5 min, and take top clear solution for injection.

(ii) *UPLC conditions*

Column: Acquity UPLC® BEH C18 1.7 μm, 2.1 × 150 mm
Flow rate: 0.4 ml/min

Injection volume: 1.0 μL
UV wavelength: 343 nm
Mobile phase A: 0.1% phosphoric acid in water
Mobile phase B: Acetonitrile
Column temperature: 45°C

Gradient:

Time (min)	A%	B%
0	85	15
7	40	60
8.0	40	60
8.5	85	15
12.0	85	15

(iii) *Results and calculation*

$$Scopoletin\ (mg/unite) = \frac{Aa \times Wstd \times Vsam \times UW}{As \times Wsam \times Vstd}$$

or

$$Scopoletin\ (\%) = \frac{Aa \times Wstd \times Vsam \times 100\%}{As \times Wsam \times Vstd}$$

Aa = Peak area of scopoletin in sample solution
As = Peak area of scopoletin in standard solution
Wstd = Weight of standard (mg)
Wsam = Weight of sample (mg)
Vsam = Total volume of sample solution (ml)
Vstd = Total volume of standard solution (ml)
UW = Unit weight (mg)

5.35 Salicylic Acid and Salicin Test Method

Willow bark contains salicin. When orally ingested, salicin is converted into salicylic acid by specialized enzymes in our digestive system. Both salicylic acid and salicin act as anti-inflammation and anti-pyretic agents.

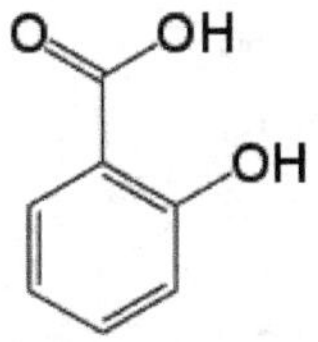

Salicylic acid

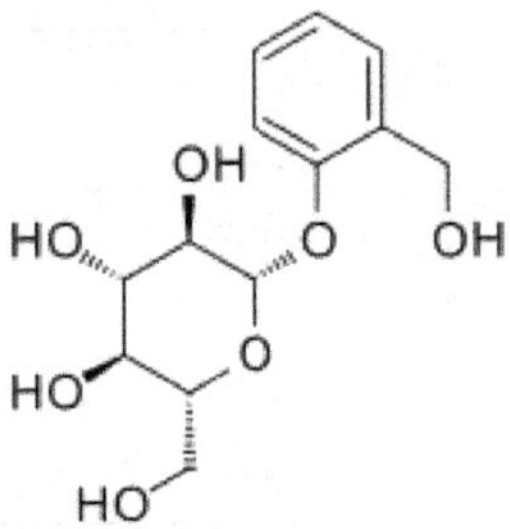

Salicin

(i) *Test procedure*

Preparation of standard solution — Accurately weigh about 10 mg of salicin and 10 mg of salicylic acid standards, and transfer it to a 100 ml volumetric flask. Add 60 ml methanol/water (30:70), and sonicate until all of the standards are dissolved. Then add methanol/water (30:70) to the volume mark, and shake well. The standard solution is ready to be injected.

Preparation of sample solution — Accurately weigh a certain amount of ground sample which contains about 10 mg salicylic acid or salicin, and transfer it to a 100 ml volumetric flask. Add 40 ml of water, and sonicate for 5 min. Then add 25 ml methanol, and sonicate for another 10 min. After the solution is cooled, fill to the volume mark with methanol/water (30:70), and shake well. Centrifuge (10,000 rpm) for 5 min, and draw the clear solution for injection.

(ii) *HPLC conditions*

Column: Phenomenex Prodigy C18 column, 5 μm, 4.6 × 250 mm
Flow rate: 1.2 ml/min
Injection volume: 10 μL
UV wavelength: 343 nm
Mobile phase A: 0.1% phosphoric acid
Mobile phase B: Acetonitrile
Column temperature: Room temperature

Gradient:

Time (min)	A%	B%
0	95	5
5.0	95	5
20	40	60
21	40	60
21.5	95	5
26.0	95	5

(iii) *Results and calculation*

$$Salicylic\,acid/salicin\ (mg/unite) = \frac{Aa \times Wstd \times Vsam \times UW}{As \times Wsam \times Vstd}$$

or

$$Salicylic\,acid/salicin\ \% = \frac{Aa \times Wstd \times Vsam \times 100\%}{As \times Wsam \times Vstd}$$

Aa = Peak area of salicylic acid/salicin in sample solution
As = Peak area of salicylic acid/salicinin in standard solution
Wstd = Weight of standard (mg)
Wsam = Weight of sample (mg)
Vsam = Total volume of sample solution (ml)
Vstd = Total volume of standard solution (ml)
UW = Unit weight (mg)

5.36 Test Method for Hydroquinone

Hydroquinone has two hydroxyl groups bonded to a benzene ring in a *para* position. It has a variety of uses principally associated with its action as a reducing agent. One application is its use in cosmetic products as a skin whitening agent, to lighten the skin.

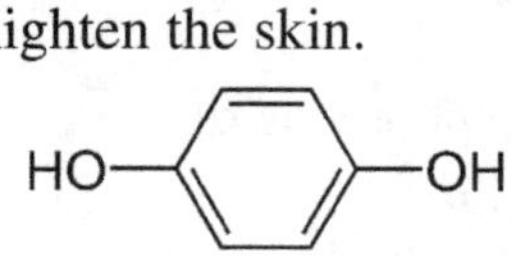

Hydroquinone

(i) *Test steps*

Preparation of standard solution — Accurately weight about 5 mg of a hydroquinone standard, and transfer it to a 100 ml volumetric flask. Add 60 ml of warm water, and vortex until the standard is completely dissolved. Then add water to the volume mark, and shake well. The solution is ready for injection.

Preparation of sample solution — Accurately weigh a certain amount of ground sample that contains about 5 mg of hydroquinone, and transfer it to a 100 ml volumetric flask. Add 60 ml of warm water, and sonicate for 10 min. After cooling, fill to volume with water, centrifuge (10,000 rpm) for 5 min, and draw the clear solution to inject.

(ii) *UPLC conditions*

Column: Acquity UPLC® HSS T3, C18 1.8 μm, 2.1 × 150 mm
Flow rate: 0.4 ml/min
Injection volume: 1.0 μL
UV wavelength: 254 nm
Mobile phase A: 0.1% phosphoric acid in water
Mobile phase B: 0.1% phosphoric acid in acetonitrile
Column temperature: 45°C

Gradient:

Time (min)	A%	B%
0	97	3
5	80	20
6.0	80	20
6.5	97	3
9.0	97	3

(iii) *Result and calculation*

$$Hydroquinone\ (mg/unite) = \frac{Aa \times Wstd \times Vsam \times UW}{As \times Wsam \times Vstd}$$

or

$$Hydroquinone\ (\%) = \frac{Aa \times Wstd \times Vsam \times 100\%}{As \times Wsam \times Vstd}$$

Aa = Peak area of hydroquinone in sample solution
As = Peak area of hydroquinone in standard solution
Wstd = Weight of standard (mg)
Wsam = Weight of sample (mg)
Vsam = Total volume of sample solution (ml)
Vstd = Total volume of standard solution (ml)
UW = Unit weight (mg)

5.37 α-Lipoic Acid Test Method

Alpha-lipoic acid is an antioxidant, and it may protect against damage to the body's cells, resulting in health benefits. These benefits may include helping with alcoholic liver disease, HIV, Alzheimer's disease, bipolar disorder, cardiac arrhythmia, high blood pressure, rheumatoid arthritis, premature labor and diabetes. To date, there is little evidence to support these claims.

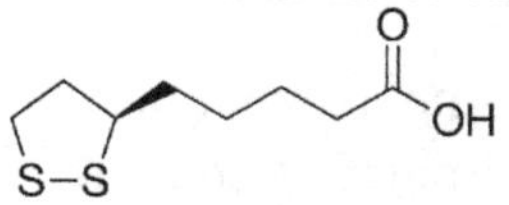

Lipoic acid

(i) *Test procedure*

Preparation of standard solution — Accurately weight 10 mg of a lipoic acid standard, and transfer it to a 100 ml volumetric flask. Add 60 ml methanol, and sonicate until standard completely dissolved. Fill with methanol to the volume mark, and shake well. This standard is ready to be injected.

Preparation of sample solution — Accurately weigh a certain amount of ground sample which contains about 10 mg of lipoic acid, and transfer it to a 100 ml volumetric flask. Add 20 ml of DMSO, and sonicate for 5 min. Then add 50 ml of methanol, and sonicate for another 15 min. After the solution is cooled, add methanol to the volume mark, and shake well. Centrifuge for 5 min, and the clear solution can be injected.

(ii) *UPLC conditions*

Column: Acquity UPLC® HSS Ts, C18 1.7 μm, 2.1 × 100 mm
Flow rate: 0.4 ml/min
Injection volume: 2.0 μL
UV wavelength: 333 nm
Mobile phase A: 0.1% phosphoric acid in water
Mobile phase B: 0.1% phosphoric acid in acetonitrile
Column temperature: 45°C

Gradient:

Time (min)	A%	B%
0	70	30
3	45	55
3.8	45	55
4.0	70	30
6.0	70	30

(iii) *Results and calculation*

$$Lipoic\,acid\,(mg/unite) = \frac{Aa \times Wstd \times Vsam \times UW}{As \times Wsam \times Vstd}$$

or

$$Lipoic\,acid\,(\%) = \frac{Aa \times Wstd \times Vsam \times 100\%}{As \times Wsam \times Vstd}$$

Aa = Peak area of lipoic acid in sample solution
As = Peak area of lipoic acid in standard solution
Wstd = Weight of standard (mg)
Wsam = Weight of sample (mg)
Vsam = Total volume of sample solution (ml)
Vstd = Total volume of standard solution (ml)
UW = Unit weight (mg)

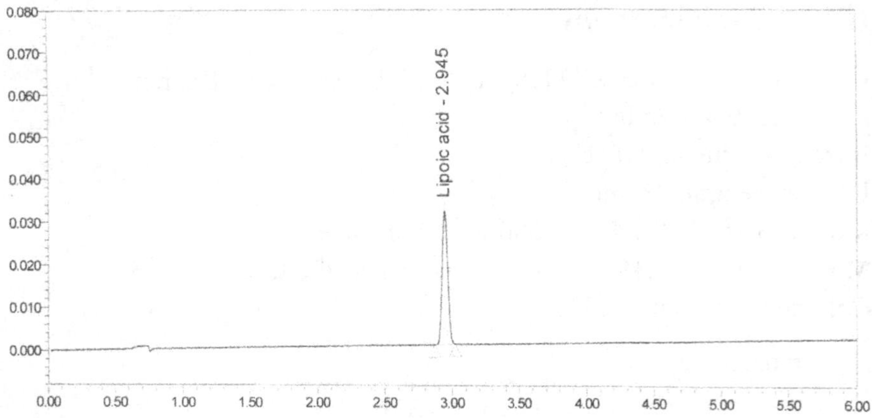

Figure 5.22: UPLC chromatogram of α-lipoic acid.

5.38 Pyridoxal-5-Phosphate Test Method

Pyridoxal-5-phosphate (P5P) is a biologically active form of vitamin B_6 (Pyridoxine).

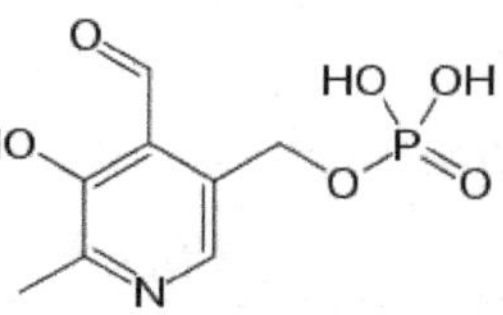

P5P

(i) *Test procedure*

Pyridoxal-5-phosphate is a multipolar molecule. Its isoelectric point is about 2.9. There are three options to consider when trying to extend the P5P peak retention time in order to reduce the opportunity for interferences.

(1) Adjust the mobile phase pH to isoelectric point 2.9, so that P5P becomes a neutral molecule. The retention time can be extended when using a reversed phase column.
(2) Add 5 mM tetra butyl ammonium chloride (TBACl) to the mobile phase A, and adjust pH ≥5. This will convert the P5P to an anion and form an ion pair with TBACl.

(3) Add 10 mM sodium hexansulfonate into mobile phase A, and adjust pH ≤ 1.5. This will convert the P5P to a cation and form an ion pair with hexansulfonate.

The most suitable option can be selected based on the actual sample being tested. Here option 1 is described:

(I) Test procedure:
Preparation of pH 2.9 buffer — Weigh 1.38 g of potassium dihydrogen phosphate (KH_2PO_4) into a 1,000 ml volumetric flask and add 600 ml of water. Sonicate until it is all dissolved. Then add 0.1 N hydrochloric acid and 0.01 N sodium hydroxide solution to adjust pH to 2.9. Fill with water to the volume mark, and shake well. Filter with a 0.2 μm filter membrane.

Preparation of standard solution — Accurately weigh about 10 mg P5P standard, and transfer it to a 100 ml volumetric flask. Add 60 ml 0.1 N hydrochloric acid, and vortex until the standard is completely dissolved. Then add 0.1 N hydrochloric acid to the volume mark and shake well. The standard is ready for injection.

Preparation of sample solution — Accurately weigh a certain amount of ground sample containing about 10 mg of P5P, and transfer it to a 100 ml volumetric flask. Add 60 ml 0.1 N hydrochloric acid, and shake for 15 min. Then sonicate for 5 min. After cooling, fill to the volume mark with 0.1 N hydrochloric acid and shake well. Centrifuge for 5 min, and take clear solution for injection.

(ii) *UPLC conditions*

Column: Acquity UPLC® HSS T3 C18 1.8 μm, 2.1 × 150 mm
Flow rate: 0.4 ml/min
Injection volume: 1 μL
UV wavelength: 295 nm
Mobile phase A: pH 2.9 buffer solution
Mobile phase B: Acetonitrile
Column temperature: 45°C

Gradient:

Time (min)	A%	B%
0	97	3
6	70	30
7.0	70	30
7.5	97	3
10.0	97	3

(iii) *Results and calculation*

$$P5P\ (mg/unite) = \frac{Aa \times Wstd \times Vsam \times UW}{As \times Wsam \times Vstd}$$

or

$$P5P\ (\%) = \frac{Aa \times Wstd \times Vsam \times 100\%}{As \times Wsam \times Vstd}$$

Aa = Peak area of P5P in sample solution
As = Peak area of P5P in standard solution
Wstd = Weight of standard (mg)
Wsam = Weight of sample (mg)
Vsam = Total volume of sample solution (ml)
Vstd = Total volume of standard solution (ml)
UW = Unit weight (mg)

5.39 Test Method for Vitamin C Palmitate

Vitamin C Palmitate is an antioxidant compound like ascorbic acid (vitamin C), but it is not the same as vitamin C. Vitamin C palmitate, or ascorbyl palmitate, is oil soluble and can be added to oil products and foods to prevent oxidation.

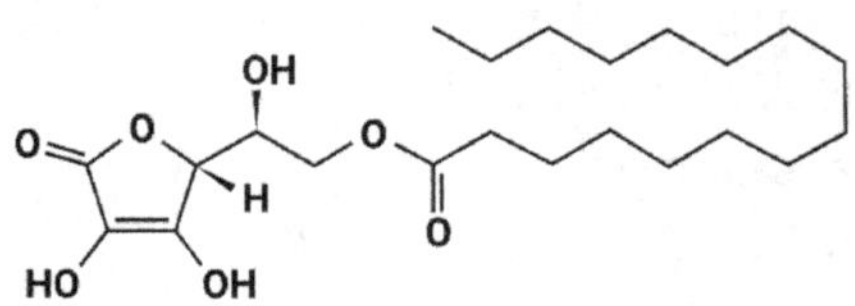

Vitamin C palmitate

(i) *Test procedure*

Preparation of standard solution — Accurately weigh about 10 mg of vitamin C palmitate standard, and transfer it to a 100 ml volumetric flask. Add 60 ml of methanol, and sonicate until the standard is completely dissolved. Then add methanol to 100 ml volume and shake well. The standard can now be injected.

Preparation of sample solution — Accurately weigh a certain amount of ground sample which contains about 10 mg of vitamin C palmitate, and transfer it to a 100 ml volumetric flask. Add 20 ml DMSO, and sonicate for 5 min. Then add 50 ml of ethanol, and sonicate for another 15 min. After the solution is cooled add methanol to the volume mark and shake well. Centrifuge (10,000 rpm) for 5 min, and take the upper clear solution for injection.

(ii) *UPLC conditions*

Column: Acquity UPLC® BEH Phenyl, 1.7 μm, 2.1 × 150 mm
Flow rate: 0.4 ml/min
Injection volume: 2 μL
UV wavelength: 243 nm
Mobile phase A: 0.1% phosphoric acid in water
Mobile phase B: 0.1% phosphoric acid in acetonitrile
Column temperature: 45°C

Gradient:

Time (min)	A%	B%
0	50	50
3.0	10	90
3.8	10	90
4.0	50	50
6.0	50	50

(iii) *Results and calculation*

$$VC\ palmitate\ (mg/unite) = \frac{Aa \times Wstd \times Vsam \times UW}{As \times Wsam \times Vstd}$$

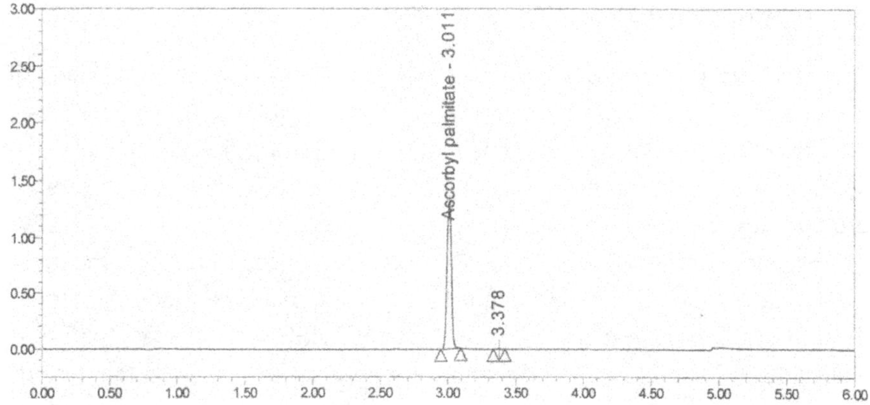

Figure 5.23: UPLC chromatogram of vitamin C palmitate.

or

$$VC\ palmitate\ (\%) = \frac{Aa \times Wstd \times Vsam \times 100\%}{As \times Wsam \times Vstd}$$

Aa = Peak area of VC palmitate in sample solution
As = Peak area of VC palmitate in standard solution
Wstd = Weight of standard (mg)
Wsam = Weight of sample (mg)
Vsam = Total volume of sample solution (ml)
Vstd = Total volume of standard solution (ml)
UW = Unit weight (mg)

5.40 Conjugated Linoleic Acid (CLA) Test Method

Conjugated linoleic acid has one pair of conjugated double bonds mainly located at 9 and 11 or 10 and 12 bond positions. CLA in dietary supplements claim multiple health benefits (such as weight loss, bodybuilding and fitness).

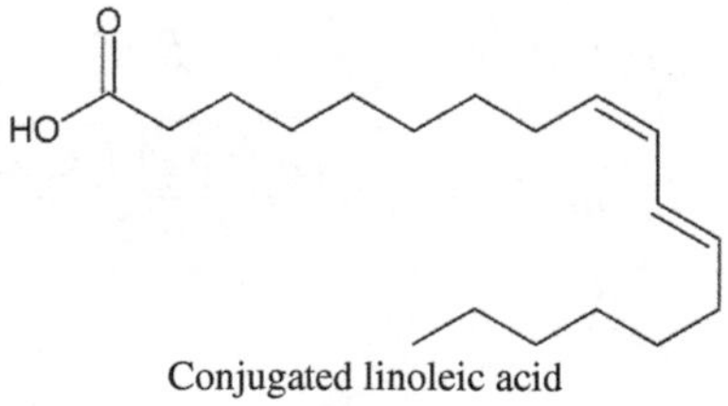

Conjugated linoleic acid

Like other fatty acids CLA can be quantified by either GC or HPLC methods. In dietary supplements CLA generally exists as a free fatty acid, so if the GC method is used, the methylation procedure is necessary for reducing the boiling point. The HPLC method can directly quantify free CLA. The following is the HPLC method.

(i) *Test procedure*

Preparation of standard solution — Accurately weigh about 100 mg of a conjugate linoleic acid standard into a 100 ml volumetric flask, and add 60 ml isopropyl alcohol. Sonicate for 2 min, and then add isopropanol to the 100 ml volume. Shake well and the standard is ready for injection.

Preparation of sample solution (for solid samples) — Accurately weigh a certain amount of ground sample that contains about 100 mg of conjugate linoleic acid, and transfer it to a 100 ml volumetric flask. Add 15 ml of DMSO, and sonicate for 5 min. Then add 60 ml IPA, and sonicate for another 15 min. After cooling add IPA to the volume mark, and shake well. Centrifuge (10,000 rpm) for 5 min, and take the upper clear liquid for injection.

Preparation of sample solution (for liquid fatty samples) — Weigh a certain amount of sample containing about 100 mg of conjugate linoleic acid into a 100 ml volumetric flask, and add 60 ml isopropyl alcohol. Sonicate for 5 min, then add isopropyl alcohol to the 100 ml volume, and shake well. Centrifuge for 5 min, and draw the clear solution for injection.

(ii) *UPLC conditions*

Column: Acquity UPLC® BEH Phenyl, 1.7 μm, 2.1 × 150 mm
Flow rate: 0.4 ml/min
Injection volume: 2 μL
UV wavelength: 232 nm
Mobile phase A: 0.1% phosphoric acid in water
Nobile phase B: Methanol
Column temperature: 45°C

Gradient:

Time (min)	A%	B%
0	35	65
4.5	5	95
5.5	5	95
6.0	35	65
8.0	35	65

(iii) *Results and calculation*

$$CLA\ (mg/unite) = \frac{Aa \times Wstd \times Vsam \times UW}{As \times Wsam \times Vstd}$$

or

$$CLA\ (\%) = \frac{Aa \times Wstd \times Vsam \times 100\%}{As \times Wsam \times Vstd}$$

Aa = Peak area of CLA in sample solution
As = Peak area of CLA in standard solution
Wstd = Weight of standard (mg)
Wsam = Weight of sample (mg)
Vsam = Total volume of sample solution (ml)
Vstd = Total volume of standard solution (ml)
UW = Unit weight (mg)

5.41 Cinnamaldehyde Test Method

Cinnamaldehyde comes from the bark of cinnamon trees, is widely used in food, beverages and dietary supplements as a flavoring.

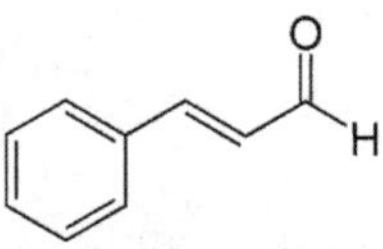

Cinnamaldehyde

Cinnamaldehyde is a non-polar compound, so revise phase chromatography (C18 column) can be used to test for it.

(i) *Test procedure*

Preparation of standard solution — Accurately weight about 5 mg of a cinnamaldehyde standard, and transfer it to a 100 ml volumetric flask. Add 60 ml methanol, and sonicate until the standard is completely dissolved. Then add methanol to the 100 ml volume and shake well. The standard is ready for injection.

Preparation of sample solution — Accurately weigh a certain amount of ground sample which contains about 5 mg of cinnamaldehyde, and transfer it to a 100 ml volumetric flask. Add 20 ml of water, and sonicate for 5 min. Then add 60 ml of ethanol, and sonicate for another 15 min. After cooling, fill to volume with methanol, and shake well. Centrifuge (10,000 rpm) for 5 min, and draw the clear solution for injection.

(ii) *UPLC conditions*

Column: Acquity UPLC® BEH C18 1.7 μm, 2.1 × 150 mm
Flow rate: 0.4 ml/min
Injection volume: 1 μL
UV wavelength: 291 nm
Mobile phase A: 0.1% phosphoric acid in water
Mobile phase B: Acetonitrile
Column temperature: 45°C

Gradient:

Time (min)	A%	B%
0	90	10
5.0	45	55
6.0	45	55
6.5	90	10
9.0	90	10

(iii) *Results and calculation*

$$Cinnamaldehyde\ (mg/unite) = \frac{Aa \times Wstd \times Vsam \times UW}{As \times Wsam \times Vstd}$$

or

$$Cinnamaldehyde\ (\%) = \frac{Aa \times Wstd \times Vsam \times 100\%}{As \times Wsam \times Vstd}$$

Aa = Peak area of cinnamaldehyde in sample solution
As = Peak area of cinnamaldehyde in standard solution
Wstd = Weight of standard (mg)
Wsam = Weight of sample (mg)
Vsam = Total volume of sample solution (ml)
Vstd = Total volume of standard solution (ml)
UW = Unit weight (mg)

5.42 Azelaic Acid Test Method

Wheat, secale, barley and other crops contain azelaic acid. Azelaic acid has anti-keratinization, anti-bacterial and other functions. Some cosmetic and dietary supplement products contain azelaic acid.

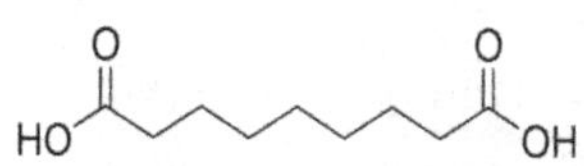

azelaic acid

(i) *Test procedure*

Preparation of standard solution — Accurately weigh about 20 mg of an azelaic acid standard, and transfer it to a 100 ml volumetric flask. Add 60 ml of ethanol, and sonicate for 2 min. Then add ethanol to the 100 ml volume and shake well. The standard solution is ready for injection.

Preparation of sample solution — Accurately weigh a certain amount of ground sample containing about 20 mg of azelaic acid, and transfer it to a 100 ml volumetric flask. Add 10 ml of water, and sonicate for 5 min. Then add 60 ml of ethanol, and sonicate for another 15 min. After cooling, add ethanol to the volume mark and shake well. Centrifuge (10,000 rpm) for 5 min, and draw the clear solution for injection.

(ii) *UPLC conditions*

Column: Acquity UPLC® HSS T3 C18 1.8 μm, 2.1 × 150 mm
Flow rate: 0.4 ml/min
Injection volume: 2 μL
UV wavelength: 211 nm
Mobile phase A: 0.1 phosphoric acid in water
Mobile phase B: Acetonitrile
Column temperature: 45°C

Gradient:

Time (min)	A%	B%
0	90	10
5.0	50	50
5.8	50	50
6.0	90	10
8.0	90	10

(iii) *Results and calculation*

$$Azelaic\,acid\ (mg/unite) = \frac{Aa \times Wstd \times Vsam \times UW}{As \times Wsam \times Vstd}$$

or

$$Azelaic\,acid\,(\%) = \frac{Aa \times Wstd \times Vsam \times 100\%}{As \times Wsam \times Vstd}$$

Aa = Peak area of azelaic acid in sample solution
As = Peak area of azelaic acid in standard solution
Wstd = Weight of standard (mg)
Wsam = Weight of sample (mg)
Vsam = Total volume of sample solution (ml)

Vstd = Total volume of standard solution (ml)
UW = Unit weight (mg)

5.43 Test Method for Polyphenols Using the Folin–Ciocalteu Method

Polyphenol solutions can react with the Folin–Ciocalteu reagent and the solution turns blue. The intensity of the color is proportional to the concentration of polyphenols and the hydroxyl group on the polyphenol molecule. The concentration of the sample solution can be calculated by comparing the absorption intensity of the sample solution with standard solution at 760 nm wavelength (blue color).

This method has some limitations with specificity and accuracy, but has been agreed upon as an industry consensus method, and is widely used.

(i) *Test procedure*

Reagent: Gallic Acid, standard
Folin-Ciocalteu reagent (2N) Sigma F9252
20% sodium carbonate solution — 50 grams of sodium carbonate anhydrous is dissolved in 250 ml of water with sonication.

Preparation of standard solution — Accurately weigh about 25 mg of a gallic acid standard, and transfer to a 50 ml volumetric flask. Add 30 ml of water to dissolve the standard, and then add water to the volume mark and shake well.

Preparation of sample solution — Accurately weigh a certain amount of sample which contains about 25 mg polyphenols, and transfer to a 50 ml volumetric flask. Add 30 ml of water, and vortex for 2 min. If needed, the sonication can be extended to 5–10 min. After cooling, add water to the volume mark and shake well. Filter 10 ml of the sample solution through a 0.45 um filter paper.

Redox reaction: Transfer 1 ml of standard solution, 1 ml of sample solutions, and 1 ml of water (blank) to three different 100 ml volumetric flasks. Add about 50 ml of water to each volumetric flask, and shake well.

Add 5 ml of Folin–Ciocalteu reagent and 15 ml of 20% sodium carbonate solution to each flask, then add water to the volume marks. Shake well and place on the lab bench for 2 h.

Use a UV/Vis spectrometer to measure absorption intensity of the aforementioned solutions at 760 nm, and then calculate the result.

$$Polyphenol\ (mg/unite) = \frac{(Aa - Ab) \times Wstd \times UW}{(As - Ab) \times Wsam}$$

or

$$Polyphenol\ (\%) = \frac{(Aa - Ab) \times Wstd \times 100\%}{(As - Ab) \times Wsam}$$

Aa = Standard solution UV/Vis absorption at 760 nm
As = Sample solution UV/Vis absorption at 760 nm
Ab = Blank solution UV/Vis absorption at 760 nm
Wstd = Weight of standard (mg)
Wsam = Weight of sample (mg)
UW = Unit weight (mg/unit)

5.44 Test Method of Proanthocyanidins

Proanthocyanidins are polymers of three or more tea polyphenols. Because of the complex structure of the original anthocyanidins, it is difficult to find individual standards to measure the individual proanthocyanidins. A common method used in industry is the Poter's method. The final results of the test method are expressed in the Poter's value (PVU).

(i) *Test procedure*

Solvent A preparation — 95 ml butanol plus 5 ml of concentrated hydrochloric acid, shake well.

Solvent B preparation — Dissolve 2 g of ferric ammonium sulfate in 100 ml of water, add 17.5 ml of concentrated hydrochloric acid, and shake well.

Sample preparation — Accurately weigh 100–120 mg sample, and transfer it to a 100 ml volumetric flask. Add 60 ml methanol, and sonicate for 10 min. After cooling, add methanol to the volume mark, and shake well. Centrifuge for 5 min, then transfer 1 ml of the clear solution to a 10 ml volumetric flask, and dilute to 10 ml with methanol.

Separately transfer 1 ml of the diluted sample solution and 1 ml of methanol (blank) to two different 10 ml test tube with screw caps. Add 6 ml of solvent A, and 0.2 ml of solvent B to each test tube, cover tightly with the lid. Mix well, and then heat in a 100°C degree water bath for 40 min. Quickly cool the test tube with cold water, and remove 1 ml solution from each tube. Place these in two different 10 ml volumetric flasks, and dilute to volume with solvent A. Shake these well. Determine the absorption intensity of the sample and blank solutions at 547 nm.

(ii) *Results and calculation*

$$Proanthocyanidins\ (PVU) = \frac{(Aa - Ab) \times 7.2 \times 10^4}{C}$$

Aa = sample solution UV/Vis absorption at 547 nm
Ab = Blank solution UV/Vis absorption at 547 nm
C = concentration of sample solution (μg/ml, total volume 1,000 ml)

This method can also be calculated using a pine bark extract reference material and the results are reported as % of pine bark extract equivalent.

$$Proanthocyanidins\ (\%\ of\ pine\,bark\,ext.) = \frac{(Aa - Ab) \times 1000}{W \times 18.4}$$

Here
Aa = Sample solution UV/Vis absorption at 547 nm
Ab = Blank solution UV/Vis absorption at 547 nm
W = Weight of sample (g)

1000 = Volume of sample solution (1,000 ml)
18.4 = Absorption value of 1 g of pine bark extract standard/1,000 (ml)

5.45 Monoglycerides Test Method

Monopalmitin, glyceryl monooleate and monosterin are commonly used emulsifiers in food and dietary supplement products.

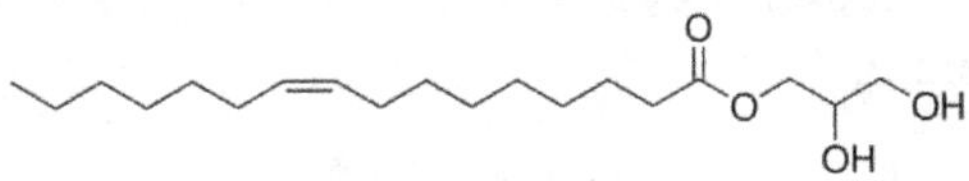

Monopalmitin

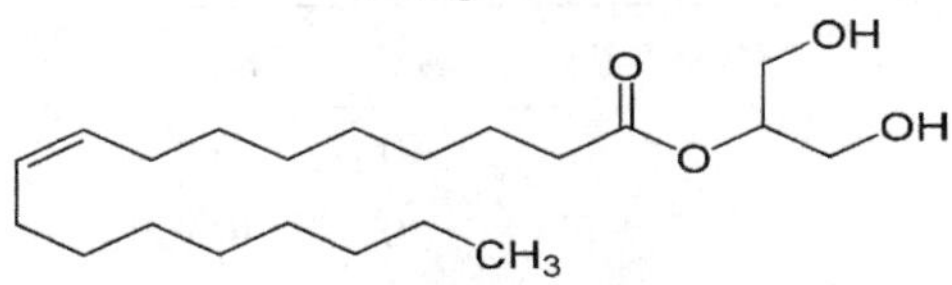

Glyceryl monooleate

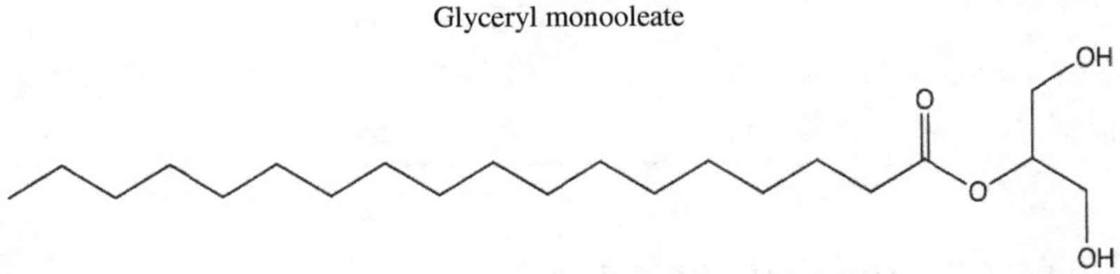

Monosterin

(i) *Test procedure*

Preparation of standard solution — In a 50 ml volumetric flask accurately weigh about 10 mg of each monopalmitin, glyceryl monooleate and monosterin. Add 30 ml of ethanol, and sonicate until all standards are completely dissolved. Fill with ethanol to the 50 ml volume and shake well. The standard can now be injected.

Preparation of sample solution — Accurately weigh a certain amount of sample containing about 10 mg of monopalmitin, or glyceryl monooleate, or monosterin, in a 50 ml volumetric flask. Add 30 ml of ethanol, and sonicate for 10 min. After cooling, add ethanol to the volume mark, and mix well. Centrifuge for 5 min, and the upper clear solution can be injected.

(ii) *UPLC conditions*

Column: Acquity UPLC® BEH C18, 1.7 μm, 2.1 × 150 mm
Flowrate: 0.4 ml/min
Injection volume: 2.0 μL
UV wavelength: 211 nm
Mobile phase A: 0.1% phosphoric acid water solution
Mobile phase B: Acetonitrile
Column temperature: 45°C

Gradient:

Time (min)	A%	B%
0	40	60
5	0	100
7.8	0	100
8.0	40	60
10.0	40	60

(iii) *Results and calculation*

$$Individual\ monoglyceride\ (mg/unite) = \frac{Aa \times Wstd \times Vsam \times UW}{As \times Wsam \times Vstd}$$

or

$$Individual\ monoglyceride\ (\%) = \frac{Aa \times Wstd \times Vsam \times 100\%}{As \times Wsam \times Vstd}$$

Aa = peak area of corresponding monoglyceride in sample solution
As = peak area of corresponding monoglyceride in standard solution
Wstd = weight of corresponding standard (mg)
Wsam = weight of sample (mg)
Vsam = Total volume of sample solution (ml)
Vstd = Total volume of standard solution (ml)
UW = Unit weight (mg/unit)

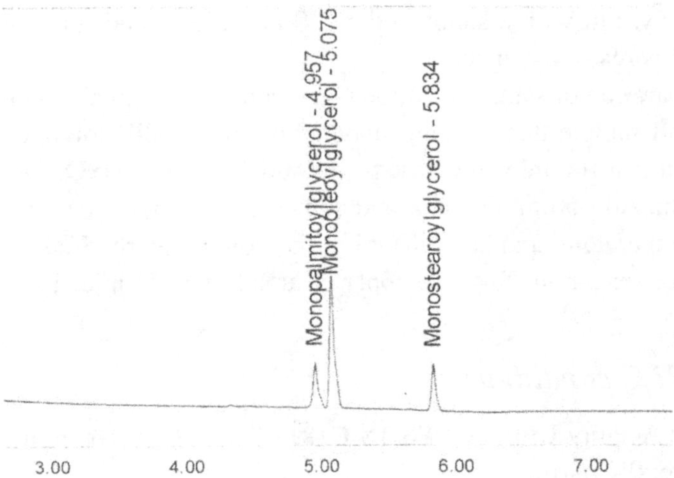

Figure 5.24: Chromatogram of monopalmitin, glyceryl monooleate and monosterin.

5.46 Diindolylmethane Test Method

3,3′-Diindolylmethane (DIM) is a compound derived from the digestion of indole-3-carbinol, and is found in cruciferous vegetables such as broccoli, brussels sprouts, cabbage and kale. 3,3-diindolylmethan may help balance the hormones in the body, and is used for preventing breast, uterine and colorectal cancer. It is also used to prevent enlarged prostate.

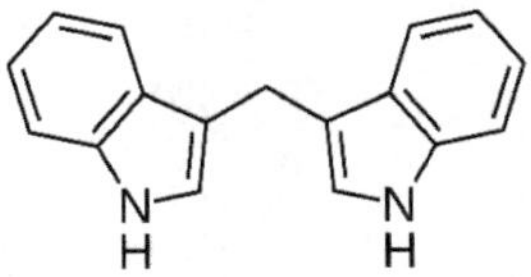

3,3-diindolylmethan

(i) *Test procedure*

Preparation of standard solution — Accurately weigh about 5 mg of a 3,3-diindolylmethan standard, and transfer it to a 100 ml volumetric flask. Add 60 ml of ethanol, and sonicate until the standard is dissolved completely. Fill with ethanol to the 100 ml volume and shake well. The standard is ready for injection.

Preparation of sample solution — Accurately weigh a certain amount of ground sample that contains about 5 mg of 3,3-diindolylmethan, and transfer it to a 100 ml volumetric flask. Add 20 ml of DMSO, and sonicate for 5 min. Add 60 ml ethanol, and sonicate for another 10 min. Cool to room temperature, and add ethanol to the volume mark. Shake well, and centrifuge for 5 min. Take the upper clear solution for injection.

(ii) *UPLC conditions*

Column: Acquity UPLC® HSS TS C18, 1.8 μm, 2.1 × 100 mm
Flow rate: 0.4 ml/min
Injection volume: 1.0 μL
UV wavelength: 282 nm
Mobile phase A: 0.1% phosphoric water solution
Mobile phase B: Acetonitrile
Column temperature: 45°C

Gradient:

Time (min)	A%	B%
0	70	30
4	20	80
4.8	20	80
5.2	70	30
8.0	70	30

(iii) *Results and calculation*

$$\text{Diindolylmethan } (mg/unite) = \frac{Aa \times Wstd \times Vsam \times UW}{As \times Wsam \times Vstd}$$

or

$$\text{Diindolylmethan } (\%) = \frac{Aa \times Wstd \times Vsam \times 100\%}{As \times Wsam \times Vstd}$$

Aa = Peak area of diindolylmethan in sample solution
As = Peak area of diindolylmethan in standard solution
$Wstd$ = Weight of standard (mg)
$Wsam$ = Weight of sample (mg)
$Vsam$ = Total volume of sample solution (ml)
$Vstd$ = Total volume of standard solution (ml)
UW = Unit weight (mg/unit)

5.47 Apigenin-7-Glycoside Test Method

Apigenin 7-glucoside is a flavonoid with anti-inflammatory and anxiolytic activities.

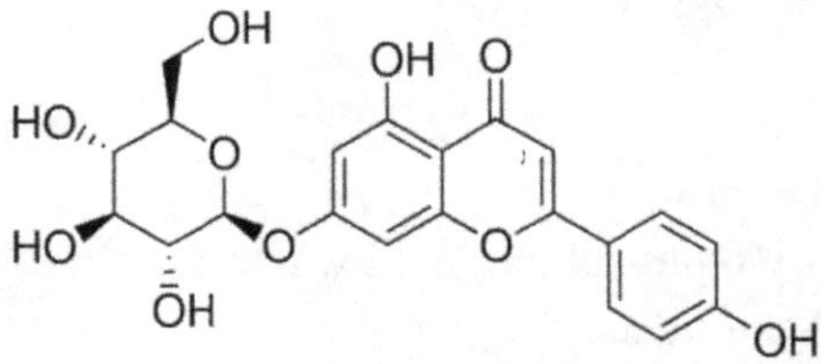

Apigenin-7-glycoside

(i) *Test procedure*

Preparation of standard solution — Accurately weigh about 5 mg of an apigenin-7-glucosin standard, and transfer it to a 100 ml volumetric flask. Add 60 ml of water, and sonicate until the standard is completely dissolved. After cooling, fill with water to the 100 ml mark and shake well. The standard is ready for injection.

Preparation of sample solution — Accurately weigh a certain amount of sample containing about 5 mg of apigenin-7-glucosin, and transfer it to a 100 ml volumetric flask. Add 60 ml of water, and sonicate for 10 min. After cooling, add water to the volume mark and shake well. Centrifuge for 5 min, and draw the clear solution for injection.

(ii) *UPLC conditions*

Column: Acquity UPLC® HSS Ts C18, 1.8 μm, 2.1 × 100 mm
Flow rate: 0.4 ml/min

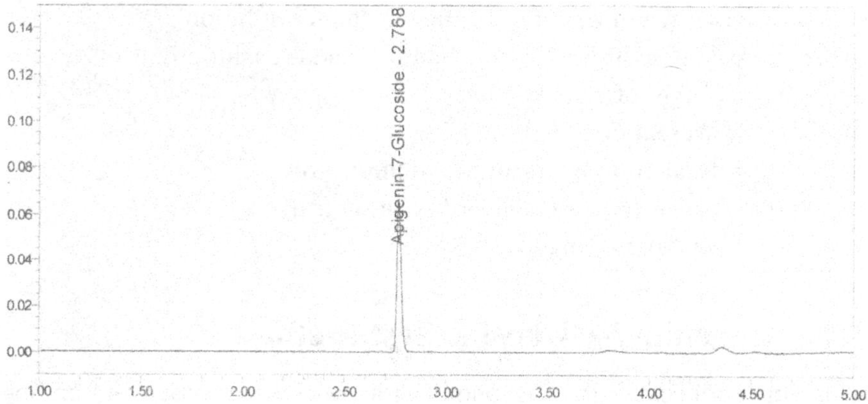

Figure 5.25: Chromatogram of apigenin -7-glucosin.

Injection volume: 1.0 μL
UV wavelength: 336 nm
Mobile phase A: 0.1% phosphoric acid water solution
Mobile phase B: Acetonitrile
Column temperature: 45°C

Gradient:

Time (min)	A%	B%
0	90	10
3	60	40
3.6	60	40
4.0	90	10
6.0	90	10

(iii) *Results and calculation*

$$Apigenin\text{-}7\text{-}glucosin\ (mg/unite) = \frac{Aa \times Wstd \times Vsam \times UW}{As \times Wsam \times Vstd}$$

or

$$Apigenin\text{-}7\text{-}glucosin\ (\%) = \frac{Aa \times Wstd \times Vsam \times 100\%}{As \times Wsam \times Vstd}$$

Aa = Peak area of apigenin-7-glucosin in sample solution
As = Peak area of apigenin-7-glucosin in standard solution
Wstd = Weight of standard (mg)
Wsam = Weight of sample (mg)
Vsam = Total volume of sample solution (ml)
Vstd = Total volume of standard solution (ml)
UW = Unit weight (mg/unit)

5.48 Para-Aminobenzoic Acid (PABA) Test Method

Para-aminobenzoic acid (PABA) helps to maintain skin and hair health. PABA is best known as a sunscreen that is applied to the skin.

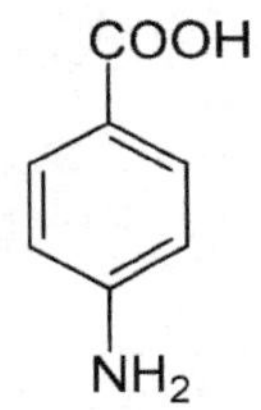

Para-aminobenzoic acid

(i) *Test procedure*

Preparation of standard solution — Accurately weigh about 5 mg of para-aminobenzoic acid standard, and transfer it to a 50 ml volumetric flask. Add 30 ml of ethanol, and sonicate until all of the standard is dissolved. After the standard is cooled, add ethanol to 50 ml mark and shake well. The standard is ready for injection.

Preparation of sample solution — Accurately weigh a certain amount of sample containing about 5 mg of para-aminobenzoic acid, and transfer it to a 50 ml volumetric flask. Add 10 ml of water, and sonicate for 5 min. Then add 30 ml ethanol, and sonicate for another 10 min. After cooling, add ethanol to the volume mark, and shake well. Centrifuge (12,000 rpm) for 5 min, and take the clear solution for injection.

(ii) *UPLC conditions*

Column: Acquity UPLC® HSS Ts C18, 1.8 μm, 2.1 × 150 mm
Flow rate: 0.4 ml/min
Injection volume: 1.0 μL
UV wavelength: 282 nm
Mobile phase A: 0.1% phosphoric acid water solution
Mobile phase B: Acetonitrile
Column temperature: 45°C

Gradient:

Time (min)	A%	B%
0	95	5
4.0	85	15
4.8	85	15
5.0	95	5
7.0	95	5

(iii) *Results and calculation*

$$PABA\ (mg/unite) = \frac{Aa \times Wstd \times Vsam \times UW}{As \times Wsam \times Vstd}$$

or

$$PABA\ (\%) = \frac{Aa \times Wstd \times Vsam \times 100\%}{As \times Wsam \times Vstd}$$

Aa = Peak area of PABA in sample solution
As = Peak area of PABA in standard solution
Wstd = Weight of standard (mg)
Wsam = Weight of sample (mg)
Vsam = Total volume of sample solution (ml)
Vstd = Total volume of standard solution (ml)
UW = Unit weight (mg/unit)

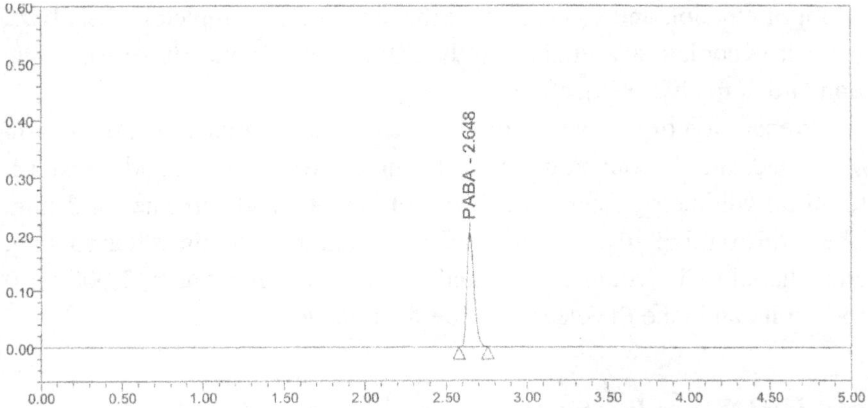

Figure 5.26: Chromatogram of PABA.

5.49 Pregnenolone Test Method

Pregnenolone is used in some countries as drug, and has some effects on the treatment of rheumatoid arthritis. Pregnenolone supplements also can help to combat age-related memory impairment, as well as protect against a variety of health conditions.

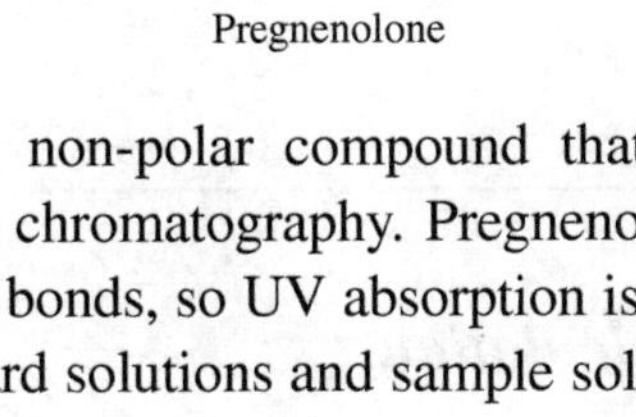

Pregnenolone

Pregnenolone is a non-polar compound that can be separated by reversed phase column chromatography. Pregnenolone contains only two non-conjugated double bonds, so UV absorption is not very sensitive. The concentration of standard solutions and sample solutions should be a little higher than normal.

(i) *Test procedure*

Preparation of standard solution — Accurately weigh about 10 mg of a pregnenolone standard, and transfer to a 50 ml volumetric flask. Add

30 ml of ethanol, and sonicate until the standard is completely dissolved. After it is cooled, add ethanol to the 50 ml volume and shake well. The standard is ready for injection.

Preparation of sample solution — Accurately weigh a certain amount of ground sample containing about 10 mg of progesterone, and transfer it to 50 ml volumetric flask. Add 10 ml of DMSO, and sonicate for 5 min. Then add 30 ml of ethanol, and sonicate for another 15 min. After cooling, add ethanol to the volume mark, and shake well. Centrifuge (12,000 rpm) for 5 min, and take the clear solution for injection.

(ii) *UPLC conditions*

Column: Acquity UPLC® BEH, C18, 1.7 μm, 2.1 × 150 mm
Flow rate: 0.4 ml/min
Injection volume: 2.0 μL
UV wavelength: 215 nm
Mobile phase A: 0.1% phosphoric acid water solution
Mobile phase B: Acetonitrile
Column temperature: 45°C

Gradient:

Time (min)	A%	B%
0	60	40
5	10	90
5.6	10	90
6.0	60	40
8.0	60	40

(iii) *Results and calculation*

$$Pregnenolone\ (mg/unite) = \frac{Aa \times Wstd \times Vsam \times UW}{As \times Wsam \times Vstd}$$

or

$$Pregnenolone\ (\%) = \frac{Aa \times Wstd \times Vsam \times 100\%}{As \times Wsam \times Vstd}$$

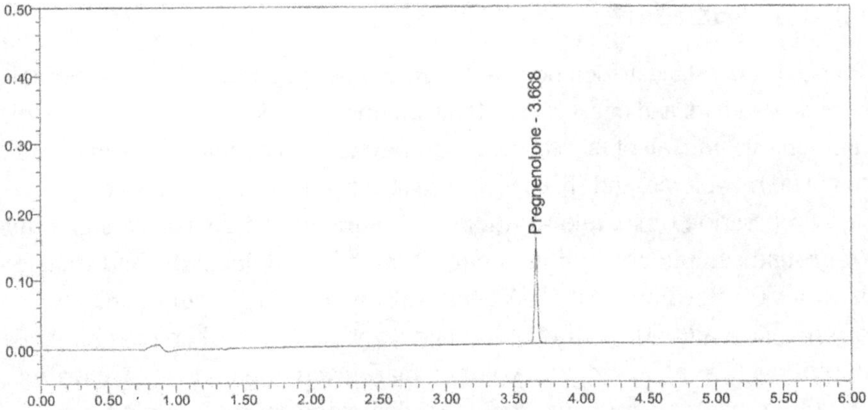

Figure 5.27: UPLC chromatogram of pregnenolone standard.

Aa = Peak area of pregnenolone in sample solution
As = Peak area of pregnenolone in standard solution
Wstd = Weight of standard (mg)
Wsam = Weight of sample (mg)
Vsam = Total volume of sample solution (ml)
Vstd = Total volume of standard solution (ml)
UW = Unit weight (mg/unit)

5.50 Perillaldehyde Test Method

Perillaldehyde can be used as a food additive, and it also can be used in dietary supplements and cosmetic products. It mainly acts as an antioxidant and gives with a calming effect. It can also help with sleep.

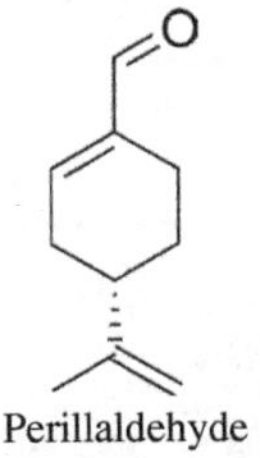

Perillaldehyde

Perillaldehyde is a non-polar compound, so a C18 column can be used to perform the test.

(i) *Test procedure*

Preparation of standard solution — Accurately weigh about 10 mg of a perillaldehyde standard, and transfer to a 50 ml volumetric flask. Add 30 ml of ethanol, and sonicate until all of the standard is dissolved. After cooling, fill with ethanol to the 50 ml volume, and shake well. The standard is ready for injection.

Preparation of sample solution — Accurately weigh a certain amount of ground sample containing about 10 mg of perillaldehyde, and transfer it to a 50 ml volumetric flask. Add 10 ml of DMSO, and sonicate for 5 min. Then add 30 ml of ethanol, and sonicate for another 15 min. After cooling add ethanol to the volume mark, and shake well. Centrifuge (12,000 rpm) for 5 min, and draw the clear solution for injection.

(ii) *UPLC conditions*

Column: Acquity UPLC® BEH, C18, 1.7 μm, 2.1 × 150 mm
Flow rate: 0.4 mg/ml
Injection volume: 2.0 μL
UV wavelength: 230 nm
Mobile phase A: 0.1% phosphoric acid water solution
Mobile phase B: Acetonitrile
Column temperature: 45°C

Gradient:

Time (min)	A%	B%
0	60	40
5	30	70
5.6	30	70
6.0	60	40
8.0	60	40

(iii) *Results san calculation*

$$Perillaldehyde\ (mg/unite) = \frac{Aa \times Wstd \times Vsam \times UW}{As \times Wsam \times Vstd}$$

or

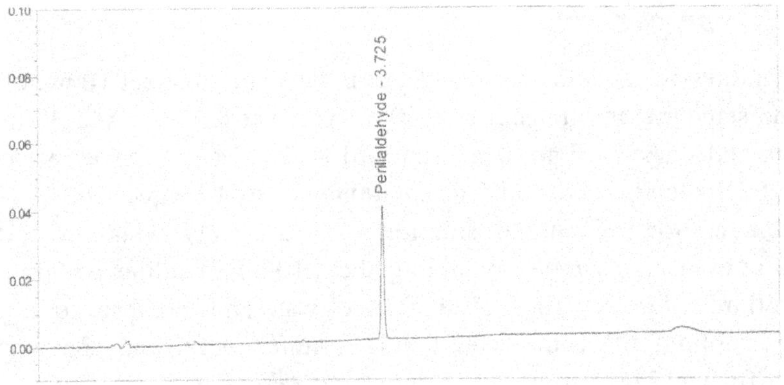

Figure 5.28: UPLC chromatogram of perillaldehyde.

$$Perillaldehyde\ (\%) = \frac{Aa \times Wstd \times Vsam \times 100\%}{As \times Wsam \times Vstd}$$

Aa = Peak area of perillaldehyde in sample solution
As = Peak area of perillaldehyde in standard solution
Wstd = Weight of standard (mg)
Wsam = Weight of sample (mg)
Vsam = Total volume of sample solution (ml)
Vstd = Total volume of standard solution (ml)
UW = Unit weight (mg/unit)

5.51 Valine Test Method

Valine is one of the eight essential amino acids in the human body. The isoelectric point of valine is 5.96. This method adjusts the pH of mobile phase to 2.0, much lower than the isoelectric point, so the valine molecules are positively charged. The retention time can be extended by using hexane sulfonate as ion pair reagent (see Chapter 1, Section 1.1.2 "Mobile phase application" section).

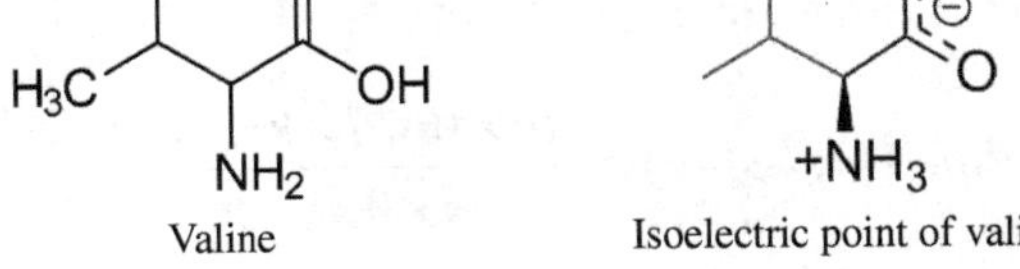

Valine

Isoelectric point of valine

(i) *Test procedure*

Preparation of standard solution — Accurately weigh about 10 mg of the valine standard, and transfer to a 50 ml volumetric flask. Add 30 ml of water, and shake until all of the standard is dissolved. Then add water to 50 ml mark, and shake well. The solution is ready for injection.

Preparation of sample solution — Accurately weigh a certain amount of ground sample containing about 10 mg of valine, and transfer to a 50 ml volumetric flask. Add 30 ml of water, and sonicate for 5 min. After cooling, fill with water to the volume mark, and shake well. Centrifuge (12,000 rpm) for 5 min, and take the clear solution for injection.

(ii) *UPLC conditions*

Column: Acquity UPLC® HSS Ts, C18, 1.7 μm, 2.1 × 150 mm
Flow rate: 0.4 ml/min
Injection volume: 2.0 μL
UV wavelength: 210 nm
Mobile phase A: 10 mM hexansulfonate, pH 2.0
Mobile phase B: Acetonitrile
Column temperature: 45°C

Gradient:

Time (min)	A%	B%
0	95	5
5.0	80	20
5.6	80	20
6.0	95	5
8.0	95	5

(iii) *Results and calculation*

$$Valine\ (mg/unite) = \frac{Aa \times Wstd \times Vsam \times UW}{As \times Wsam \times Vstd}$$

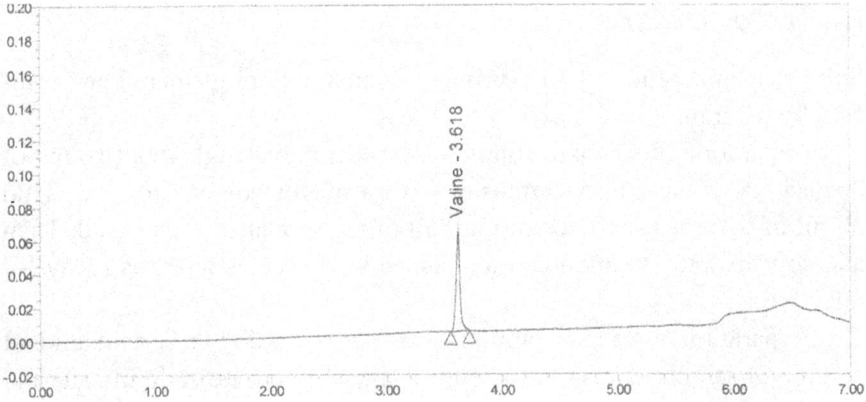

Figure 5.29: UPLC chromatogram of valine.

or

$$Valine\ (\%) = \frac{Aa \times Wstd \times Vsam \times 100\%}{As \times Wsam \times Vstd}$$

Aa = Peak area of valine in sample solution
As = Peak area of valine in standard solution
$Wstd$ = Weight of standard (mg)
$Wsam$ = Weight of sample (mg)
$Vsam$ = Total volume of sample solution (ml)
$Vstd$ = Total volume of standard solution (ml)
UW = Unit weight (mg/unit)

5.52 Docusate Test Method

Docusate is a surfactant used in pharmaceutical products and dietary supplements to help dissolve active compounds. Docusate also can be used as a stool softener in dietary supplements.

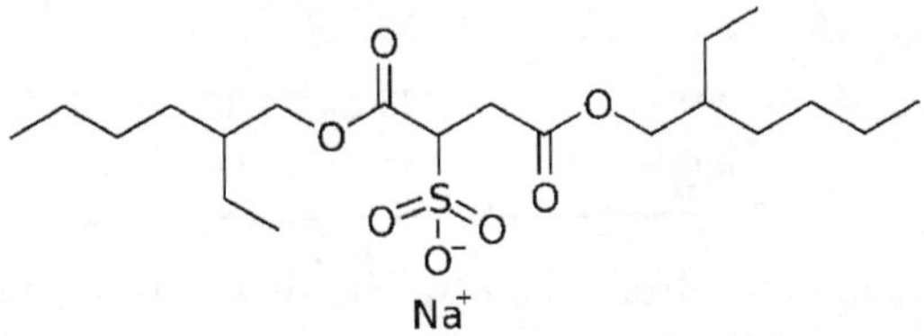

Docusate sodium salt

(i) *Test procedure*

Solvent 1 preparation — In 200 ml water mix 200 ml methanol and sonicate for 10 min.

Preparation of standard solution — Accurately weigh about 10 mg of docusate sodium salt, and transfer it to a 50 ml volumetric flask. Add 30 ml of solvent 1, and vortex until all of the standard is dissolved. Then add solvent 1 to volume mark and shake well. The standard is ready for injection.

Preparation of sample solution — Accurately weight a certain amount of ground sample containing about 10 mg of docusate sodium salt, and transfer it to a 50 ml volumetric flask. Add 30 ml of solvent 1, and sonicate for 5 min. After cooling add solvent 1 to the volume mark and shake well. Centrifuge (12,000 rpm) for 5 min, and draw the clear solution for injection.

(ii) *UPLC conditions*

Column: Acquity UPLC® BEH, C18, 1.7 μm, 2.1 × 150 mm
Flow rate: 0.4 ml/min
Injection volume: 2.0 μL
UV wavelength: 216 nm
Mobile phase A: 0.1% trifluoroacetic acid water solution
Mobile phase B: Acetonitrile
Column temperature: 45°C

Gradient:

Time (min)	A%	B%
0	70	30
3.0	25	75
3.8	25	75
4.0	70	30
6.0	70	30

Note: Docusate is a sulfonic acid, which is a strong acid. This method uses a strong acid, trifluoroacetic acid aqueous solution, in the mobile

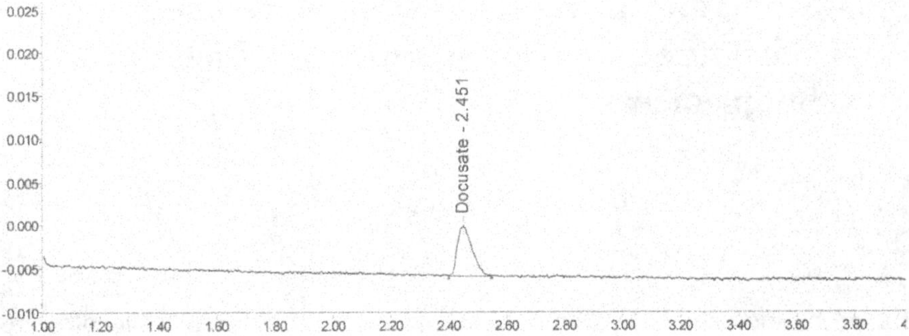

Figure 5.30: UPLC chromatogram of docusate.

phase to reduce the polarity of the docusate, and to extend the retention time. But from the above chromatogram it can be seen that the peak shape is not very good. It may be because the pH is not low enough. So, using an ion pair reagent (such as tetrabutyl ammonium salt) is recommended. This will form ion pairs with docusate to improve the peak shape, as well to extend the retention time. The pH can also be adjusted to 3–5 (see Chapter 1, Section 1.1.2 "Mobile phase application").

(iii) *Results and calculation*

$$Docusate\ (mg/unite) = \frac{Aa \times Wstd \times Vsam \times UW}{As \times Wsam \times Vstd}$$

or

$$Docusate\ (\%) = \frac{Aa \times Wstd \times Vsam \times 100\%}{As \times Wsam \times Vstd}$$

Aa = Peak area of docusate in sample solution
As = Peak area of docusate in standard solution
Wstd = Weight of standard (mg)
Wsam = Weight of sample (mg)
Vsam = Total volume of sample solution (ml)
Vstd = Total volume of standard solution (ml)
UW = Unit weight (mg/unit)

5.53 Simultaneous Determination of Betaine, Carnitine and Acetyl-carnitine in Dietary Supplements

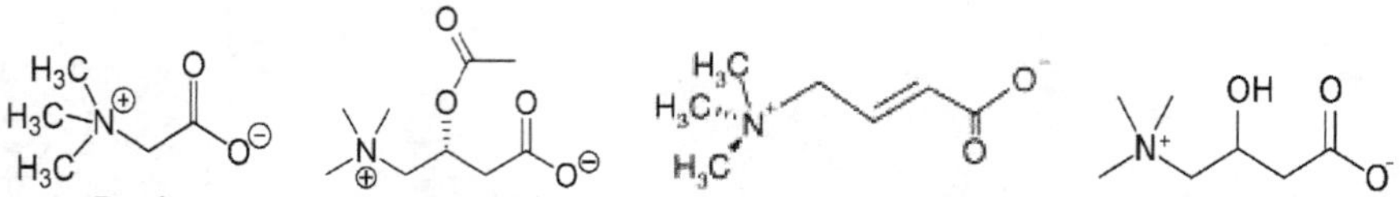

Betain Acetyl-carnitine Crotonoylbetain Carnitine

From the molecular structures it can be seen that the four molecules are alkaline. In a low pH solution, the simplest way to handle this is to add anions (such as hexansulfonate) into the mobile phase, so that the alkaline cations can form an ion pair, and extend the retention time (see Chapter 1, Section 1.1.2 "Mobile phase application"). However, the ion pairing method cannot separate carnitine and crotonoylbetain. Crotonoylbetain is a by-product of carnitine; crotonoylbetain contains a pair of conjugate double bonds, so the intensity of UV absorption at 210 nm is about 200 times higher than that of carnitine. This means if a pure carnitine contains 0.5% of crotonoylbetain, and cannot be separated chromatographically, then the results measured may be 200% of the actual content.

In order to separate all four of the aforementioned compounds, ion exchange column is used. Cation exchange columns with an aqueous solution of ammonia chloride mix with acetonitrile as mobile phase, and can be used to separate the cations that are being tested. At low pH, ammonia chloride is dissociated into NH_4^+ and Cl^-. NH_4^+ ions and the cations of analytes are competitors in the cation exchange column, thereby increasing the concentration of NH_4^+ ions, and can make the alkaline analytes elude sooner. Therefore, adjusting the concentration of NH_4^+ in the mobile phase can make the ions being tested get better retention times and improved separation (see Chapter 1, Section 1.1.2 "Mobile phase application").

(i) *Test procedure*

Preparation of crotonoylbetain stock solution — Accurately weigh about 5 mg of a crotonoylbetain standard, and transfer to a 25 ml volumetric flask. Add water to dissolve the standard and fill with water to the 25 ml volume, and shake this solution well.

Preparation of standard solution — Accurately weigh about 20 mg of each of betain, acetylcarnine and carnitine standards, and transfer them to a 50 ml volumetric flask. Add 30 ml of water, and shake until all of standards are dissolved. Then add 0.5 ml of the crotonoylbetain stock solution, add fill with water to volume mark. Shake well, and the standard solution is ready for injection.

Preparation of sample solution — Accurately weigh a certain amount of ground sample containing about 20 mg of carnitine, or acetyl carnitine, or betain, and transfer it to a 50 ml volumetric flask. Add 30 ml of water, and sonicate for 10 min. Cool to room temperature, and fill with water to the volume mark. Shake well, and then centrifuge (12,000 rpm) for 5 min. Draw the clear solution for injection.

(ii) *HPLC conditions*

Column: Supelcosil LC-SCX, 5 μm, 4.6 mm × 250 mm
Flow rate: 1.5 ml/min
Injection volume: 20.0 μL
UV wavelength: 210 nm
Mobile phase A: 10 mM potassium phosphate, 20 mM ammonia chloride, adjust pH to 2.0
Mobile phase B: Acetonitrile
Mobile phase A: Mobile phase B = 25%:75%

(iii) *Results and calculation*

$$Analyte\ (mg/unite) = \frac{Aa \times Wstd \times Vsam \times UW}{As \times Wsam \times Vstd}$$

or

$$Analyte\ (\%) = \frac{Aa \times Wstd \times Vsam \times 100\%}{As \times Wsam \times Vstd}$$

Aa = peak area of corresponding analyte in sample solution
As = peak area of corresponding analyte in standard solution
Wstd = weight of corresponding standard (mg)

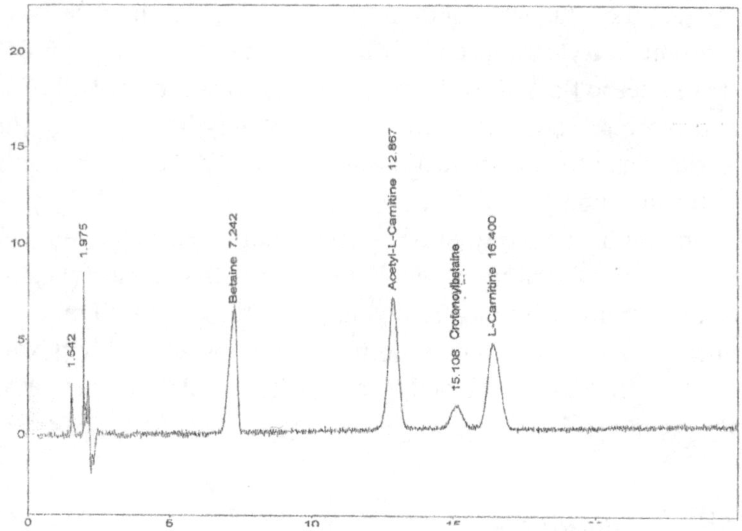

Figure 5.31: Chromatogram of betaine, acetyl-carnitine, crotonoylbetaine and carnitine.

Wsam = weight of sample (mg)
Vsam = Total volume of sample solution (ml)
Vstd = Total volume of standard solution (ml)
UW = Unit weight (mg/unit)

5.54 L-Dihydroxyphenylalanine (L-DOPA) Test Method

L-dopa is a precursor to dopamine and has an auxiliary effect on the treatment of Parkinson's disease.

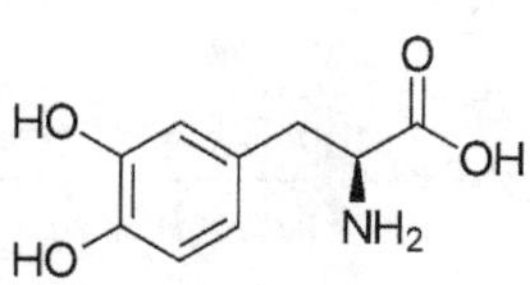

L-DOPA

The isoelectric point of L-dopa is 5.7. At a low pH (pH < 5.7–1, see Chapter 1, Section 1.2) the molecule is positively charged. By adding an anion (such as hexansulfonate sodium) to the mobile phase, a neutral ion pair can be formed which will extend the peak retention time with a reversed phase column.

(i) *Test procedure*

Preparation of standard solution — Accurately weigh about 10 mg of L-dopa standard, and transfer it to a 100 ml volumetric flask. Add 60 ml 0.1 N hydrochloric acid solution, and vortex until the standard is completely dissolved. Then fill the flask to the 100 ml volume with 0.1 N hydrochloric acid. Shake well, and the standard solution can be injected.

Preparation of sample solution — Accurately weight a certain amount of ground sample containing about 10 mg of L-dopa, and transfer it to a 100 ml volumetric flask. Add 60 ml 0.1N hydrochloric acid and sonicate for 10 min. After cooling, add 0.1 N hydrochloric acid to the volume mark and shake well. Centrifuge (12,000 rpm) for 5 min and take the clear solution for injection.

(ii) *HPLC conditions*

Column: Supelcosil Discovery RP-Amide C16 column, 4.6 × 150 mm
Flow rate: 1.1 ml/min
Injection volume: 20.0 μL
UV wavelength: 280 nm
Mobile phase A: 10 mM hexansulfonate sodium, pH 2.5 water solution
Mobile phase B: Acetonitrile
Column temperature: Room temperature

Gradient:

Time (min)	A%	B%
0	98	2
10	85	15
12	85	15
12.5	98	2
18	98	2

(iii) *Results and calculation*

$$\text{L-dopa } (mg/unite) = \frac{Aa \times Wstd \times Vsam \times UW}{As \times Wsam \times Vstd}$$

or

$$\text{L-dopa } (\%) = \frac{Aa \times Wstd \times Vsam \times 100\%}{As \times Wsam \times Vstd}$$

Aa = Peak area of L-dopa in sample solution
As = Peak area of L-dopa in standard solution
Wstd = Weight of standard (mg)
Wsam = Weight of sample (mg)
Vsam = Total volume of sample solution (ml)
Vstd = Total volume of standard solution (ml)
UW = Unit weight (mg/unit)

5.55 Lecithin Test Method

Lecithin mainly consists of phosphatidylcholine (PC), phosphatidylethanolamine (PE), phosphatidylinositol (PI) and phosphatidtserine (PS). In dietary supplements, usually phosphatidylcholine (PC) and phosphatidtserine (PS) are the most commonly used. This method only describes the quantitative testing method for PC and PS.

Both the PC and PS have one end that is polar and the other end is non-polar. Since the carbon chains at the non-polar end are particularly long, the non-polarity is very strong. This makes these compounds difficult to elute out of a reversed phase column. This method uses a normal phase separation column to quantitatively test PC and PS.

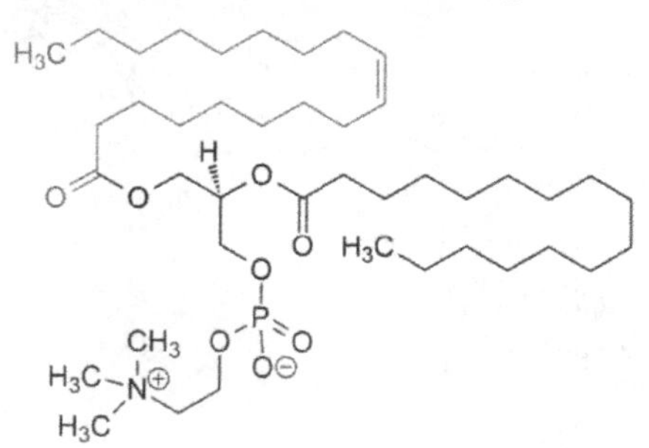

PC

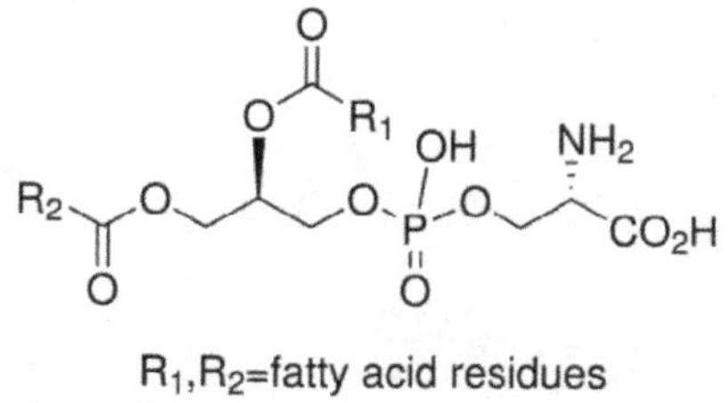

PS

Theoretically, fatty acids in lecithin molecules are extremely varied, and molecular weight is not a constant. In most cases, however, the chromatograms only show a single peak. This may be caused by the selectivity of solvents used to extract lecithin in the manufacturing process, or the subsequent purification processes that are used to yield a narrow range molecule.

(i) *Test procedure*

Preparation of standard solution — Accurately weigh about 20 mg of a phosphatidylcholine or a phosphatidylserine standard as needed, and transfer it to a 25 ml volumetric flask. Add 10 ml of chloroform, and sonicate until all of the standard is dissolved. Cool the solution to room temperature, and add ethanol to the 25 ml volume, and shake well. The standard solution is ready for injection.

Preparation of sample solution — Accurately weigh a certain amount of ground sample containing about 20 mg of phosphatidylcholine or phosphatidylserine, and transfer to 25 ml volumetric flask. Add 10 ml of warm water, and sonicate for 5 min. Centrifuge to remove as much water as possible, then add 10 ml of chloroform and 5 ml ethanol. Sonicate for 10 min, and then cool. Add ethanol to the volume mark, and after shaking, centrifuge (12,000 rpm) for 5 min. Draw the clear solution to make injections.

(ii) *HPLC conditions*

Column: Supelcosil LC-SCX, 5 um, 250 × 4.6 mm
Flow rate: 1.0 ml/min
Injection volume: 15 μL
UV wavelength: 215 nm
Mobile phase A: 650 ml of pH 3.5 buffer (50 mM KH_2PO_4, add phosphoric acid to pH 3.5), mix with 350 ml of acetonitrile
Mobile phase B: Methanol
Column temperature: Room temperature
Mobile phase A:mobile phase B = 20:80

(iii) *Result and calculation*

$$PC/PS\ (mg/unite) = \frac{Aa \times Wstd \times Vsam \times UW}{As \times Wsam \times Vstd}$$

or

$$PC/PS\ (\%) = \frac{Aa \times Wstd \times Vsam \times 100\%}{As \times Wsam \times Vstd}$$

Aa = Peak area of PC/PS in sample solution
As = Peak area of PC/PS in standard solution
$Wstd$ = Weight of standard (mg)
$Wsam$ = Weight of sample (mg)
$Vsam$ = Total volume of sample solution (ml)
$Vstd$ = Total volume of standard solution (ml)
UW = Unit weight (mg/unit)

5.56 Cynarin Test Method

Cynarin is one of the active ingredients found in artichokes. It boosts liver vitality and promotes the elimination of toxins from the liver (such as ammonia produced by digestive proteins). Cynarin also promotes the regeneration of liver cells to enhance the secretion of bile and the digestion of fat.

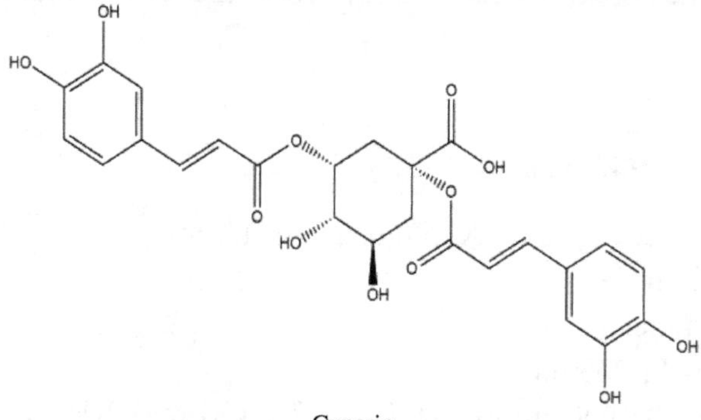

Cynarin

(i) *Test procedure*

Preparation of standard solution — Accurately weigh 10 mg of a cynarin standard, and transfer it to a 100 ml volumetric flask. Add 60 ml of methanol, and vortex until all the standard is dissolved. Then add methanol to the 100 ml volume mark, shake well, and the standard solution is ready for injection.

Preparation of sample solution — Accurately weigh a certain amount of ground sample containing about 10 mg of cynarin, and transfer it to a 100 ml volumetric flask. Add 15 ml of water, and sonicate for 5 min. Then add 60 ml of ethanol, and sonicate for another 10 min. After the solution is cooled, add methanol to the volume mark, and shake well. Centrifuge (12,000 rpm) for 5 min, and draw the clear solution for injection.

(ii) *HPLC conditions*

Colum: Acquity BEH C18, 1.7 μm, 2.1 × 150 mm
Flow rate: 0.4 ml/mi
Injection volume: 1 μL
UV wavelength: 322 nm
Mobile phase A: 0.1% phosphoric acid water solution
Mobile phase B: Acetonitrile
Column temperature: 45°C

Gradient:

Time (min)	A%	B%
0	90	10
3	75	25
3.6	75	25
4.0	90	10
6.0	90	10

(iii) *Results and calculation*

$$\text{Cynarin } (mg/unite) = \frac{Aa \times Wstd \times Vsam \times UW}{As \times Wsam \times Vstd}$$

or

$$\text{Cynarin } (\%) = \frac{Aa \times Wstd \times Vsam \times 100\%}{As \times Wsam \times Vstd}$$

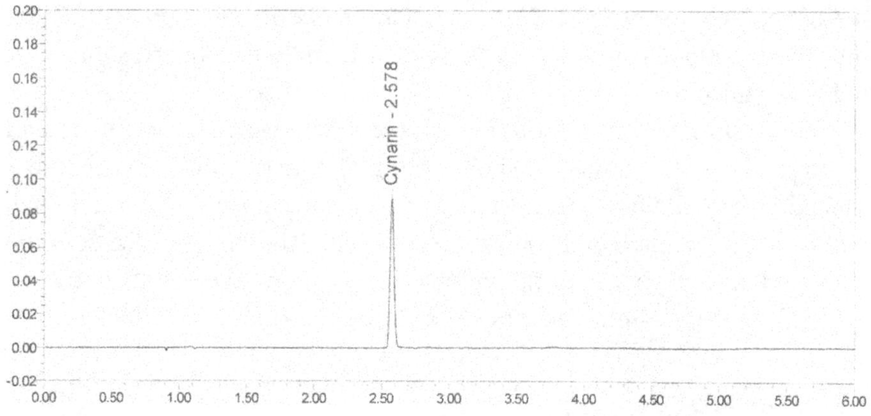

Figure 5.32: Chromatogram of cynarin.

Aa = Peak area of cynarin in sample solution
As = Peak area of cynarin in standard solution
Wstd = Weight of standard (mg)
Wsam = Weight of sample (mg)
Vsam = Total volume of sample solution (ml)
Vstd = Total volume of standard solution (ml)
UW = Unit weight (mg/unit)

5.57 Disodium Uridine-5′-Monophosphate Test Method

Disodium uridine-5′-monophosphate is a component in human breast milk. It is added to infant milk powder to make it resemble breast milk more closely. It has been shown to improve immunity, and it is used in dietary supplements for that effect.

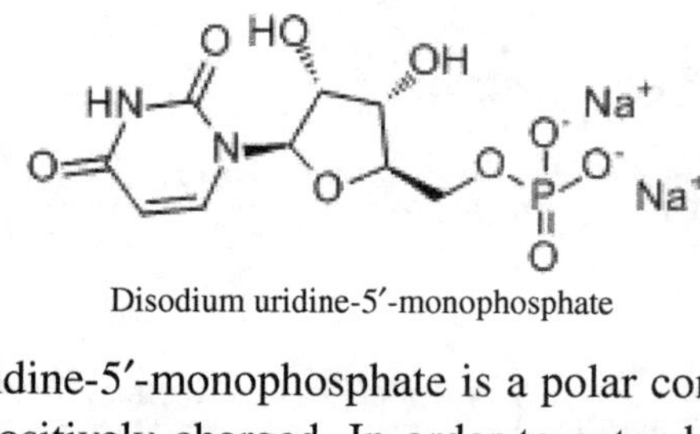

Disodium uridine-5′-monophosphate

Disodium uridine-5′-monophosphate is a polar compound; therefore, at low pH it is positively charged. In order to extend the peak retention time in a reversed phase column, this method adds hexane sulfonate sodium salt into the mobile phase. This forms a neutral ion pair with the disodium uridine-5′-monophosphate molecule, and extends the retention time (see Chapter 1, Section 1.1.2 "Mobile Phases application").

(i) *Test procedure*

Preparation of standard solution — Accurately weigh about 10 mg of a disodium uridine-5′-monophosphate standard, and transfer it to a 100 ml volumetric flask. Add 60 ml of water, and shake until the standard is completely dissolved. Then fill with water to the volume mark, and shake well. The standard solution is ready for injection.

Preparation of sample solution — Weigh a certain amount of ground sample containing about 10 mg of disodium uridine-5′-monophosphate, and transfer it to a 100 ml volumetric flask. Add 60 ml of water, and shake for 10 min. Then sonicate for 5 min, and cool. Add water to the volume mark, and shake well. Centrifuge (12,000 rpm) for 5 min, and draw the clear solution for injection.

If the sample contains proteins, salts such as NaCl or K_2SO_4, it can be used to denaturation the sample.

(ii) *UPLC conditions*

Column: Acquity HSS T3 C18, 1.8 μm, 2.1 × 150 mm
Flow rate: 0.4 ml/min
Injection volume: 1 μL
UV wavelength: 262 nm
Mobile phase: 10 mM hexansulfonate sodium, pH 1.5 water solution
Column temperature: 45°C

Note: In the Figure 5.33 chromatogram, the retention time of uridine-5′-monophosphate peak is not long enough. It could easily be interfered. One suggestion could be is to use a cation exchange column that combines with a mobile phase containing counter ion NH_4^+ to regulate the peak retention time (see Chapter 1, Section 1.1.2 "Mobile phase application").

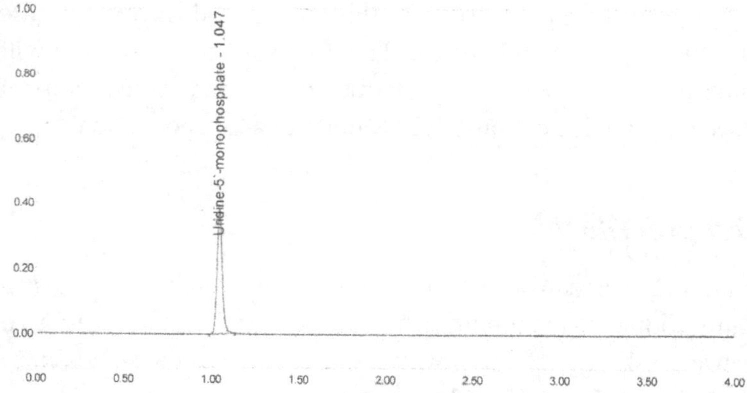

Figure 5.33: UPLC chromatogram of disodium uridine-5′-monophosphate.

(iii) *Results and calculation*

$$Uridinemonophosphate\ (mg/unite) = \frac{Aa \times Wstd \times Vsam \times UW}{As \times Wsam \times Vstd}$$

or

$$Uridinemonophosphate\ (\%) = \frac{Aa \times Wstd \times Vsam \times 100\%}{As \times Wsam \times Vstd}$$

Aa = Peak area of uridine-5′-monophosphate in sample solution
As = Peak area of uridine-5′-monophosphate in standard solution
Wstd = Weight of standard (mg)
Wsam = Weight of sample (mg)
Vsam = Total volume of sample solution (ml)
Vstd = Total volume of standard solution (ml)
UW = Unit weight (mg/unit)

5.58 N-Acetyl-Glucosamine Test Method

N-acetyl-glucosamine is often used as a complementary supplement for the treatment of arthritis. Unlike glucosamine, there is a double bond in n-acetyl-glucosamine molecule. Thus, it can be monitored using a UV detector. In addition, n-acetyl-glucosamine is a polar compound, so there is no interaction with reversed phase HPLC columns. However, because the molecule contains an amide group, it will be positively charged under acidic conditions; therefore, it can be separated and quantified by using a cation-exchange column combined with UV detector.

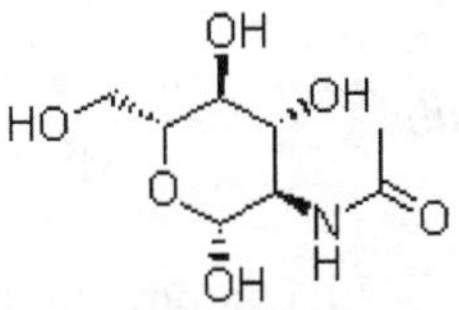

N-acetyl-glucosamine

(i) *Test procedure*

Preparation of standard solution — Accurately weigh about 20 mg of an n-acetyl-glucosamine standard, and transfer it to a 50 ml volumetric flask. Add 30 ml of water, and sonicate until the standard is completely dissolved. Then add water to the volume mark, and shake well. The standard can now be injected.

Preparation of sample solution — Accurately weigh a certain amount of ground sample containing about 20 mg of n-acetyl-glucosamine, and transfer it to a 50 ml volumetric flask. Add 30 ml of water, and sonicate for 10 min. After the solution is cooled, add water to the volume mark and shake well. Centrifuge (12,000 rpm) for 5 min, and draw the clear solution for injection.

(ii) *HPLC conditions*

Column: Suplcosil LC-SCX 4.6 × 250 mm
Flow rate: 1.2 ml/min
Injection volume: 20 μL
UV wavelength: 210 nm
Mobile phase A: 0.02 mole KH_2PO_4, adjust pH to 2.0 with phosphoric acid
Mobile phase B: Acetonitrile
Mobile phase A: Mobile phase B is 20:80
Column temperature: Room temperature

(iii) *Results and calculation*

$$Acetyl\text{-}glucosamine\ (mg/unite) = \frac{Aa \times Wstd \times Vsam \times UW}{As \times Wsam \times Vstd}$$

or

$$Acetyl\text{-}glucosamine\ (\%) = \frac{Aa \times Wstd \times Vsam \times 100\%}{As \times Wsam \times Vstd}$$

Aa = Peak area of acetyl-glucosamine in sample solution
As = Peak area of acetyl-glucosamine in standard solution
Wstd = Weight of standard (mg)
Wsam = Weight of sample (mg)
Vsam = Total volume of sample solution (ml)
Vstd = Total volume of standard solution (ml)
UW = Unit weight (mg/unit)

5.59 Creatine Test Method

Creatine can quickly provide human energy, improve muscle strength and endurance. It can also prevent fatigue, so it is often used in sports nutrition products.

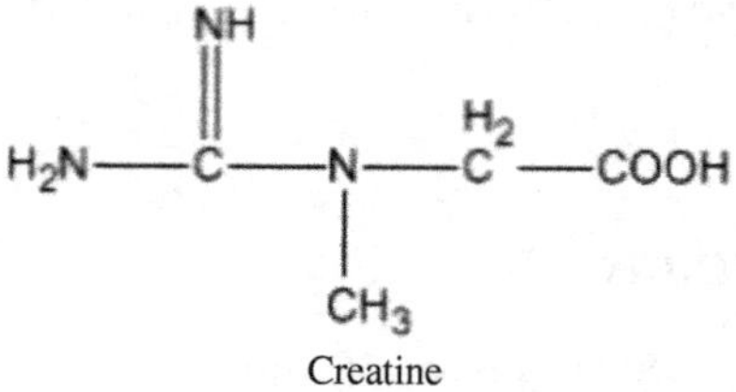

Creatine

According to the molecular structure, creatine is a multipolar molecule, so regulating pH can change the polarity. The isoelectric point of creatine is around 11.0, so the aqueous solution at pH less than 11–1 = 10 (see Chapter 1, Section 1.1.2 "Mobile phase application") is positively charged. This method reduces the pH of the mobile phase to 2, and then separates creatine with a cation exchange column.

(i) *Test procedure*

Preparation of standard solution — Accurately weigh about 20 mg of a creatine standard, and transfer it to a 50 ml volumetric flask. Add 30 ml of water, and shake until the standard is dissolved. Then add water to the volume mark, shake well, and the standard can be injected.

Preparation of sample solution — Accurately weigh a certain amount of ground sample containing about 20 mg of creatine, and transfer it to a 50 ml volumetric flask. Add 30 ml of water, and sonicate for 5 min. After cooling, fill with water to the volume mark and shake well. Centrifuge (12,000 rpm) for 5 min, and draw clear solution for injection.

(ii) *HPLC conditions*

Column: Suplcosil LC-SCX 4.6 × 250 mm
Flow rate: 1.5 ml/min
Injection volume: 20 μL
UV wavelength: 210 nm
Column temperature: Room temperature
Mobile phase A: 10 mM KH_2PO_4, adjust pH to 2.0 with phosphoric acid
Mobile phase B: Acetonitrile
Mobile phase A: Mobile phase B is 25:75.

(iii) *Results and calculation*

$$Creatine\ (mg/unite) = \frac{Aa \times Wstd \times Vsam \times UW}{As \times Wsam \times Vstd}$$

or

$$Creatine\ (\%) = \frac{Aa \times Wstd \times Vsam \times 100\%}{As \times Wsam \times Vstd}$$

Aa = Peak area of creatine in sample solution
As = Peak area of creatine in standard solution
Wstd = Weight of standard (mg)
Wsam = Weight of sample (mg)
Vsam = Total volume of sample solution (ml)

Vstd = Total volume of standard solution (ml)
UW = Unit weight (mg/unit)

5.60 Glutathione Test Method

Glutathione is a tripeptide compound formed by polymerizing glutamate, cysteine and glycine. These are the most important low-molecule thiols in mammalian cells for regulating antioxidant stress. Glutathione is used in dietary supplements and functional food and widely as an antioxidant, for removal of free radicals, for detoxification, to enhance immunity, to delay aging and for other functions.

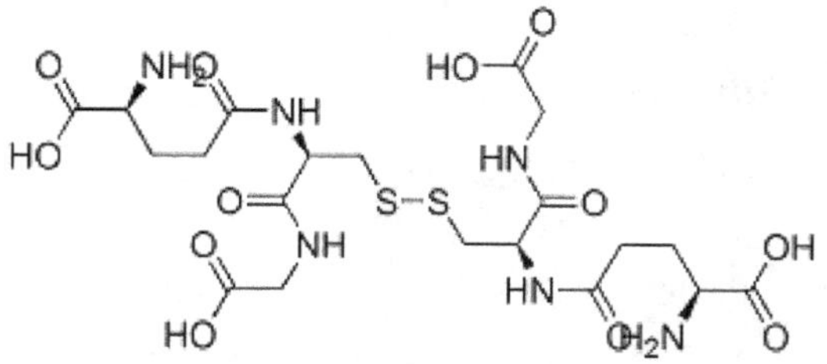

Glutathione

Glutathione is a multipolar compound with an isoelectric point of 5.93. This method reduces the pH of the mobile phase to 2.0, making the glutathione molecule positively charged. Then the glutathione is separated with a cation exchange column (see Chapter 1, Section 1.1.2 "Mobile phase application").

(i) *Test procedure*

Preparation of standard solution — Accurately weigh about 20 mg of a glutathione standard, and transfer it to a 50 ml volumetric flask. Add 30 ml of water, and sonicate it until the standard is completely dissolved. Then add water to the volume mark and shake well. The standard solution can be injected now.

Preparation of sample solution — Accurately weigh a certain amount of ground sample containing about 20 mg of glutathione, and transfer it to a 50 ml volumetric flask. Add 30 ml of water, and sonicate for 5 min. After cooling, fill with water to the volume mark and shake well. Centrifuge (12,000 rpm) for 5 min, and draw the clear solution for injection.

(ii) *HPLC conditions*

Column: Suplcosil LC-SCX 4.6 × 250 mm
Flow rate: 1.5 ml/min
Injection volume: 20 μL
UV wavelength: 210 nm
Column temperature: Room temperature
Mobile phase A: 10 mM KH_2PO_4, adjust pH to 2.0 with phosphoric acid
Mobile phase B: Acetonitrile
Mobile phase A Mobile phase B is 25:75.

(iii) *Results and calculation*

$$\text{Glutathione } (mg/unite) = \frac{Aa \times Wstd \times Vsam \times UW}{As \times Wsam \times Vstd}$$

or

$$\text{Glutathione } (\%) = \frac{Aa \times Wstd \times Vsam \times 100\%}{As \times Wsam \times Vstd}$$

Aa = Peak area of glutathione in sample solution
As = Peak area of glutathione in standard solution
$Wstd$ = Weight of standard (mg)
$Wsam$ = Weight of sample (mg)
$Vsam$ = Total volume of sample solution (ml)
$Vstd$ = Total volume of standard solution (ml)
UW = Unit weight (mg/unit)

5.61 Octacosanol Test Method

Octacosanol functions as an anti-fatigue agent and as an endurance enhancer. Octacosanol can be extracted from sugarcane wax or other plants. In these products, small quantities of linoceryl alcohol, hexacosanol, heptacosanol and triacosanol are also found. These are thought to have similar functions. For this reason, these compounds are also included in the test.

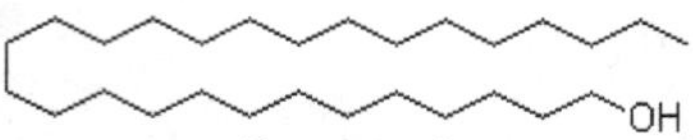

Octacosanol

Octacosanol is a non-polar compound, and it is not easy to elute with revered phase liquid chromatography. Also, octacosanol does not have strong UV absorption, so HPLC-UV cannot be used to test octacosanol. Octacosanol does have a low boiling point (around 225°C), and GC-FID can be used for testing.

(i) *Test procedure*

Preparation of the internal stand solution — Accurately weigh about 20 mg of cholestane, and dissolve in 10 ml of tetrahydrofuran. Then dilute with tetrahydrofuran 5 times, and set this standard aside.

Preparation of standard solution — Accurately weigh about 5 mg of each linoceryl alcohol, hexacosanol, heptacosanol and triacosanol; and 15 mg of octacosanol standard. Transfer these to a 10 ml volumetric flask, add 6 ml of the internal standard solution. Sonicate until all the standards are dissolved. After cooling use the internal standard solution to fill the flask to volume mark, and shake well. The standard solution is ready to be injected.

Preparation of sample solution — Accurately weigh a certain amount of ground sample containing about 15 mg of octacosanol, and transfer it to a 15 ml volumetric flask. Accurately transfer 6 ml of the internal standard solution to the flask, and sonicate for 5 min. After the solution is cooled, accurately add 4 ml of internal standard solution and shake well. Centrifuge (12,000 rpm) for 5 min, and draw the clear solution for injection.

(ii) *GC-FID conditions*

Capillary column: Restek RTX-5, 30 m × 0.25 mm, 0.25 nm
Carry gas flow rate: 1.0 ml/min (nitrogen)
Injection volume: 1 μL
Temperature of injector: 300°C
Temperature of detector: 300°C

Oven temperature: 200°C for one minute, 12°C/min increasing rate to 320°C, holding for 15 min, Finish.

(iii) *Results and calculation*

$$Octacosanol\ (\%) = \frac{Cs \times PARu \times Vu \times 100\%}{PARs \times Wu}$$

$$Other\ individual\ alkanols\ (\%) = \frac{Cs \times PARu \times Vu \times 100\%}{PARs \times Wu}$$

Cs = Concentration of corresponding alkanol in standard solution (mg/ml)
PARu = Peak area ratio of corresponding alkanol/internal standard in sample solution
PARs = Peak area ratio of corresponding alkanol/internal standard in standard solution
Vu = Total volume of sample solution (ml)
Wu = Weigh of sample (mg)

5.62 Inositol Test Method

Inositol, sometimes referred to as vitamin B_8, occurs naturally in foods such as fruits, beans, grains and nuts. It is also produced in the human body and can be synthesized in a laboratory. Inositol may have mental health benefits, and may help prevent diabetes. It also may help lower cholesterol, and promote healthy hair growth, and prevent hair loss.

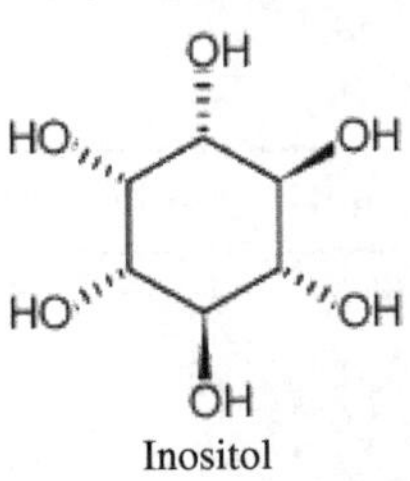

Inositol

Inositol is a polar compound, and it does not contain any double bonds, and has no characteristic UV absorption. Therefore, reversed phase chromatography-UV methods are not suitable for inositol analysis.

Inositol can be separated and measured using ion exchange chromatography with electrochemical detection.

(i) *Test procedure*

Standard preparation — Accurately weigh about 10 mg of an inositol standard, and transfer it to a 100 ml volumetric flask. Add 60 ml of water, and sonicate for 5 min. After the solution is cooled, add water to volume mark, and shake and mix well. Transfer 1 ml of the solution to another 100 ml volumetric flask, and dilute with water to the volume mark. Shake well, and the standard solution is ready for injection.

Sample preparation — Accurately weigh certain amount of ground sample which contains about 10 mg of inositol, and transfer it to a 100 ml volumetric flask. Add 60 ml of water, and sonicate for 10 min. After cooling fill with water to the volume mark, and shake well. Centrifuge (10,000 rpm) for 5 min, and transfer 1 ml of the clear solution to a 100 ml volumetric flask. Dilute to volume with water, and shake well. The sample solution is ready for injection.

(ii) *IC conditions*

Column: CarboPac® SA 10, 4 × 250 mm
Detector: Electrochemical detector
Flow Rate: 1 mL/min
Mobile Phase A: 200 mM NaOH
Mobile Phase B: DI water
Run Time: 15 min

Gradient:

Time	A%	B%
Initial	95.0	5.0
1.00	95.0	5.0
9.00	75.0	25.0
10.00	75.0	25.0
10.50	95.0	5.0
15.00	95.0	5.0

(iii) *Results and calculation*

$$Inositol\ (mg/unite) = \frac{Aa \times Wstd \times Vsam \times UW}{As \times Wsam \times Vstd}$$

or

$$Inositol\ (\%) = \frac{Aa \times Wstd \times Vsam \times 100\%}{As \times Wsam \times Vstd}$$

Aa = Peak area of inositol in sample solution
As = Peak area of inositol in standard solution
$Wstd$ = Weight of standard (mg)
$Wsam$ = Weight of sample (mg)
$Vsam$ = Total volume of sample solution (ml)
$Vstd$ = Total volume of standard solution (ml)
UW = Unit weight (mg/unit)

5.63 Methylparaben and Propylparaben Test Method

Methylparaben and propylparaben are commonly used as preservatives in food, dietary supplements and cosmetics. In some countries and regions there are strict usage restrictions, so accurate testing of the content of methylparaben and propylparaben is important.

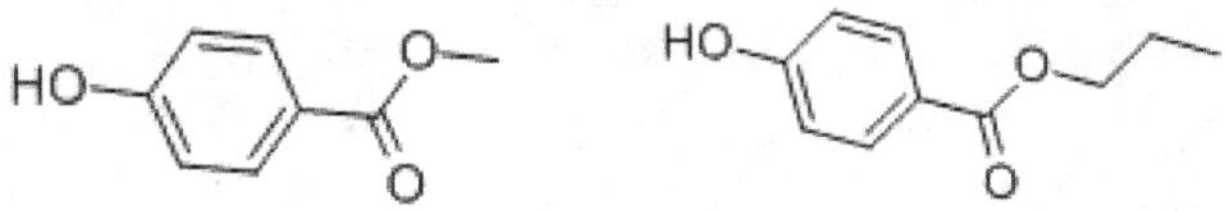

Methylparaben Propylparaben

From the molecular structures it can be seen that propylparaben contains two more methane groups than methylparaben, so a reversed phase HPLC column can separate them well.

(i) *Test procedure*

Preparation of standard solution — Accurately weigh about 10 mg of a methylparaben and 10 mg a propylparaben standard, and transfer both to a 100 ml volumetric flask. Add 60 ml of methanol, and sonicate for 5 min.

After cooling, add methanol to the volume mark, and shake well. This solution is ready to be injected.

Preparation of sample solution — Accurately weigh a certain amount of ground sample containing about 10 mg of methylparaben or propylparaben, and transfer it to a 100 ml volumetric flask. Add methanol 60 ml, and sonicate 15 min. After cooling add methanol to the volume mark, and shake well. Centrifuge (12,000 rpm) for 5 min, and draw the clear solution for injection.

(ii) *HPLC conditions*

Column: Supelco Discovery C18 4.6 × 150 mm,
Flow rate: 1.1 ml/min
Injection volume: 15 μL
UV wavelength: 260 nm
Mobile phase A: 0.1% phosphoric acid water solution
Mobile phase B: Acetonitrile
Column temperature: Room temperature

Gradient:

Time (min)	A%	B%
0	80	20
1.0	80	20
14.0	25	75
16.5	25	75
17.0	80	20
25.0	80	20 End

(iii) *Results and calculation*

$$Methylparaben/propylparaben\ (mg/unite) = \frac{Aa \times Wstd \times Vsam \times UW}{As \times Wsam \times Vstd}$$

or

$$Methylparaben/propylparaben\ (\%) = \frac{Aa \times Wstd \times Vsam \times 100\%}{As \times Wsam \times Vstd}$$

Aa = Peak area of methylparaben/propylparaben in sample solution
As = Peak area of methylparaben/propylparaben in standard solution
Wstd = Weight of standard (mg)
Wsam = Weight of sample (mg)
Vsam = Total volume of sample solution (ml)
Vstd = Total volume of standard solution (ml)
UW = Unit weight (mg/unit)

Index

CPSIA information can be obtained
at www.ICGtesting.com
Printed in the USA
BVHW052235250522
638186BV00002B/14

9 789811 249242